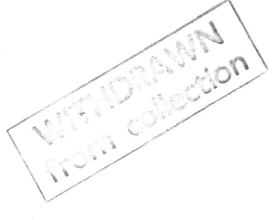
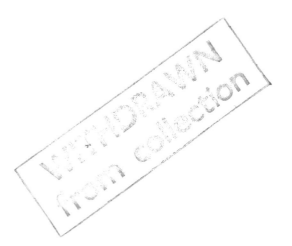

Essentials of Veterinary Parasitology

Edited by

Hany M. Elsheikha and Naveed Ahmed Khan

School of Veterinary Medicine and Science
University of Nottingham
Loughborough
UK

 Caister Academic Press

Caister Academic Press
Norfolk, UK

www.caister.com

British Library Cataloguing-in-Publication Data
A catalogue record for this book is available from the British Library

ISBN: 978-1-904455-79-0 (paperback) and 978-1-904455-80-6 (hardback)

Cover image adapted from Figure 9.6

Printed and bound in Great Britain

This book is dedicated to veterinary students and practising veterinarians, for whom it was written

and

to scientists in the field who have advanced our knowledge, without whose dedication and assistance this book would not have been possible

Current Books of Interest

Contents

Contributors

David J. Bartley
Moredun Research Institute
Penicuik
Scotland
UK

Dave.Bartley@moredun.ac.uk

Gerald C. Coles
School of Clinical Veterinary Science
University of Bristol
Langford
Bristol
UK

Gerald.C.Coles@bristol.ac.uk

Hany M. Elsheikha
School of Veterinary Medicine and Science
University of Nottingham
Loughborough
UK

Hany.Elsheikha@nottingham.ac.uk

Scott D. Fitzgerald
Diagnostic Center for Population and Animal Health
Michigan State University
Lansing, MI
USA

Fitzgerald@dcpah.msu.edu

Neil Foster
School of Veterinary Medicine and Science
University of Nottingham
Loughborough
UK

N.Foster@nottingham.ac.uk

Timothy G. Geary
Institute of Parasitology
McGill University
Montreal, QC
Canada

timothy.g.geary@mcgill.ca

Ray M. Kaplan
Department of Infectious Diseases
College of Veterinary Medicine
University of Georgia
Athens, GA
USA

rkaplan@uga.edu

Naveed A. Khan
School of Veterinary Medicine and Science
University of Nottingham
Loughborough
UK

Naveed.Khan@nottingham.ac.uk

Steven McOrist
School of Veterinary Medicine and Science
University of Nottingham
Loughborough
UK

Steven.Mcorist@nottingham.ac.uk

Heinz Sager
Novartis Animal Health
Novartis Centre de Recherche
Sante Animale SA
Switzerland

heinz.sager@novartis.com

Philip J. Skuce
Moredun Research Institute
Penicuik
Scotland
UK

Philip.Skuce@moredun.ac.uk

Preface

As new research and clinical experience broaden our knowledge of parasites, the need for a concise, clinically oriented parasitology textbook becomes necessary. The first edition of this book provides a complete guide that covers all the essentials of veterinary parasitology for use in a busy practice setting and crowded curriculum. Its composition has taken into consideration the increasing sophistication of veterinary parasitology, and the difficulty of adequately covering many emerging topics.

For students, this book provides a solid foundation for exploring the various aspects of parasitic diseases, including clinical features, laboratory findings, differential diagnosis, and therapeutic options. All topics covered in this book are relevant to parasitologists, zoologists, biologists and veterinarians in general practice who examine many patients in the first instance. Many details of less common parasitic diseases have been omitted *deliberately*, with emphasis placed on epidemiology, choice of logical diagnostic methods, proven treatment and effective prevention strategies. For practitioners, this book provides concise yet substantial guidelines on the diagnosis and treatment of a range of important parasitic diseases to facilitate the care of the patients, and can be used as a resource for continuing veterinary education.

A logical building-block approach supplies what students and veterinarians need to know in an easy-to-use, memorable format. Many illustrations are included both for the information of the student and general practitioner, but also for use in client education. Material is presented in a progressive manner, from basic principles and concepts in parasitology to systematic description of major parasitic diseases affecting livestock and companion animals, ending with principles of parasitic diseases diagnosis and control.

For purposes of readability, references are omitted from the text, but each chapter ends with an updated list of relevant books, review articles, and selected research papers for readers who wish to pursue specific topics.

Authored by elite clinical and basic researchers at the forefront of veterinary and medical parasitology, the book presents a powerful and comprehensive synthesis of current research and clinical practices on veterinary parasitology.

Hany M. Elsheikha and Naveed A. Khan
University of Nottingham, UK

Editors' Note

Therapeutics is an ever-changing field. Readers of this book are advised to check the most current product information provided by the manufacturer of each drug to verify the recommended dose, the method and duration of administration, and adverse effects. It is the responsibility of attending practitioners to be familiar with the laws governing drugs in their practice areas. Both clients and clinicians should be cognizant of and take steps to reduce drug residues in food animals. Neither the publisher nor the editors assume any liability of any injury and/or damage to persons or property with the use of material(s) contained in this book. The mention of trade names or commercial products in this book is soley for the purpose of specific information and does not imply recommendation or endorsement by the publisher or authors.

Section I

Nature and Characteristics of Parasitism

Introductory Parasitology

Hany M. Elsheikha and Naveed A. Khan

We tend to think of parasites as a nuisance, but they are in fact very serious disease-causing agents. Despite advances of veterinary medicine, parasitic diseases have remained a major cause of morbidity, mortality and economic losses worldwide. With the increasing burden of parasites on human and animal suffering, study of 'parasitology' has become an important and rapidly growing discipline of science. Veterinarians' awareness of parasitic diseases is undoubtedly more critical now than at any time in the history of veterinary medical practice. This chapter provides a short introduction to parasites and their unique properties.

What is a parasite?

In simple terms, parasite is an organism that is metabolically and physiologically dependent on another organism. Parasite exploits the host for development and survivability during one or more stages of its life cycle. All parasites are eukaryotic, but some are unicellular and others are multicellular. They range in size from tiny protozoa as small as 1–2 μm in diameter (= the size of many bacteria) to arthropods or tapeworms that can measure several metres in length. In some cases, two or more parasites can occur in the same host and this phenomenon is known as polyparasitism.

Types of parasites

Based on site of infection, parasites can be divided into ecto- and endoparasites. External or ectoparasites feed or live on the body surface of the host. They either suck the blood and lymph or feed upon feather, hair, skin and its secretions. Most of ectoparasites are arthropods, i.e. invertebrates with jointed legs and hard external skeletons, e.g. lice, ticks, fleas, bugs, flies and mosquitoes. Internal or endo-parasites live inside the host. Based on the site of infection, they can be divided further: for example, enteric parasites such as *Ascaris* spp. that occupy the digestive tract; haemoparasites such as *Babesia* are found in blood and blood forming organs; venereal parasites such as *Trichomonas* in cattle and *Trypanosoma equiperdum* in equines cause infections of the reproductive organs.

Based on their life cycle, parasites can be divided into facultative or obligatory parasites. Facultative parasites can live freely and complete their life cycle without the need of a host and only under certain conditions; they enter the body of the host and produce infection, e.g. *Strongyloides* worms or free-living amoebae. In contrast, obligatory parasites must enter their host to complete their life cycle, e.g. *Plasmodium* spp. Obligatory parasites can be further divided into monoxenus or heteroxenous groups according to the number of hosts needed to complete their life cycles. Monoxenus parasites (*Ascaris*, *Eimeria*) need one host to complete their life cycle while heteroxenous parasites (*Fasciola*) need two or more hosts for their development.

Parasites may exist in one of the following forms:

- Permanent parasites spend most of their life cycle in association with their hosts, e.g. *Entamoeba histolytica*, liver flukes, *Taenia* spp.
- Temporary parasites visit their hosts occasionally and at intermittent times for taking their meal, e.g. mosquitoes, bugs.
- Periodic or seasonal parasites are found on the body of their hosts during a certain time of the year, e.g. *Oestrus ovis*, mosquitoes.
- Incidental parasites are found in hosts other than their normal hosts, e.g. *Dipylidium caninum*.
- Erratic parasites are found in their normal hosts but in unusual organs or tissues in which they are not adapted to live, e.g. *Heterophyes*, *Fasciola* spp.
- Specific parasites have adapted to live in a specific host and within a certain part of the body, e.g. *Taenia saginata* in small intestine of humans while its larval stage (*Cysticecus bovis*) is found in the musculature of cattle.

Classification of parasites

Scientific nomenclature assigns each parasite two names; the genus name is the first name and is always capitalized, followed by species name that is not capitalized. Both names are underlined or italicized. Normally, after a scientific name has been mentioned once, it can be abbreviated with the initial of the genus followed by the species name. The taxonomic classification scheme places parasites within a phylum, class, order, family, genus and species (Table 1.1).

Table 1.1 Example of parasite nomenclature

Phylum	Arthropoda
Class	Arachnida
Order	Ixodida
Family	Ixodidae
Genus	*Ixodes*
Species	*I. ricinus* (Linnaeus 1758)

Veterinarians should become familiar with both the common and the scientific names of parasite (e.g. barber's pole worms = *Heamonchus contortus*). Each parasite species has a preferred site (i.e. site of predilection) within the host body. In many cases, organ of the preference provides common names of some parasites, such as the eyeworm (*Thelazia*), the ligament worm (*Onchocerca*) and the intestinal threadworm (*Strongyloides*). The ability to discriminate between distinct groups of parasites and to communicate with a common language about parasites in the context of disease is essential for clinical parasitologists and for veterinarians caring for patients. In general, parasites are categorized into two major divisions, protozoa and metazoa.

Protozoa

The term protozoan is derived from 'proto' meaning 'first' and 'zoa' meaning 'animal'. Protozoa are 'first animals', which generally describes their animal-like nutrition. Protozoa are the largest group of single-celled, microscopic organisms, with more than 20,000 species, that are found in all aspects of life. Protozoa are single-cell (unicellular) eukaryotic organisms. Protozoa are widely distributed in various environments from favourable rainforests to sandy beaches to the bottoms of oceans to snow-covered mountains. They range in size from 2 μm to 25 cm. Their protoplasm is enclosed by a cell membrane and contains numerous organelles, including a membrane-bound nucleus, an endoplasmic reticulum, food storage granules, and contractile and digestive vacuoles. Their morphology is varied, and their physiology and metabolism are adapted to their needs. Protozoa are mostly aerobic and contain mitochondria to generate energy, although many intestinal protozoa are capable of anaerobic growth. The anaerobes lack recognizable mitochondria but may contain hydrogenosomes, mitosomes or glycosomes instead. Organs of motility vary from simple cytoplasmic extensions or pseudopods to more complex structures such as flagella or cilia. Protozoa reproduce asexually by binary fission (parent cell mitotically divides into two daughter cells), multiple fission, also known as schizogony (parent cell divides into several daughter cells), budding, and spore formation, or sexually by conjugation (two cells join, exchange nuclei and produce progeny by budding or fission). Some protozoa produce gametes (gametocytes, i.e. haploid sex cells), which fuse to form a diploid zygote. From more than 20,000 species of protozoa, only a handful cause human and animal diseases. However, these few are a major burden on human health and have a severe economic impact. The mechanisms by which the protozoa affect the body systems may be direct damage to the tissue (e.g. toxoplasmosis) or through a systemic inflammatory response by haematogenous dissemination (e.g. malaria).

Classification of protozoa based on mode of locomotion

Before the availability of molecular tools, taxonomists divided the protozoa into five groups, based on the organisms' mode of locomotion as follows.

Phylum Sarcomastigophora

This phylum includes the subphylum Sarcodina (amoebae) and Mastigophora (flagellates). Locomotion of amoebae is accomplished by the extrusion of pseudopodia 'false feet', whereas flagellates move by the lashing of their whip-like flagella. The number and position of flagella vary in different species. Examples include *Entamoeba* spp. and *Trypanosoma* spp.(Fig. 1.1).

Phylum Ciliophora

Ciliophora consists of the ciliates, which include a variety of free-living and symbiotic species. The fundamental feature of these protozoa is the presence of cilia, along the whole of the cellular membrane or at specific locations, which are used both for movement and for food capture. Examples include *Balantidium coli*. Cilia are structurally similar to flagella but are usually shorter and more rounded (Fig. 1.2). Some ciliates are multinucleate.

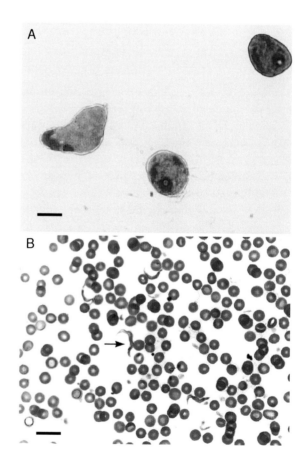

Figure 1.1 (A) *Entamoeba histolytica* trophozoite (agent of Amebiasis); (B) *Trypanosoma cruzi* trypomastigote in a thin blood smear stained with Giemsa (agent of American Trypanosomiasis). Scale bars = 10μm.

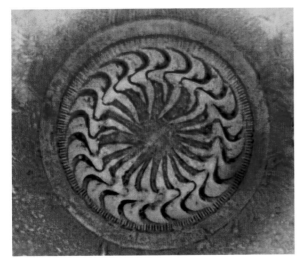

Figure 1.2 Silver nitrate-stained specimen of *Trichodina* sp. from skin of a *Tilapia* fish.

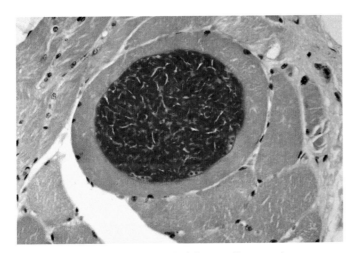

Figure 1.3 *Sarcocystis* sp. cyst in feline cardiac muscle.

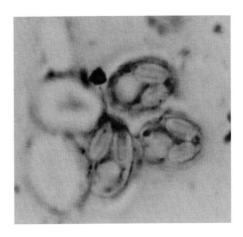

Figure 1.4 *Myxospora* spores from a cyst in the fin of a fish.

Phylum Myxozoa

The phylum Myxozoa is an entirely endoparasitic group of organisms which produce complex spores. Some myxozoan species are highly pathogenic, parasitizing both freshwater and marine fishes, in which the development culminates in myxosporean-type spores with one to several polar capsules (Fig. 1.4). Spores of some Myxozoan species have been incidentally found in patients with diarrhoeal illness and/or associated with immunosuppression.

Classification of protozoa based on ribosomal RNA sequencing

The aforementioned scheme is based on the organisms' locomotion and does not reflect any genetic relatedness. Based on nucleotide sequencing of the small subunit ribosomal RNA (SSU rRNA) gene, protozoa are reclassified into several groups (Fig. 1.5).

Parabasala

Protozoa placed in this group lack mitochondria, contain a single nucleus and a parabasal body, which is a Golgi body-like structure. Examples include *Trychonympha* and *Trichomonas*.

Cercozoa

Cercozoa is a group of amoebae with thread-like pseudopodia. These include foraminifera containing a porous shell, composed of calcium carbonate. Pseudopodia extend through holes in the shell. These may be microscopic or several centimetres in diameter. Commonly, foraminifera live on the ocean floor.

Radiolaria

Radiolaria is a group of amoebae that also have thread-like pseudopodia. The organisms have ornate shells composed of silica and live in marine waters as part of plankton. The pseudopodia of radiolarians radiate from the central body like spokes of a spherical wheel.

Phylum Apicomplexa (Sporozoa)

These protozoa are obligate intracellular parasites with one unique characteristic, the presence of an 'apical complex', i.e. an intracytoplasmic specialized organelles at their apical end that produces hydrolytic enzymes that are crucial for the parasite invasion and exit from host cells. Some Apicomplexa species have the capacity to produce tissue cysts (Fig. 1.3).

Phylum Microspora

Microspora are small intracellular obligate parasites that differ significantly in structure from the Apicomplexa. They lack organs such as mitochondria and Golgi apparatus. Their life cycle consists of an infective extracellular phase and a multiplication phase in the host cell, with spores, as the infecting forms. These spores have a complex tubular extrusion mechanism (polar tubule) used to inject the infective material (sporoplasm) into the cytoplasm of the host cells. They cause diseases in humans and animals, as well as invertebrates. *Encephalitozoon* species are reported from humans especially AIDS patients.

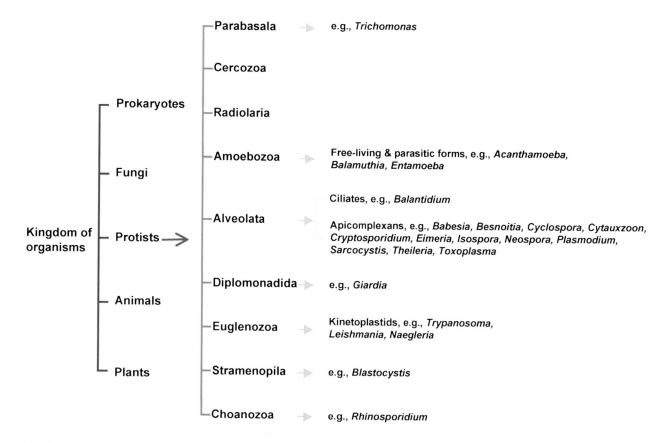

Figure 1.5 The present classification scheme of protists, based largely on their genetic relatedness.

Amoebozoa

This is the third group of amoebae that can be distinguished from the other two groups by having lobe-shaped pseudopodia and no shells. Examples include *Acanthamoeba*, *Balamuthia* and *Entamoeba*. In addition, slime moulds are also included in this group (previously thought to be fungi), based on lobe-shaped pseudopodia, no cell wall (cell wall is present in fungi), and feeding. Slime moulds can be further divided into cellular slime moulds such as *Dictyostelium* and acellular slime moulds (also known as plasmodial slime moulds) that are characterized by filaments of cytoplasm that creep as amoebae and may contain millions of nuclei.

Alveolata

Protozoa in this group contain small membrane-bound cavities known as alveoli beneath their cell surface, although the function of these structures remains unclear. This group is further divided into three subgroups: (i) ciliates such as *Balantidium coli*, (ii) Apicomplexans such as *Plasmodium*, *Cryptosporidium parvum*, *Toxoplasma gondii*, *Babesia microti* and *Isospora belli*, and (iii) dinoflagellates, which are phototrophic, such as *Gymnodinium* and *Gonyaulax*.

Diplomonadida

Protozoa in this taxon lack mitochondria, Golgi bodies and peroxisomes. The organisms have two equal-sized nuclei and multiple flagella, for example *Giardia*.

Euglenozoa

This group is further subdivided into two groups.

i   The euglenids are photoautotrophic unicellular microbes with chloroplasts containing pigments (historically thought to be plants). However, they possess flagella, lack cell wall and are chemoheterotrophic phagocytes (in the dark), for example *Euglena*.
ii The kinetoplastids have a single large mitochondrion that contains a unique region of mitochondrial DNA, called a kinetoplast. Kinetoplastids live inside animals and some are pathogenic, for example *Trypanosoma* and *Leishmania*.

Stramenopila

This group is a complex assemblage of 'botanical' protists with both heterotrophic and photosynthetic representatives. The evolutionary history of this group is unclear. Generally, the organisms included in this group are slime nets, water moulds and brown algae, and are characterized by possessing flagella. Recent molecular phylogenetic studies revealed that *Blastocystis* belongs to this group.

It is important to indicate that no single classification scheme has gained universal support and future studies will almost certainly dictate changes in the above scheme. The representative protozoal pathogens that are covered in this book are indicated in Chapter 7.

Metazoa

Metazoa are classified within the kingdom Animalia. They are multicellular organisms in which life functions occur in cellular structures organized as tissue and organ systems. The majority of metazoan parasites that affect animals and humans are encompassed within two major groups: the helminths 'worms' and the arthropods (insects, ticks, and the like).

Helminths (endoparasites)

Helminths are complex, multicellular organisms that are significantly larger than the protozoan parasites, ranging in size from a few millimetres to more than 10 m. The external surface of some worms is covered with a protective cuticle, which is acellular and may be smooth or contains ridges, spines, scales or tubercles. Frequently, helminths possess elaborate attachment organs, such as hooks, suckers, teeth or plates. These structures are usually located anteriorly and are useful in species identification. Typically, helminths have primitive nervous and excretory systems. Some have alimentary tracts; however, none has a circulatory system. The helminths are separated into three parasitic phyla: Nemathelminthes, Platyhelminthes and Acanthocephala. Growth and life cycles of parasites within each group are generally distinct from those of the other two groups.

Phylum Nemathelminthes

Nematoda is the major parasitic class in this phylum. Nematodes are by far the most economically important internal parasites of domestic animals. Nematodes are also called roundworms because they have non-segmented cylindrical bodies (Fig. 1.6) covered by a tough skin called a cuticle. They have separate sexes and complete digestive system. The nematodes may inhabit the intestine or infect the blood and tissue. The nematode life cycle encompasses three stages (egg, larval and adult stages). The larval stage can be subdivided into:

i   First-stage larva (L1), which develops within the eggs and hatches out. This larva sheds it external cuticle to grow to the next stage. The shedding of this outer layer is called 'moulting' or 'ecdysis'. Shedding of the cuticle occurs by deposition of a new cuticle and exsheathment of the old one.

ii Second-stage larva (L2), which eventually moults into the next stage.

iii Third-stage larva (L3) is the infective stage as it infects the definitive host.

iv Fourth-stage larva (L4) occurs when the third stage exsheaths within the definitive host. The initial signal for triggering each moult is determined by specific stimuli, which can be host molecules or environmental triggers.

Males of certain nematode species use certain structures, such as copulatory bursa and spicules, during mating (Fig. 1.7). Bursa is a posterior expansion of the cuticle or skin, which is bell-shaped, or funnel-shaped and supported by finger-like projections called rays. Spicules are used by the male to hold open the vulva of the female during mating. The shape and configuration of the male bursa and spicules vary from one species to another and are used to identify different nematodes. The mouth area may be specialized for attaching to or feeding on the host. For example, the kidney worm, *Stephanurus dentatus*, has six teeth in its mouth to perform such functions. See Chapter 4 for details.

Phylum Platyhelminthes

Members of this phylum have flattened bodies, which are either leaf-like (class: Trematoda) or resemble ribbon segments (class: Cestoda). In general, the flatworm's life cycle has three stages: egg, larva and adult. Most adult parasitic trematodes produce damage of economic importance in some geographic areas, while adult tapeworms are usually of minor importance.

Trematodes (flukes)

Trematodes are flat, leaf-shaped worms (Fig. 1.8). In many areas of the world, the liver fluke causes heavy losses in farm animal production. Trematodes are hermaphroditic, with male and female sex organs in a single body except the schistosomes, which have separate sexes. Their digestive systems are incomplete and have oral opening and sac-like intestinal tubes but no anus. Their life cycle is complex; snails serve as first intermediate hosts and other aquatic animals or plants as second intermediate hosts.

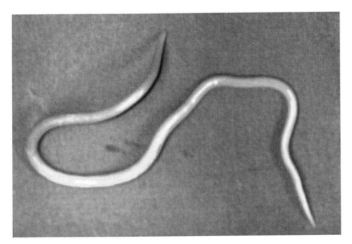

Figure 1.6 Adult ascarid nematode of cattle.

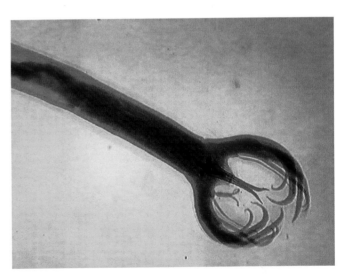

Figure 1.7 Copulatory bursa of *Haemonchus contortus*.

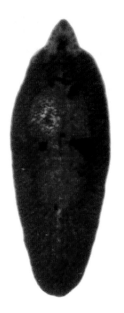

Figure 1.8 Adult *Fasciola hepatica* (digenetic trematode).

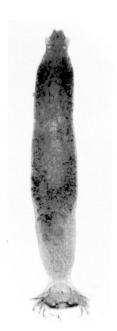

Figure 1.9 Monogenetic trematode isolated from the gills of a fish.

Class Trematoda is further divided into two orders based on the number of hosts required for the completion of the life cycle into monogenetic trematodes and digenetic trematodes. The *monogenetic trematodes* (Fig. 1.9) require a single host to complete their life cycles. They are ectoparasites of fish, amphibians, and reptiles and have a direct life cycle. *Digenetic trematodes* require two hosts to complete their life cycle (Fig. 1.10). Adult flukes reside in the predilection site in the definitive host and lay eggs that pass in the faeces. The larval form hatches from the egg when optimal

moisture and temperature exist and penetrates the snail host. Finally, during the infective stage the adults leave the snail host and infect the definitive host. See Chapter 6 for details.

Cestodes (Tapeworms)

Cestodes of veterinary importance are classified into two main orders: Pseudophyllidea (tapeworms of carnivores) and Cyclophyllidea (important tapeworms of humans and animals). Cestodes are commonly called tapeworms because they may

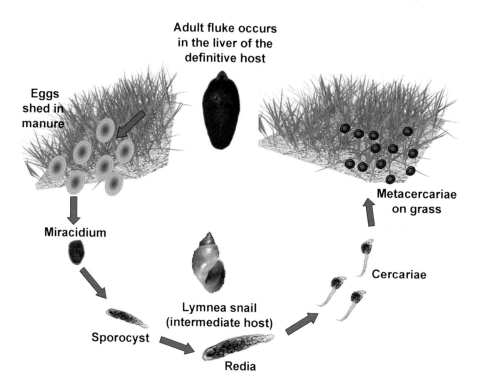

Figure 1.10 Life cycle of *Fasciola* spp. as an example of digenetic trematodes.

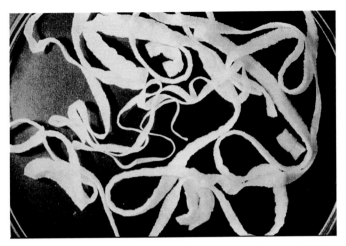

Figure 1.11 Adult cestode (tapeworm). (Image kindly supplied by Jerzy Behnke, University of Nottingham.)

reach a length of several meters in some species. Cestodes are flat, ribbon-like worms (Fig. 1.11). They have no digestive tract, but absorb nourishment directly through their tegument from the gut contents of the host animal. The tapeworm has a head, called a 'scolex', and a body made of many segments (band-like) called 'proglottids'. Each mature proglottid is a complete functional unit, incorporating a digestive system, organs of both sexes (hermaphroditic), and other organs. The life cycles of cestodes are complex and require one or more intermediate hosts. Adult tapeworms are endoparasites, and inhabit the small intestine of the principal host or, with *Thysanosoma* spp., have access to the intestine. The intermediate host harbours the larval, immature, asexual stages of the parasite. See Chapter 5 for details.

Phylum Acanthocephala

Acanthocephalans are found in many species of fish, amphibians, birds, and mammals. Several morphological characteristics serve to separate acanthocephalans from other parasitic worms, but probably the most notable is the presence of an anterior, protrusible proboscis that is usually covered with hooks. It is this characteristic that gives the acanthocephalans their common name, the 'thorny-headed worms'. The life cycles of all acanthocephalans appear to follow the same basic pattern. The adult acanthocephalans occur in the intestine of the definitive host. The sexes are separate i.e. they are dioecious, and the females produce eggs that are passed in the host's faeces. The eggs are ingested by an intermediate host, an arthropod in which the parasite goes through several developmental or juvenile stages. The definitive host is infected with the parasite when it eats an intermediate host containing the parasite.

Arthropoda (ectoparasites)

Members of the phylum Arthropoda constitute the largest group of organisms in the kingdom Animalia. Arthropods are complex, multicellular organisms that may be involved directly in causing an invasive or a superficial disease process or indirectly as intermediate hosts and vectors of many infectious agents, including protozoan and metazoan parasites. Arthropods are important

external parasites whose outer shell is composed of chitin, a polysaccharide that some chemotherapeutic products are designed to inhibit. Some arthropods emerge from eggs resembling adults except for minor differences and these are known as ametabola, e.g. Cyclops. However, the majority of arthropods hatch from eggs in a form different from that of adult and must undergo morphological and developmental changes (i.e. metamorphosis) to reach adult stage. Such arthropods are known as metabola. These are further divided into two groups: holometabola (complete metamorphosis), where each stage differs markedly from others in morphology (in particular size and genital organs), feeding habits and types of food, e.g. flies and fleas (Fig. 1.12); and hemimetabola (incomplete metamorphosis), in which there are slight changes in feeding habits and morphology between different stages, e.g. lice, mites, ticks (Fig. 1.13).

The ectoparasites of domesticated animals are generally members of the phylum Arthropoda. There are many different types of ectoparasites, including ticks, mites, fleas, lice, blood-sucking flies, and myiasis-inducing flies. Some are host specific, whereas others infect any number of animals. Diagnosis is generally based on the external morphological appearance, with the use of taxonomic keys. Control is often difficult, sometimes necessitating treatment of the premises and prevention by prohibiting interaction with infected animals (e.g. companion animals with fleas, ticks, or lice). Within the phylum Arthropoda, there are two major classes, namely Arachnida and Insecta, which are of particular veterinary medical importance.

Class Arachnida

These include vectors for microbial diseases (mites and ticks) or act as venomous animals that bite (spiders) or sting (scorpions). Arachnids are ectoparasitic organisms whose body is composed of head and abdomen. Metamorphosis is incomplete. The arachnid life cycle has four stages, namely egg, larva, nymph and adult. Unlike insects, arachnids have no wings or antennae, and adults have four pairs of legs (Fig. 1.14), compared with three pairs for insects. The larval arachnid is unusual because it has only six legs. Arachnids' mouth part consists of five elongated structures, namely a pair of chelicerae, a pair of pedipalps and a central hypostome armed with backward-projecting teeth. There are two major families of ticks, the Argasidae, or soft ticks, and the Ixodidae, or hard ticks (Table 1.2).

Class Insecta

Insects are both ecto- and endoparasites and include aquatic and terrestrial forms. They have three pairs of legs and three body parts; head, thorax and abdomen (Fig. 1.15). The mouth consists of five elongated organs, namely labrum epipharynx, hyopharynx, two mandibles, two maxillae and the labium. Wings and antennae are present in most of insects. An insect's life cycle has four stages: egg, larva, pupa and adult. Development may be complete (e.g. flies) or incomplete (e.g. lice, bugs, cockroaches). Flies are classified according to the habits of the females. *Oviparous* females, e.g. the house fly, lay immature eggs in early stage of development and hatching occurs after a certain period. *Viviparous (Larviparous)* females lay larvae, e.g. the flesh fly. *Pupiparous* females lay

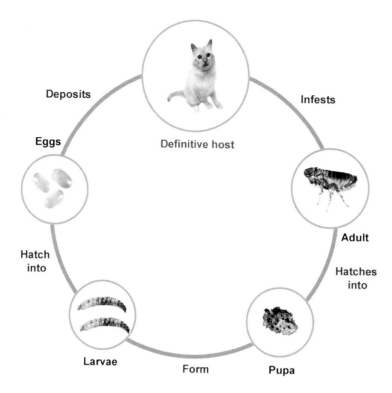

Figure 1.12 Life cycle of fleas with complete metamorphosis.

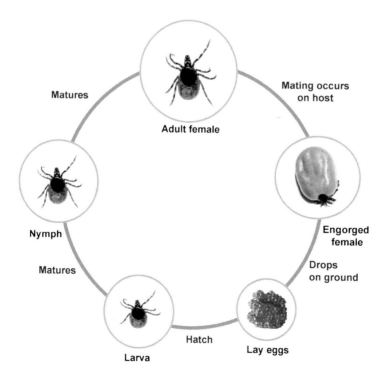

Figure 1.13 Life cycle of ticks with incomplete metamorphosis.

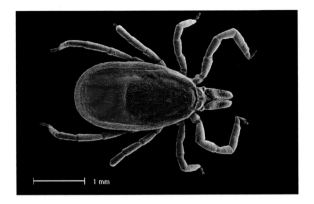

Figure 1.14 A photograph of a female hard tick showing scutum partly covering the dorsum. (Image kindly supplied by Novartis Animal Health Inc., Switzerland.)

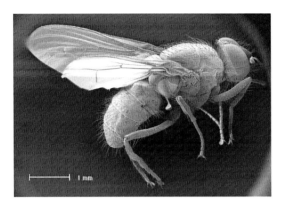

Figure 1.15 Adult *Haematobia irritans*, the horn fly. (Image kindly supplied by Novartis Animal Health Inc., Switzerland.)

Table 1.2 Comparison between soft ticks and hard ticks

Family	Argasidae	Ixodidae
Common name	Called 'soft ticks' because they lack the scutum	Called 'hard ticks' because of the hard dorsal scutum
Scutum	Absent	Present and covers whole dorsal surface of male and anterior portion of female
Sexual dimorphism	Slight	Marked
Sexual differentiation	Difficult	Easy by scutum
Mouth parts	In nymph and adult are ventrally situated and never protrude anteriorly, or seen from dorsal view	Protrude anteriorly and easily visible from dorsal view
Festoons	Absent	Present posteriorly
Eyes	Absent, but when present, they are located on the lateral margin of the body	Present on the edges of the scutum
Spiracles	Anterior to the fourth coxa	Posterior to the fourth coxa
Habits	Temporary ectoparasites of birds and mammals; attack host to feed at night only	Permanent ectoparasites of most animals. They suck blood during day and night and never leave host except for egg laying or for developing to the next stage
Nymphal stages	More than one nymphal stage (4–5)	One nymphal stage only
Eggs	Female lays multiple, small batches of eggs in between several blood meals	Female lays a single, large batch of eggs, then die

well-developed larvae which convert into pupa rapidly after deposition, e.g. *Glossina*, *Hippobosca*. Of veterinary medical importance are the many insects that serve as vectors for microbial diseases including mosquitoes, fleas, flies, lice, and bugs, or as venomous animals that sting such as bees, wasps and ants.

Subphylum Crustacea

Crustacea consists of aquatic forms, such as crabs, crayfish, shrimp, and copepods. The latter include species which cause direct damage to the host, e.g. the crustacean copepod *Lambroglena* spp. (Fig. 1.16). Several are used as intermediate hosts in life cycles of various helminths, e.g. *Diphylobothrium latum*.

Pentastomida (endoparasites)

Pentastomids share features with Arthropoda, but is usually regarded as an independent phylum. The pentastomids (tongue worms) are respiratory endoparasites of reptiles, birds, and mammals. Adult pentastomids are white and cylindrical or flattened parasites that possess two distinct body regions: an anterior cephalothorax and an abdomen. Life cycle is indirect (i.e. involves an intermediate host). Diagnosis may be made by finding the eggs in the faeces or respiratory secretions. There is currently no effective treatment for pentastomid infestations. Humans can act as intermediate hosts, becoming infected by having their hands contaminated from the faeces or saliva of the reptile, and accidentally ingesting the eggs. In some cases infected patients develop localized inflammation.

What is a host?

A host is a person, an animal or other living organism that affords subsistence or lodgement to the parasite under natural conditions, but, at the same time, suffers from the harm or injury caused by that parasite. Some parasites pass successive stages in alternate hosts of different species. Hosts may be divided based on the role they play in the life cycle of parasite into the following types:

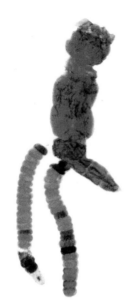

Figure 1.16 Adult *Lamproglena* isolated from the gills of a Tilapia fish.

- The *definitive or final host* is a host in which the parasite attains its sexual maturity. This is most often the vertebrate host, e.g. humans, dogs and cats are final hosts for *Heterophyes heterophyes* (intestinal fluke).
- The *intermediate host* is a host that provides the parasite with a temporary environment for completion of immature stages of its life cycle, but one in which only the asexual or immature stages of the parasite occur. Some parasites need more than one intermediate host to complete their life cycle. So intermediate hosts may be:
  - *first intermediate host,* in which the early larval stages are formed, e.g. *Pirinella conica* snail is the 1st intermediate host for *H. heterophyes*
  - *second intermediate host,* which harbour the later developmental or larval stages, e.g. Fish (*Mugil, Tilapia*) is the 2nd intermediate host for *H. heterophyes.*
- The *transport host* is a host that is unnecessary for the parasite to complete any stage of its life cycle and is merely used to carry the non-developing parasite for sometimes to the next host without further development, e.g. earth worm may ingest eggs or larvae and disseminate them as they pass through its gut.
- A *paratenic host* is a potential intermediate host in which there is no development of the immature parasite; the host does not favour or hinder the parasite in the completion of its life cycle. The parasite may exist for longer periods here than in a transport host.
- A *reservoir host* is an infected definitive host serving as a source from which other animals or humans can become infected and never suffer from such association, e.g. antelopes infected with *Trypanosoma* of cattle.
- A *carrier host* is a natural definitive host carrying the parasite without the appearance of any pathological lesions or disease manifestations and at the same time it can spread the infection to other hosts, e.g. *Trichomonas foetus* in bulls.

- A *vector* is an agent of transmission. When the final or intermediate host that delivers the infectious agents to the animal or human is an arthropod it is defined as vector, e.g. ticks act as a vector host for *Babesia* and mosquitoes act as a vector for malaria.
- *Paratenesis* is the passage of an infective-stage larva by a transport or paratenic host to the definitive host; the larva does not undergo essential development within the transport host, but is maintained in its infective stage from one season of transmission to another.

With respect to susceptibility to parasites, different types of hosts are recognized.

- *Tolerant hosts* are easily parasitized with certain species of parasites.
- *Refractory hosts* are difficult to be parasitized.
- *Natural hosts* are frequently parasitized by certain species of parasites.
- *Foreign hosts* occasionally become parasitized.
- *Accidental hosts* are very seldom to be parasitized with a certain species of parasite.
- *Provisional or temporary hosts* may become infected but throw off the infection after a short time.

Spectrum of host–parasite interaction

For successful control and treatment of parasitic diseases, an understanding of the nature and types of the host–parasite interactions is essential. The spectrum of possible interactions among hosts and parasites may appear too complex for analysis. However, it is constructive to simplify the variables and consider only the general domains of these interactions. To illustrate this principal, four host–parasite relationships whereby parasites interact with the hosts are outlined (Table 1.3).

Why we study parasites

Most parasites are true disease-causing agents and are capable of causing significant damage to the host.

Parasites cause animal disease

Parasites cause severe economic losses in animals predominantly due to lost productivity in livestock world-wide. Clinical signs associated with parasitism include anaemia (Fig. 1.17A), diarrhoea (Fig. 1.17B), hypoproteinaemia, vomiting and life-threatening obstruction of vital body organs. These signs are frequently associated with weight loss and loss of condition and, if left untreated, infection can result in mortality. Many of the parasites responsible for important diseases are acquired by the consumption of contaminated food or water, or are transmitted by arthropod vectors. The control and prevention of each parasitic disease discussed in this book are provided in the following chapters. The adverse effects of parasites on their host can be due to a direct harmful effects caused by the parasite or caused by the over response of host's body to the intruder parasite. The type of damage may vary between different parasites. In Great Britain, the

Table 1.3 Common patterns of host–parasite relationships

Type	Description	Example
Parasitism	Obligatory association between two distinct organisms (the parasite and the host), where the parasite lives on the expense of the host and at the same time causing a damage (pathological lesions or disease condition) to the host	Relationship between intestinal round worms and a dog
Symbiosis (sym = together, bios = life)	Obligatory relationship between two organisms in which both gain benefits while living alone for each being impossible (i.e. have complementary needs)	Flagellates in the gut of termites
Commensalism (com = together, mensa = table)	This occurs when one member of the associating pair, usually the smaller, receives all the benefit and the other member is neither benefited nor harmed. The basis for a commensalistic relationship between two organisms may be space, substrate, defence, shelter, transportation, or food. If the association is merely a passive transportation of the commensal by the host it is called phoresy	*Entamoeba coli* lives in colon of humans
Mutualism	This facultative relationship occurs between two organisms when each member of the symbiotic relationship benefits the other	Relationship between ungulates and their ciliates

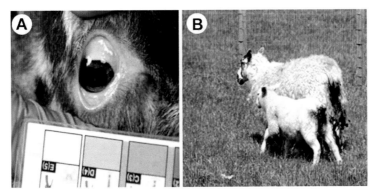

Figure 1.17 Some clinical signs associated with gastrointestinal parasitic infections in ruminants: (A) anaemia, (B) diarrhoea. (Image kindly supplied by Dave Bartley, Moredun Research Institute.)

cost of all parasitic diseases was estimated in 2005 to be around £84 million.

Endoparasites (protozoa and worms) use various mechanisms to induce pathological damages in the hosts including:

- *compete for nutrients* – some parasites ingest nutrients meant for the host, compromising the host's ability to thrive, or even survive, e.g. *Ascaris* and tapeworms;
- *feeding on the surrounding tissues* – e.g. *Entamoeba histolytica*, *Syngamus trachae*;
- *ingestion of blood and lymph* – leading to severe anaemia, e.g. *Haemonchus contortus* and ancylostomes;
- *sucking of blood* – with subsequent anaemia and/or transmission of other disease agents, e.g. mosquitoes and ticks;
- *destruction of large number of erythrocytes* – e.g. *Plasmodium* and *Babesia*;
- *toxic secretions and excretions of the parasite* – e.g. *Plasmodium*, *Trypanosoma*, and roundworms secrete proteases that destroy tissue;
- *tissue damage* – this may be due to direct penetration or destruction of epithelial cells, e.g. enteric coccidiosis;
- *formation of tumours* – e.g. *Habronema* spp., *Spirocerca lupi*, and *Schistosoma* spp.;
- *obstruction of a vital organ* – *Fasciola* spp. in the bile ducts, *Filariasis* in camel obstructs the spermatic artery, and massive ascarid infections can block the intestines;

- *traumatic inflammatory condition* – due to the presence of suckers, hooks or teeth as well as the migration of the parasite or its larval stage inside the host, e.g. *Ancylostoma* spp., *Taenia* spp., and migration of trematode larvae;
- *disruption of metabolic function* – via increasing abomasal pH, e.g. *Ostertagia ostertagi* and *Haemoncus contortus*;
- *the parasite or its larval stages may carry other pathogens* – such as bacteria while penetrating the host tissues, e.g. *Clostridium novyi* with the larval stages of *Fasciola* spp.

Ectoparasites, besides playing a very impotent role in the transmission of various infectious agents, they can produce certain diseases and affections including:

- *myiasis* – caused by invasion of live host tissue by larvae of *Hypoderma*, *Gastrophilus* and *Lucilia*;
- *mange* – caused by certain mites that cause severe damage of the skin and wool with economic losses;
- *dermatitis* – a skin irritation and inflammatory manifestations result from the bite of mosquitoes, fleas, lice or bed-bugs or the invasion of the skin with myiasis producing flies as *Dermatobia*;
- *poisoning* – the poison may be introduced into the body during the bite, e.g. cone-nosed bugs or through a sting, e.g. scorpions;
- *allergy* – sensitivity to the excretions of insects, e.g. the bite of mosquitoes, bed bugs, wasps or bees;

- *entomophobia* (the fear from insects) – animals become excited on hearing the sound of some insects. The animals do not feed; try to hide from the insect resulting in low production (e.g. *Oestrus ovis* in sheep) or force itself against a fence leading to injuries (*Hypoderma* fly in cattle);
- *irritation* – caused by the egg-laying behaviour of female *Oxyuris equi* will cause the animal to rub itself against the wall or any objects in the stable and injuries itself.

Parasites and public health

Parasitic diseases represent a major global public health problem because many parasitic infections are zoonotic, transmitted between animals and humans. These infections are always of concern to the public and to certain occupational groups who come into daily contact with exotic, wild, and/or domesticated animals. Although parasites have a limited host range, they can and do spread across species barriers. Parasite zoonoses can cause a variety of symptoms in humans, from skin irritation caused by flea bites, to death from multi-organ failure as seen in advanced Lyme disease. Some parasites are human specific, but others may be incidental i.e. accidentally-infecting humans. Because some of the common parasites that infect animals also infect humans, especially young children, pregnant women, and immunosuppressed individuals, they pose a public health risk and veterinarians have a responsibility to inform their clients about a parasite's zoonotic potential. The great majority of these diseases are in relation with the faecal contamination of soil, the general level of hygiene and the food practices and meat-related products. Hence, control of most of zoonotic parasitic diseases requires strict attention to personal hygiene and avoidance of contaminated materials. The public health implications of each parasitic disease discussed in this book are provided in the following chapters.

Social burden of parasites

The World Health Organization ranks five parasitic diseases, namely malaria, schistosomiasis, amoebiasis, hookworm infection, and African trypanosomiasis among the top 20 microbial causes of human death in the world. The migrations and tourism help spread tropical diseases outside their geographical range. Additionally, parasitic infections may play a role in the spread and establishment of bacterial, viral, and fungal pathogens. For example, free-living *Acanthamoeba* is known to host microbes such as viruses, bacteria, yeast and other protozoa which may help in their transmission to the susceptible hosts. Some of the parasites have only recently been identified as a major threat to human health. For example, *Cryptosporidium* was originally described in the 19th century, but has recently been associated with serious human infections in AIDS patients. It was responsible for causing disease in 400,000 people in an outbreak in Milwaukee, USA, in 1993. Other examples include *Pneumocystis*, the leading cause of death in AIDS patients.

What can we do?

It has become patently obvious that the continued complacency towards the parasitic diseases has made everyone vulnerable to the emerging and re-emerging parasitic diseases. It must be understood that parasitic diseases are a common target that continues to seriously threaten the human species. Parasitic agents from all over the world has a common objective, i.e. to target other living organisms to ensure the survival of their species. We must have early warning systems in place to prevent the spread of parasitic diseases, as well as rapidly increase the arsenal of drugs for our urgent needs and develop alternative strategies for therapeutic interventions. The urgent needs are as follows:

1 Seriously ill hosts may be infected with more than one parasite and the diagnosis is difficult. Thus combined therapy should prove highly effective.
2 Increased awareness and better feeding practices will significantly reduce the risk of parasitic diseases.
3 Early diagnosis is of crucial value for the successful treatment of parasitic diseases.
4 Identification of the risk factors should enhance our ability to interfere with the parasitic diseases. For example, malaria is spread by mosquitoes and the use of bed-nets during sleep should help reduce the number of malaria-associated deaths.
5 Availability of drugs: as indicated above, millions of people/animals in developing countries are dying needlessly from diseases that could be easily treated with inexpensive drugs. Access of these drugs to the needy can help develop these communities.
6 Education of sexually transmitted diseases, hygiene and their associated risks.
7 Mass immunizations have proven effective in eradicating smallpox and similar approaches for parasitic diseases should be the objective.
8 Strengthen health services and delivery systems in developing countries.
9 Expansion of surveillance systems to alert the unexpected outbreaks, the emergence of new diseases and increased drug resistance.
10 Need to develop novel drugs as well as to slow the rate of drug resistance.
11 Development of diagnostic tools, new drugs and vaccines that can further improve our ability to target parasitic diseases.
12 To eliminate or reduce the risk of arthropod-borne diseases, it is necessary to control the environment, reservoirs of infection and the vectors. This would include control of water and food, carriers of disease agents, and the protection of animals and humans from the infection. Where possible and practical, the reservoirs and arthropod vectors of disease should be destroyed and measures should be undertaken to make the environment unfavourable for their propagation, such as draining swamps and spraying insecticides.

Perspectives

Parasitic diseases of animals cause serious economic losses by reducing animal performance and productivity, in many cases have fatal consequences. Parasitic diseases also represent major global health problems. African sleeping sickness, malaria, leishmaniosis, Chagas disease, and schistosomiasis are some examples of parasitic diseases that cause millions of deaths annually, and present an immense social and economic burden. For successful control and treatment of parasitic diseases, knowledge of the type and nature of harm and damage caused by parasitic infections is fundamental.

Further reading

Boreham, R.E., Hendrick, S., O'Donoghue, P.J. and Stenzel, D.J. (1998). Incidental finding of *Myxobolus* spores (Protozoa:Myxozoa) in stool samples from patients with gastrointestinal symptoms. J. Clin. Microbiol. *36*, 3728–3730.

Canning, E.U. and Lom, J. (1986). The Microsporidia of Vertebrates (Academic Press, Inc., New York).

Cavalier-Smith, T. (1993). Kingdom protozoa and its 18 phyla. Microbiol. Rev. *57*, 953–994.

Elsheikha, H.M. (2007). Heterophyosis: risk of ectopic infection. Vet. Parasitol. *147*, 341–342.

Elsheikha, H.M. and Sheashaa, H.A. (2007). Epidemiology, pathophysiology, management and outcome of renal dysfunction associated with plasmodia infection. Parasitol. Res. *101*, 1183–1190.

Levine, N.D., Corliss, J.O. and Cox, F.E.G., Deroux, G., Grain, G., Honigberg, B.M., Leedale, G.F., Loeblich, A.R., Lom, J., Lynn, D., *et al.* (1980). A newly revised classification of the protozoa. J. Protozool. *27*, 37–58.

MacKenzie, W.R., Hoxie, N.J., Proctor, M.E., Gradus, M.S., Blair, K.A., Peterson, D.E., Kazmierczak, J.J., Addiss, D.G., Fox, K.R., Rose, J.B., *et al.* (1994). A massive outbreak in Milwaukee of *Cryptosporidium* infection transmitted through the public water supply. N. Engl. J. Med. *331*, 161–167.

Moncada, L.I., López, M.C., Murcia, M.I., Nicholls, S., León, F., Guío, O.L. and Corredor, A. (2001). *Myxobolus* sp., another opportunistic parasite in immunosuppressed patients? J. Clin. Microbiol. *39*, 1938–1940.

Nieuwhof, G.J., Bishop, S.C. (2005). Costs of the major endemic diseases of sheep in Great Britain and the potential benefits of reduction in disease impact. Anim. Sci. *81*, 23–29.

Petney, T.N. and Andrews, R.H. (1998). Multiparasite communities in animals and humans: frequency, structure and pathogenic significance. Int. J. Parasitol. *28*, 377–393.

Sutherst, R.W. (2004). Global change and human vulnerability to vector-borne diseases. Clin. Microbiol. Rev. *17*, 136–173.

Vora, N. (2008). Impact of anthropogenic environmental alterations on vector-borne diseases. Medscape J. Med. *10*, 238.

Principles of Parasite Infection

2

Hany M. Elsheikha and Naveed A. Khan

Introduction

How do parasites establish themselves inside their hosts is one of the most intriguing questions in parasitology. Given the diversity that exists among parasites, it is not surprising that the mechanics of parasitic infections are highly variable. The diverse strategies that pathogenic parasites use to infect their hosts have become better understood by means of molecular techniques that have allowed the identification of parasitic genes and virulence factors which are crucial to disease establishment and progression. Despite all this progress, predicting the transmission of any parasitic disease remains a challenge (Table 2.1). This chapter addresses the interplay between parasites and their host organisms, introduces the fundamentals of parasite infection, and provides an overview of the multiple determinants — related to the parasite, the host, and the environment — that influence the parasite's capacity to cause a disease at the cellular and population levels.

What can life cycles tell us?

Life cycle is a description of the life history of the parasite (from egg or larva to sexual maturity and reproduction) including its entire links to vertebrates and other hosts. The life cycles of parasites can be complex; with some parasites establish a permanent relationship with certain hosts and others go through a series of developmental stages in a succession of hosts. Life cycle of the parasite can be divided into growth and maturation, reproduction and transmission phases. Life cycle can be direct or indirect. *Direct life cycle*: the infective stage of the parasite (such as a cyst, egg or larva) released by one host is directly taken up (often ingested) by another host, in which the parasite grows and matures (Fig. 2.1). *Indirect life cycle* is one in which the parasite requires one or more additional host, often belonging to a different phylum, to complete its development (Fig. 2.2) and are difficult to control. Even if the definitive host is treated, the life cycle will continue because the parasite may be present in the untreated intermediate host, and this will permit reinfection of the definitive host.

Treatment, including selection of the proper drug and appropriate control measures, always requires a thorough knowledge of the biology of each parasite. Veterinarians need to know what stage of a parasite's life cycle is spent on the animal they are treating because it influences diagnostic assays and what products will be most effective for treatment and prevention. Parasites have diverse patterns of life cycles. The life cycle, or developmental stages, of a parasite differs depending on the group to which it belongs. The life cycle of nematodes encompasses five developmental stages, three of these are free-living (i.e. periods of a parasite's life outside the host). Some nematodes, such as the strongyle of ruminants and horses, produce eggs that pass with faeces into the environment. A first-stage larva develops within each egg and hatches to become free-living. This first-stage larva grows and moults (sheds the skin or cuticle) to a second-stage larva, which then grows and moults into a third-stage larva (the infective stage). This infective stage larva is usually ingested and develops into a fourth-stage larva and finally into a fifth-stage larva within the host. Some nematodes possess some modifications of this general life cycle. For example, hookworm larvae generally penetrate the skin and circulate in the host's tissue before completing their development in the small intestine. Others, such as roundworms and whipworms, develop the infective stage within the eggs, which do not hatch until they are ingested by the host. Other nematodes, such as *Strongyloides* spp., have first-stage larvae in the eggs when passed. In the light of these facts, knowledge of the life cycles

Table 2.1 Fundamental questions of parasite pathogenesis

At the host level

How does the parasite infect the host?

What is the initial host response?

How does parasite replication occur?

What organs or tissues are infected?

Does infection disseminate to other organs in the host's body?

How is parasite shed and transmitted?

At the parasite level

How does a parasite enter the host cells?

How does the infection alter the body function?

Is the infection cleared from the host or is a persistent infection established?

How is the parasite transmitted to other hosts?

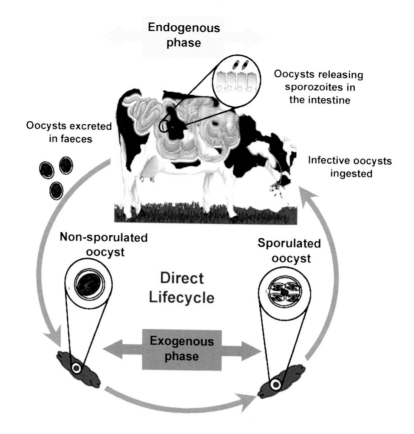

Figure 2.1 General life cycle of *Eimeria*, the agent of coccidiosis.

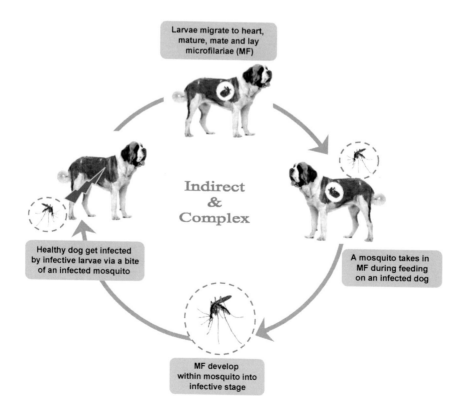

Figure 2.2 Life cycle of *Dirofilaria immitis*, the agent of heartworm disease.

contributes to the effectiveness of parasite control by permitting development of well-timed control programmes.

The infection mechanisms of parasites are highly variable and include phases outwith and within the same host in case of direct life cycles or different phases in different hosts in case of indirect life cycles. To understand the infection process we will analyse the phases of infection i.e. chain of infection.

Parasite pathogenesis

Parasites command our attention because of their association with many animal and human diseases. The step by step process by which parasites cause disease is called parasite pathogenesis. To study this process, we must investigate not only the relationships of parasites with specific host cells that they infect but also the consequences of infection to the host organism. The nature of parasitic infection depends on the ability of the parasite to spread in and among host, the parasite's ability of entering the host body, the responses of the host defence systems, the effects of parasite replication on host cells, and the parasite's ability to survive in reservoir hosts or in the environment. All these factors are collectively known as chain of infection (Fig. 2.3).

Parasite agent

Whether parasites cause an infection or an infestation depends on what part of the host's body they inhabit. Parasites that live on their host are called ectoparasites (external parasites), and their presence is called an *infestation*. They may live on the surface or in pores of the skin, or they may attach themselves to the animal's hair. Some external parasites spend only a short time on the host; others stay a life time. Lice and ticks are an example of a parasite that infest. Parasites that live in their hosts are called endoparasites (internal parasites); their presence is called an *infection*. Each type of endoparasite occupies a particular niche within the body. Tapeworms and hookworms are an example of an endoparasite

that infect or live in the gut. Most diseases caused by parasites are the result of infection; that is, the development of disease requires multiplication of the parasite in host tissues. Whether infection or infestation, parasites must remain metabolically dependent on the host.

Environment and reservoir

A fundamental part of understanding parasite infection chain and host–parasite interactions is to understand the exogenous phase of parasite infection, such as the strategies of host finding and host manipulation by parasites, as well as parasite mechanisms of adaptation outside the host.

Mechanics of host findings

We need to remember that parasites spend some of their life outside the host in the environment or in other reservoir hosts, and host finding deals with everything involved in getting into (or onto) a new host. There are three main mechanisms by which the parasite encounters a host.

Passive methods of host finding

In this type, the parasites find a host by simply waiting for a host to find them. This mode of transmission applies to coccidian oocysts, parasitic worm eggs and larval stages in some species. Larval stages present in intermediate hosts or vectors may also be transmitted passively.

Active methods of host finding

Some parasites are mobile and seek their next host actively. Significant mobility on land is restricted to the parasitic arthropods, e.g. fleas possess well-developed legs to jump onto passing hosts. Nematodes have limited mobility and use it primarily to place themselves in habitats where they are likely to come in contact with hosts. For examples, strongyle larvae climb and accumulate in a drop of water on the tip of the grass and wait to be ingested by the grazing sheep.

Transmission by vectors or intermediate hosts

Some parasites enter vectors passively, as the vectors are feeding. The parasite then undergoes some development or replication in the vector. When the vector seeks out a new host to feed on, it introduces the parasites it is harbouring. Blood-feeding insects are the most common vectors, e.g. mosquitoes transmit many apicomplexan protozoans, such as *Plasmodium*. Parasites may enter intermediate hosts actively or passively. Once inside they usually transform into a stage that can persist for long periods, until that host is eaten by another animal that can serve as a second intermediate host or definitive host, e.g. the intestinal fluke *H. heterophyes* uses snail as a first intermediate host, fish as a second intermediate host, and fish-eating mammals as a definitive host.

Manipulation of intermediate hosts

Induced alteration of host behaviour is a widespread transmission strategy among some parasites. Understanding how it works is an exciting challenge from both a mechanistic and an evolutionary perspective. There are key examples of the mechanisms by which

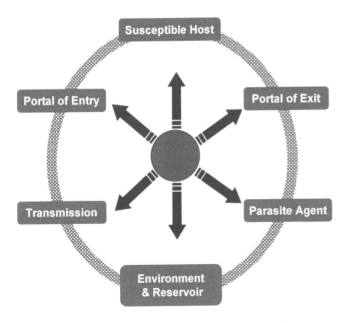

Figure 2.3 Factors involved in the parasite infection cycle.

parasites are known to control/manipulate the behaviour of their hosts. The first example is the parasitic helminth *Dicrocoelium dendriticum* (lancet liver fluke). This fluke typically lives in the bile duct of the liver of grazing animals (and sometimes humans). It has a typical trematode (fluke) life cycle, but with three different hosts. Interestingly, it alters the behaviour of one of the intermediate hosts (ants), making it more likely to reach the next host. The second example is the protozoan *Toxoplasma gondii*, which lives and reproduces in the cat's intestines, leading to formation and shedding of the oocysts in the cat faeces. After a few days the oocysts mature and become ready to infect their next animal host, which is rodent (rat or mouse). After ingesting the oocysts the parasite then goes into the bloodstream and takes up residence in various places in the rodent's body as an immature form. The life cycle will be completed when the cat eats an infected rat. The problem is that rodents are naturally afraid of cats and will avoid them at all costs. But, after become infected with *T. gondii* they become hyperactive and less afraid of cats. This lack of cat fear makes infected rats more likely to be eaten by a cat. Thus, the life cycle continues. More interestingly, research on *T. gondii* in humans suggests that chronic infection causes subtle behavioural, personality, and psychological changes in infected people.

Environmental adaptation

During the early phase of the infection process before invading the host tissue, the development of parasites greatly depends on favourable environmental conditions such as, temperature, surface moisture, relative humidity, soil salinity, oxygen and direct sunlight. The life cycle, ecology, and bionomics of pre-infective and infective larval stages of strongyle nematodes is a good model of nematode parasite adaptation to the environment. In regard to the pre-infective larval stage, the eggs of the parasite are passed in the faeces, in early stages of segmentation. Eggs are thin-shelled, composed of an outer chitinous shell and an inner delicate vitelline membrane. Embryonation commences immediately but is dependent on suitable environmental conditions mentioned above. Fully embryonated eggs hatch to release a first free-living stage within a day at about 26°C. Development to the first larval stage may be inhibited by several factors. Temperature and lack of moisture are the two critical ones. After hatching from the eggs the larvae are in the first stage (L1) and are characterized by having a rhabditiform oesophagus. They feed mainly on bacteria for a short while, and moult for the first time by shedding the cuticle and transforming into the second-stage larva (L2) which has a less rhabditiform oesophagus than L1. When L2 moults to form the third-stage larva (L3), the old cuticle of the L2 is separated off, but it is not shed; it remains as protective sheath round the L3. This sheathed L3 has a filariform oesophagus. Infection occurs by ingestion of infective larvae (ensheathed L3). Liberation of the infective larva from the retained sheath of the second-stage larva (exsheathment) occurs in the host's gut.

Behaviour of the infective L3 is different from that of the earlier pre-infective stages. It does not feed and survive on the reserve food granules stored in its intestinal cells. The larva does not actively enter the host, but is swallowed with herbages, or sometimes water. However, L3 larvae respond to a number of external stimuli that increase the possibility of finding a host. The larva is negatively geotropic, so it crawls up blades of grass or other herbage. Also, it is positively phototropic to a mild light, but is repelled by strong sunlight. So, the larvae will crawl up the blades of the grass or other herbages only in early morning, towards the evening and at other times of the day in dull weather. At night some of the larvae may descend to the soil. Moisture is necessary for these migrations, as the larvae are unable to crawl on a dry surface. There is a certain level of response to heat; migration is more active in warm than in cold weather. Some larvae may penetrate the soil, where they survive more readily than on the surface. In loose sandy soil, they are able to move easily and to penetrate deeper than in clay soil. Taking all these factors together, the length of life of a larva in a pasture is favourably affected by moisture, shade and a relatively low temperature and under such conditions some larvae may live for a year or longer in the soil.

How do parasites spread?

The first event in the parasite life cycle is the transmission. Mode of transmission of parasites varies based on their location on the host's body. Parasitic diseases are transmitted from one host to another via exposure to contaminated environment or infected host (Fig. 2.4).

Contact transmission

This may involve direct contact with the infected host or indirect contact via sharing of an inert infected object (e.g. mange).

Vehicle transmission

This may be airborne (dust particles), waterborne (streams or swimming pools) or food-borne (e.g. uncooked meat).

Vector transmission

Ectoparasites (Arthropods) serve as a vector for transmitting infectious agents (protozoa, bacteria, viruses) to the animals. Arthropods' capacity to transmit diseases can vary from one animal or from a locality to another. The transmission may occur either through biting or contaminating food. The transmitted infectious agents have a complex biological relationship with the insect, as well as the host. Arthropods can serve as a site of maturation for the parasite, and passage through the insect is crucial step in the natural life cycle of the infectious agent (e.g. *Dirofilaria immitis*, canine heartworm cannot be transmitted to a new host without passing through a mosquito).

Mechanical transmission

Mechanical transmission occurs either externally by the feet, body hairs, or by proboscis, or occurs internally by swallowing the infective material which passes through the alimentary canal unchanged, e.g. transmission of *Entamoeba histolytica* cysts by the house fly from excreta to food. Another example is the transmission of *Trypanosoma evansi* by *Tabanus*. This transmission does not require multiplication or development of the infectious agents within the arthropod.

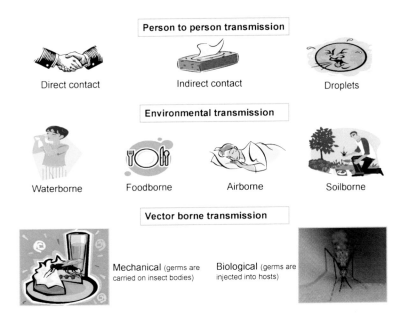

Figure 2.4 Means of transmission of parasites.

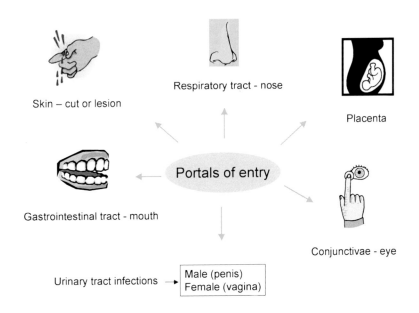

Figure 2.5 Portal of parasite entry to the host body.

Biological transmission

Biological transmission causes the pathogens to undergo certain changes as increase in number or develop to other stages or undergo a special cycle while inside the body of the arthropod vector. Transmission may be by injection of saliva during biting or by regurgitation, or deposition on the skin of faeces or other material capable of crossing through the bite wound or through an area of trauma from rubbing or scratching. Different types of biological transmission exist. These include:

- *Propagative.* The pathogen increases in number only without any cycle in the arthropod, e.g. endemic typhus by lice and plague by fleas.
- *Cyclopropagative.* The pathogen undergoes a certain cycle inside the body of arthropod and at the same time increase in number, e.g. malaria in mosquitoes and *Leishmania* in sand flies.
- *Cyclodevelopmental.* The pathogen undergoes a certain cycle inside the arthropod and at the same time develop to further stages but there is no increase in the pathogen number, e.g. *Filaria* spp. in mosquitoes.
- *Transovarian.* Similar to cyclopropagative type but differs in that the pathogens are transmitted to the offspring by invading the ovaries of arthropod and then infect the ova, e.g. *Babesia* by ticks. In this type, the infectious agent is passed vertically to succeeding generations of arthropods.
- *Trans-stadial.* Transmission involves the passage of the parasitic agent from one stage of the life cycle to another, as nymph to adult.

How do parasites enter the host body?

Given the access and/or opportunity parasites can attack nearly all tissues/organs of the host body. Some produce infections at their portals of entry and may disseminate to other organs (Fig. 2.5) to produce multiple infections, while others only can cause tissue/organ-specific infections. Below are examples of major portals of entry for parasitic diseases. It is noteworthy that many potential pathogens may reside in their host as part of the normal flora and produce infections under specific conditions such as the weak immune system. There are four major portals of entry: (i) skin, e.g. *Schistosoma, Ancylostoma,* (ii) mucosal membranes (respiratory tract, e.g. *Entrobius;* gastrointestinal tract, e.g. *Fasciola;* urogenital tract e.g. *Trichomonas foetus* in cattle, *Trypanosoma equiperdum* in equines), (iii) placenta (intrauterine transmission), e.g. *Toxocara canis, T. vitulorum, T. gondii,* (iv) transmammary transmission through the mother's milk to its offspring, e.g. *Toxocara canis* and *Ancylostoma caninum.*

Infection of a susceptible host

Infection will not be established without the presence of a susceptible host who is capable of being infected. The parasitic phase inside the host's body is complex and well-coordinated. It starts with exposure to parasite, followed by adherence, invasion, and colonization in specific host cells or organs, followed by evasion of the host immune responses, replication and secretion of toxic substances, leading to tissue damage. A summary of how parasites cause disease is illustrated (Fig. 2.6).

Exposure to parasites

Protozoa and helminths are always acquired from an *exogenous source*, and hence, they have evolved numerous ways to enter the body of the host. The most common mode of entry is oral ingestion or direct penetration through the skin or mucous membranes of different body systems. At this initial stage of parasitic disease process the *route of exposure* and *inoculum size* are critical factors that determine the outcome of host–parasite interactions. For instance, pathogenic strains of *Entamoeba histolytica* are unlikely to cause disease on exposure to intact skin but may cause severe dysentery after oral ingestion. Likewise, whereas an individual may acquire malaria by a single bite of an infected female mosquito, large inocula are usually necessary to produce coccidiosis.

Adherence and colonization

Most parasitic infections are initiated by the attachment of the parasite to host tissues, followed by replication to establish colonization. *E. histolytica* is a good model for the importance of adhesions in disease mechanism. The pathogenesis of invasive amebiasis requires adherence of amoebae to the clonic mucous layer, parasite attachment to and lysis of enteric epithelium and inflammatory and other immune responses. Another example is *Giardia intestinalis* which uses a ventral disk to attach to the intestinal epithelium by a clasping or suction mechanism. In helminths, there are many examples of mechanisms of attachment, such as the hookworms *Necator americanus* and *Ancylostoma caninum* which use mechanical and biting proboscis (mouth parts) to adhere to enteric mucous layer; the liver (*Fasciola*) and intestinal (*Paramphistomum*) flukes use acetabulum, which is a muscular

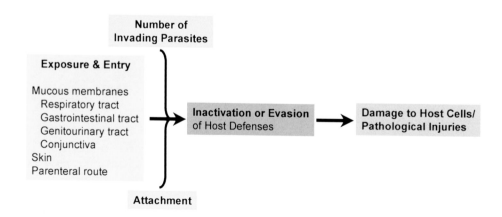

Figure 2.6 Important stages of parasite mechanism of pathogenicity.

sucker on the ventral or terminal region of the body, and is often ringed by small spines. In cestodes, scolex, the main organ of attachment, is located at the anterior end and can be armed with suckers and an array of different building hooks.

After attaching to specific cell or tissue type, the parasite may undergo replication to establish infection as the next step in the disease process. Most protozoan parasites replicate intracellularly or extracellularly in the host, whereas replication is generally not observed among helminths. Pathogenic parasites vary greatly in the extent to which they colonize the host animal. Some parasites use unique strategies for colonizing the host tissue, e.g. larvae of important gastrointestinal nematodes are able to undergo a period of arrested development (hypobiosis) inside the host, where larvae become metabolically inactive for a period that may last several months. Larvae usually arrest at times of the year when conditions in the environment are least favourable for development and survival of eggs and larvae, and resume development when climatic conditions become favourable for transmission. The role of hypobiosis in the epidemiology of gastrointestinal trichostrongylid nematodes is well documented especially in the temperate regions of the world. It was initially thought that hypobiosis was solely induced by host resistance to worm infection, but more recent studies have shown that environmental changes may play a more significant role. Hypobiosis is also of importance in overwintering of the bovine lungworm *Dictyocaulus viviparus*.

Inactivation and evasion of host defences

Although the cell and tissue damage are often enough to initiate clinical manifestation, the parasite must be able to evade the host's immune defence system for the disease process to be maintained. Parasites elicit humoral and cell-mediated immune responses; however, parasites are well evolved at avoiding these defence mechanisms. Some parasites can shift antigenic expression, such as that observed with the African trypanosomes. Many protozoan parasites evade the immune response by assuming an intracellular location, e.g. *Toxoplasm agondii* reside in macrophages and dendrite cells and use them as a shuttle to reach its destination in the brain. Parasites can also disrupt the host immune defences. Indeed, immunosuppression of the host has been observed during the course of some parasitic infections. However, it is not clear if the suppression is parasite specific or generalized. Certain helminths, such as *Schsitosoma mansoni*, may also produce proteases that can degrade antibodies.

Replication and tissue damage

Parasites initiate disease process by invading normally sterile and intact tissue with subsequent replication and destruction. The most common forms of direct damage from helminthic parasites are those resulting from mechanical blockage of internal organs (e.g. *Ascaris* spp., tapeworms), from the effects of pressure exerted by the growing parasite stage (e.g. hydatid cyst, cysticercosis), or from migration of helminthic larvae through tissue (e.g. visceral larva migrans). Some progress has been made in identifying factors that are critical to parasite virulence and the pathogenesis of the diseases they produce. Among the most widely studied of these factors are parasite-derived proteases. These proteases can play a variety of roles in establishing, maintaining, and exacerbating an infection. Proteases play key roles in tissue invasion, immune evasion, and anticoagulation for parasitic helminths (e.g. hookworms). Many helminth parasites release inhibitors of proteases that are believed to downregulate host immune and inflammatory responses. In protozoa, proteases of *Leishmania* and *Entamoeba* have critical roles in invasion and manipulation of host immune responses. Toxic products elaborated by parasites are also responsible for at least some aspects of pathology. For example, hydrolytic enzymes, collagenase, and elastase are secreted by schistosomes (cercariae), *Strongyloides* spp., hookworms, *E. histolytica*, African trypanosomes and *Plasmodium falciparum*.

The manifestations of parasitic disease are due not only to the mechanical or chemical tissue damage produced by the parasite, but also to the host responses to the presence of the parasite. During a parasitic infection, host cell products such as cytokines and lymphokines are released from activated immune cells. These mediators influence the action of other cells and may contribute directly to the pathogenesis of parasite infections. For example, cellular hypersensitivity is observed in many protozoan (*Trypanosoma cruzi* infection, leishmaniasis, malaria) and helminthic (schistosomiasis) diseases. Immunopathological reactions can range from acute anaphylactic reactions to delayed cell-mediated hypersensitivity reactions. Parasitic infections are long-lived, as such, many inflammatory changes become irreversible, leading to functional alterations in tissues, e.g. hyperplasia of the bile ducts secondary to the presence of liver flukes and extensive fibrosis leading to hepatic dysfunction. Also, chronic inflammatory changes around parasites such as *Schistosoma haematobium* have been linked to induction of carcinomatous changes in the urinary bladder of affected hosts.

Clinical parasitological periods

There are some critical clinical parasitological periods related to the host or the parasite during the course of an infection (Fig. 2.7). Periods concerning the parasite include:

- the *prepatent period*, which begins from the time of infection with the infective stage till the appearance of diagnostic stages, such as eggs, larvae, and cysts;
- the *patent period*, during which the parasite could be detected by diagnostic laboratory methods till the disappearance of the parasite.

Periods concerning the host include:

- the *incubation period*, which lasts from the time of an infection until the onset of clinical signs and usually longer than the prepatent period;
- the *period of signs*, during which the disease symptoms could be clinically recognized, such as high temperature, diarrhoea, coughing, etc.;
- the *convalescence period*, which follows the disappearance of clinical signs till the complete throw off the parasite;
- the *period of relapse*, during which the signs reappear again without reinfection, e.g. malaria in mammals.

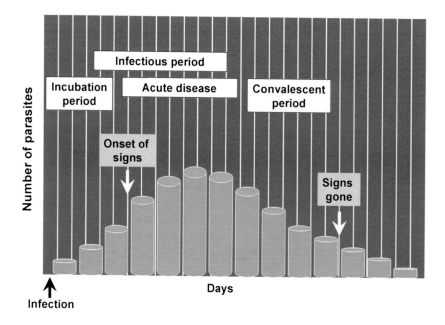

Figure 2.7 Disease course showing critical parasitological periods.

Portal of exit

There are many way for the parasite agent to escape from the body of the host. These include faeces, urine, sexual secretions, mucous discharges, blood, and draining wounds.

Factors affecting the host–parasite interaction

The association of a particular species of host with a particular species of parasite depends on factors related to parasite, to the host, and to the environment. These factors are important and must be considered when discussing parasite pathogenicity.

Host factors

Many host factors influence pathogenesis, including genetic characteristics of the host (i.e. species, breed, organ specificity, tissue specificity, and cell receptor types). Other factors include host immunity, age, stress, hormonal level, nutritional status, health condition and concurrent infection. Host and parasite must live in the same geographical region. The habit of the host must be such as to bring it into proper contact with the infective stage of the concerned parasite.

Parasite factors

Parasite-related factors associated with parasite pathogenicity include the infective dose and routes of exposure, means of attachment, the ability to cross anatomic barriers, level of cell and tissue damage, mechanisms of disruption, and evasion of host defences. The presence of protozoa and their waste products often contribute to the clinical features of the disease. Some protozoa, such as *Plasmodium* malaria invade host cells and reproduce within red blood cells, causing their rupture. *Toxoplasma* attaches to macrophages and gains entry by phagocytosis. Other protozoa, such as *Giardia*, attaches to host cells and digest the intestinal cells and tissue fluids. Other protozoa can evade host defences and cause disease for very long periods of time, e.g. *Trypanosoma* can alter its outer antigenic coat, which can't be recognized by the host immune cells. Some of the helminths use the host tissues for their own growth or produce large parasitic masses; the resulting cellular damage evokes the signs, e.g. filarial nematodes. This parasite blocks lymphatic circulation, leading to an accumulation of lymph and causing swelling of the limbs and other body regions. Importantly, the life cycle of the parasite must be such that its infective stage is reached when and where the susceptible host is available to be parasitized, e.g. blood parasites are transmitted between vertebrate hosts when the vector arthropod host feeds on the blood of infected vertebrate host.

Role of the environment

Parasitic disease can be considered as an ecological phenomenon. Indeed, it is assumed that the environment is the driving force for the disease process and exerts considerable influence over the incidence of diseases. Climate plays a crucial role in determining patterns of disease and the weather can influence the day-to-day changes in the life cycle of the parasite. Presently, there is a broad consensus among scientists that the global climate is changing. Climatologists have identified upward trends in global temperatures. In the UK, all available predictions also indicate that, over the next decade, the weather in the UK will feature greater extremes of climatic conditions, with a trend towards drier, warmer summers and milder, wetter winters. These changes will obviously impact on the transmission and epidemiology of many parasitic diseases of man and animals, directly or indirectly. Parasites in free existence are usually required to undergo one or more developmental stages before they can infect a host. In general, high temperatures accelerate the rate of development and shorten the life cycle of the parasite. Humidity, rainfall, surface water and precipitation are all factors which can influence the rate of development. Unless these conditions are favourable, the parasite may be unable to commence or complete development. The liver fluke (fascioliasis) and gastrointestinal nematode parasites of ruminants are key endemic diseases that can be markedly affected by a changing climate, as they possess free-living larval stages and, in the case of flukes, intermediate hosts also are free-living snails in the environment. The ability of larval stages of some nematodes (e.g. *Nematodirus, Ostertagia, Haemonchus*) to overwinter on pasture or survive arrested within the host has the potential to alter the epidemiology of these infections and cause unexpected clinical disease. Seriously, climate changes can also affect the vector populations, and thus, the introduction and dissemination of serious infectious diseases.

The environmental factors play an important role in disease epidemiology and therefore forecasting. Forecasting schemes, when successful, should provide the veterinarians and farmers with the information necessary to provide cost-effective means of protecting animals from the ravages of parasitic infections. Much research is expended on capturing meteorological information and relating disease outbreaks to weather criteria. The basic systems consider only rainfall, its frequency and intensity; the more sophisticated include temperature (both maximum, minimum and mean), humidity, wind speed, direction and hours of sunshine. The duration of these events and the period in which they fall, e.g. during night or day, are also important elements of data requirement. It is worth pointing out that the host, and the nature of host's resistance, whether it is absent, partial or total, will affect the speed of development of the parasitic disease and therefore will interact with any forecasting scheme. Hence, understanding the main components of the 'disease tetrahedron' (Fig. 2.8), the dynamic interaction between determinants belong to the host, parasite, environment and human activity is essential for devising suitable forecasting systems. The importance of understanding the relationships between all the above variables became apparent during the warble fly eradication campaign in the UK.

How do parasite populations evolve?

To put the process of evolution of parasites in perspective, it is important to have a basic understanding of host–parasite interactions. A fundamental principle of parasite biology and evolution is the ability of a parasitic agent to maintain itself over evolutionary time via mechanisms of transmission that ensure that at least some minimal percentage of infected hosts pass the infection on to another host. An infection will spread if each infected host infects more than one new host before dying or clearing the infection. Every time a host dies or clears an infection by becoming resistant, all of the parasites die. This represents extinction of this particular clone of parasite, unless before that event some of these parasites have successfully colonized a new host. Thus, the parasites that exist today are ones that have an unbroken history of successful transfer before host death or immune clearance. That does not mean that every infected host has spread its infection to another; rather, it means that among all infected hosts at a given time, at least one successfully transferred the parasite to another host.

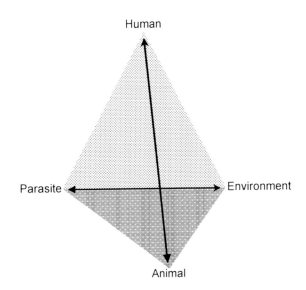

Figure 2.8 The epidemiological 'Disease tetrahedron' framework for infectious disease transmission illustrating the dynamic interactions between environment, parasite, host and human's activity.

Commensalism is believed to be the optimal end point for host and parasite relationship, and parasite species that coexist peacefully with their hosts have the best chance of long-term survival. This means that severe parasitic disease represents a lack of coadaptation between parasites and their hosts. However, from an evolutionary standpoint the dynamic of host–parasite interaction and the outcome of the disease process that occurs within a species can be attributed to gene frequencies. For example, parasites whose genetic make-up results in benign diseases by coding for low level of proliferation may lose out to those whose genetic constitution results in more severe disease through higher levels of multiplication. Also, highly productive parasites may reach susceptible hosts sooner than the less productive rivals and they may stimulate an immune response that precludes the latter's invasion. Competition may also occur inside infected hosts, resulting in transmission of the more highly productive genotypes and in the stimulation of a strong immune response (or host death) that reduces or eliminates the rivals' chances of transmission. Understanding disease dynamics at the population level is how we investigate these and other features of the disease process. Studying the evolution of parasite pathogenicity will inform the development of rational treatment strategies.

When diagnosing and treating an animal with a parasitic disease, it is important to know the parasite's host range. Some parasites are unique to one host and are called species specific. For example, *Dictyocaulus arnfieldi*, the lungworm, infects horses and donkeys, whereas another species of the same genus, *D. viviparus*, infects cattle. Other parasites are generalist and have evolved to cross the host species barrier and infect/infest every host they encounter in their environment. For example, *Trichostrongylus axei* may infect cattle, sheep, and horses. This type of information helps veterinarians rule out or in other parasites.

Perspectives

The relationships of parasites and their hosts are in constant flux. In this chapter we addressed the basic concepts of how a parasitic infection is established in a host. However, our understanding of the parasite pathogenesis is compounded by the complexity and dynamics of the host–parasite interactions. Some parasites are host specific, whereas others are evolved to be generalist and capable of infesting or infecting a broad range of hosts. Modes of transmission vary considerably from simple, direct transmission to a complex life cycle involving the use of an intermediate host or transport host or specific environmental conditions. The interplay between host and parasite is an ongoing process and if we are to make any headway in developing new drugs or vaccines for parasitic diseases, it is clear that our understanding of the pathogenesis of these pathogens must be more advanced than it is today. The study of parasite pathogenesis will evolve rapidly as new technology for working with animals as well as tracking and identifying parasite agents, progress. It will be exciting to read about how the modern molecular technologies reveal the genes and perhaps selection pressures that drove the evolution of parasitic defences in different animal species.

Further reading

Elsheikha, H.M. and Khan, N.A. (2010). Protozoa traversal of the blood–brain barrier to invade the central nervous system. FEMS Microbiol. Rev. 34, 532–553.

Eastick, F.A. and Elsheikha, H.M. (2010). Stress-driven stage transformation of Neospora caninum. Parasitol Res. 106, 1009–1014.

Jones, K.E., Patel, N.G., Levy, M.A., Storeygard, A., Balk, D., Gittleman, J.L., Daszak, P. (2008). Global trends in emerging infectious diseases. Nature 451, 990–993.

Lambert, H., Hitziger, N., Dellacasa, I., Svensson, M. and Barragan, A. (2006). Induction of dendritic cell migration upon Toxoplasma gondii infection potentiates parasite dissemination. Cell Microbiol. 8, 1611–1623.

McKerrow, J.H., Caffrey, C., Kelly, B., Loke, P. and Sajid, M. (2006). Proteases in parasitic diseases. Annu. Rev. Pathol. 1, 497–536.

Murray, H.W. (1983). How protozoa evade intracellular killing. Ann. Intern. Med. 98, 1016.

O'Connor, L.J., Walkden-Brown, S.W. and Kahn, L.P. (2006). Ecology of the free-living stages of major trichostrongylid parasites of sheep. Vet. Parasitol. 142, 1–15.

Sibley, L.D. (2004). Intracellular parasite invasion strategies. Science 304, 248–253.

The Immune Defences of The Host

Neil Foster and Hany M. Elsheikha

3

Introduction

In addition to the host's behaviour and physiology, immunity is another important host factor that influences the host–parasite interactions. The immune system is one of the most complex and diverse body components. This system recognizes parasite antigens as 'non-self' (foreign) and an immune response to these parasites is then initiated. It is difficult to generalize about the mechanisms of anti-parasite immunity because there are many different parasites that have different forms, which reside in different tissues of the animal body and in some cases may reside in different host species. Parasites have also evolved very elaborate mechanisms to escape attack by the host immune system. In this chapter we describe the range of defences the mammalian body possess to combat parasitic infections.

Mechanisms of immunity

Immune defence against invading parasites include two major components; innate (non-specific) and acquired (specific) immunity. Other factors also prevent parasitic disease, or in some way hinder infection, these include: tissue barriers and their secretions. For example, the skin as a barrier and the secretion of sebum, by the sebaceous glands, onto its surface t and the secretion of mucus, via the goblet cells, onto mucosal surfaces. Parasites may also be incompatible with a particular host, for example they may express receptors which are needed to bind to the cells of one species but not another species.

Innate immunity

The innate immune system must have evolved much earlier than the adaptive immune system since it is found in both invertebrate animals, which are devoid of an adaptive immune system, and vertebrates, which have both innate and adaptive immune systems. The innate immune system comprises of a number of different cell types (all of which derive from myeloid pre-cursors in bone marrow) and the complement system (a group of plasma proteins which directly or indirectly affect the clearance of pathogens). During parasitic diseases granulocytes, such as eosinophils, mast cells and basophils, are activated to produce toxic enzymes and oxygen and nitrogen radicals which may damage parasite membranes. Neutrophils (another type of granulocyte) are not usually activated by parasites but may be involved in killing the vulnerable extracellular phases of intracellular parasites. Neutrophils are also associated with infection by filarial nematodes such as *Dirofilaria immitis* (canine heartworm) but this is probably due to co-infection with a bacterial species (*Wolbachia* spp.) which are thought to have a mutualistic association with filarial nematodes. Other innate immune cells which may kill parasites are blood monocytes and tissue macrophages (which are derived from monocytes). These cells are phagocytic and can engulf protozoan parasites which are then killed intracellularly by toxic oxygen and nitrogen radicals. However, some innate immune cells can also present antigens to lymphocytes and this process is a crucial step towards development of adaptive immunity and immune memory. Antigen-presenting cells (APCs) include macrophages and dendritic cells (DCs), and to a much lesser degree blood monocytes. Signals provided by APCs also direct the nature of the immune response by inducing development of pro-inflammatory or anti-inflammatory T cell subsets.

Phagocytosis and opsonization

Many innate immune cells ingest protozoan pathogens by a process known as phagocytosis (literally eating cells) and collectively these cells are known as phagocytes. These include granulocytic neutrophils and eosinophils and also non-granulocytic macrophages, dendritic cells and monocytes. During this process the immune cell membrane engages parasite and completely envelopes it by the formation of the phagosome. The phagosome fuses with intracellular lysosomes (to form a phagolysosome) which contains toxic enzymes such as lysozyme and toxic oxygen and nitrogen radicals which kill the internalized parasite. Phagocytosis is greatly enhanced if the parasite is first coated with antibody or complement which binds to antibody or complement receptors on the surface of the phagocyte, this process is known as opsonization and complement and antibodies that are utilized in this way are known as opsonins.

Acquired immunity

The acquired (or adaptive) immune response to parasites involves the specific recognition of parasite antigens by lymphocytes. The response by the acquired immune system develops much less rapidly than the innate immune response but culminates in the subsequent activation of parasite-specific effector cells and antibodies, and the generation of memory cells (dormant populations of parasite-specific lymphocytes which will be rapidly activated following secondary exposure to the parasite). The principal cell types involved in this arm of the immune system are T and B lymphocytes and antibody-secreting plasma cells. Adaptive immunity is however linked to innate immunity by innate antigen-presenting cells, such as dendritic cells and macrophages, which process and present antigens to lymphocytes in conjunction with relevant major histocompatibility complex (MHC) molecules. Lymphocyte populations consist of two major types, cytotoxic T lymphocytes (CTL), which express CD8 on their surface, and helper T (Th) lymphocytes, which express CD4 instead of CD8 on their surface.

Major histocompatibility complex (MHC)

Resolution of parasitic infections via the adaptive immune system first requires processing of the parasite antigens by antigen-presenting cells (APC). Phagocytosis of an exogenous parasite or parasite antigen is followed by processing of the antigen prior to its presentation, in association with MHCII on the cell membrane of the APC. This antigen–MHCII complex is recognized by Th lymphocytes. Endogenous antigens are processed by endogenous pathways in phagocytes and are presented in association with MCHI molecules which will be recognized by antigen-specific CTLs. Since lymphocytes have this absolute MHC requirement they are said to be MHC-restricted cells.

Cell-mediated immunity

T helper (Th) lymphocytes are the principal orchestrators of the immune response because they are needed for activation of important effector cells. Effector cells include cytotoxic T lymphocytes (CTL) and antibody producing B cells and plasma cells.

However, some Th cell types (Th1 cells) also stimulate innate immunity by increasing phagocytosis and the magnitude of biochemical killing pathways within these phagocytes. The activation of Th cells occurs early in the immune pathway and requires at least two signals. One signal is provided by binding of the T cell antigen receptor to the class II MHC–antigen complex on the APC. The second signal is provided by binding of co-stimulatory molecules such as the B7 family (CD80 and CD86) on the APC surface to CD28 on the T cell membrane. Subsequent activation of CTL and B lymphocytes is dependent upon cytokines which are secreted by activated Th lymphocytes early in infection. The major function of the CTL is to kill cells that express foreign antigens in association with MHCI. This interaction of CTL with infected target cell includes the binding of Fas ligand (FasL) on the surface of the CTL with Fas on the surface of the target cell. Fas/FasL interaction induces production of a protein (Perforin) by the CTL which creates pores in the target cell membrane. The CTL then produces another enzyme (Granzyme) which enters the pores and activates caspase pathways within the target cell. Activation of these caspase pathways induces apoptosis of the target cell. Natural killer cells also kill target cells by this mechanism. However, although NK cells are lymphoid in origin they are not MHC restricted and the biology of NK cells, therefore, resembles that of both lymphoid and myeloid immune cells.

Cytokine-mediated immunoregulation

Although our understanding of immune regulation is incomplete, many thousands of studies have suggested that Th (CD4+) populations consist of different Th subsets which have different effects on the immune response. This Th paradigm indicates that during an immune response naïve (Th0) lymphocytes may differentiate into two distinct subsets (Th1 or Th2) which can be defined by the patterns of cytokines they produce and the immunological effect they orchestrate (Fig. 3.1). Whether Th0 cells

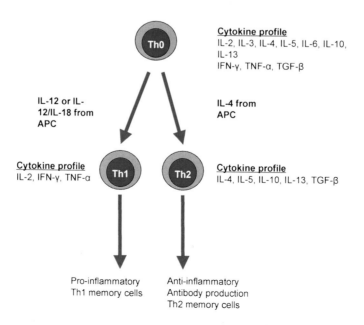

Figure 3.1 Differentiation of Th0 lymphocytes to Th1 or Th2 lymphocytes as characterized by cytokine profile.

differentiate into Th1 or Th2 subsets is dependent upon cytokine signals received by the APC (in particular DCs). Production of IL-12 or synergistic production of IL-12 and IL-18 by DCs will induce development of T helper type 1 (Th1) lymphocytes while production of cytokines such as IL-4 will induce T helper type 2 (Th2) lymphocytes.

Differentiation of Th1 lymphocytes has been shown to be preferentially stimulated by intracellular parasites (protozoa) which induce IL-12 and IL-18 production from APCs. The production of Th1 cytokines, such as interferon gamma (IFN-γ) and Tumour necrosis factor alpha (TNF-α) activates macrophages, NK cells and cytotoxic T cells which are required for suppression and/or clearance of these intracellular parasites. Characteristic production of the serum antibody immunoglobulin G subtype 2 (IgG2) also occurs during Th1 dominated immune responses and this antibody is important during the immune response to some parasites (discussed later).

Differentiation of Th2 lymphocytes occurs preferentially due to infection by extracellular pathogens (parasitic worms). The Th2 pathway inhibits Th1 activity and activates the humoral (antibody) immune system via the production of cytokines, which promote B lymphocyte growth and differentiation (such as IL-4) and production of IgG1 (IL-4), IgA (IL-5) and IgE (IL-4 and IL-13). The Th2 response also stimulates effector cells that use these antibody isotypes or are activated by Th2 cytokines. For example, mast cells and basophils will degranulate if IgE, bound to their surface, subsequently binds parasite antigen, while IL-5 (a Th2 cytokine) induces degranulation of eosinophils.

Humoral immunity (antibody response) to parasites

B lymphocytes express MHCII and can therefore present antigens to T lymphocytes. However, the most important function of B lymphocytes involves the production parasite-specific antibodies. Antibody production occurs when immunoglobulin M (IgM) is shed from the surface of B lymphocytes following antigen binding. These B cells will differentiate into plasma cells which will then produce increased concentrations of IgM. However, for a robust antibody response B lymphocytes need to be stimulated by Th2 cytokines. Th2 cytokines (such as IL-4) not only increase

B lymphocyte differentiation and IgM production by plasma cells but also alter the class of antibody produced by plasma cells. This 'class switching' ensures that appropriate antibody classes are produced according to the type of infection.

In mammals five antibody classes (or isotypes) exist. IgM exists as a monomer on the surface of B lymphocytes (the B cell receptor) and as a pentamer when secreted in circulation). IgG constitutes 75% of the circulating antibody and exists as different subclasses, with IgG1 production being dependent upon Th2 cytokines and IgG2 production being dependent upon Th1 cytokine production (note this relationship may be different in some species). IgE mediates mast cell and basophil degranulation and is upregulated by plasma cells which are induced to class switch to IgE by Th2 cytokines (IL-4 and IL-13). IgA exists in two different forms (secretory and non-secretory), with secretory IgA being an important antibody in mucosal secretions, colostrum and milk. Class switching to IgA production is also stimulated by Th2 cytokines which include IL-5. IgD is found predominantly on the surface of mature B lymphocytes and may have some function in B lymphocyte maturation.

Immunological memory

A primary immune response requires that antigenic material is processed by APCs and presented to lymphocytes in association with MHC. Initially this leads to a relatively weak immune response with upregulation of IgM in serum after about 1 week (the lag or latent phase). During this period, activation of T and B lymphocytes takes place and results in the exponential phase, which marks a rapid increase in the quantity of antibodies in the circulation and antibody class switching. In serum, class switching (known as seroconversion) is measured by a reduction in IgM and a significant increase in IgG (Fig. 3.2), while IgA and IgE may also be synthesized and measured in serum and mucosal tissues. After an interval during which the IgG concentration remains relatively constant, because synthesis and degradation are occurring at approximately equal rates, the antibody concentration gradually decline as synthesis of new antibody wanes. However, if the animal subsequently encounters the same antigen a rapid secondary immune response occurs in

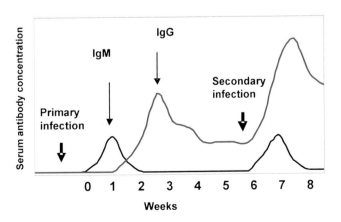

Figure 3.2 Relative IgM and IgG concentrations in serum following primary and secondary infection. During parasitic infections mucosal IgA and IgE are very important.

which very significant concentrations of class switched antibodies are produced (IgG in serum). This phenomenon is known as the amnestic (memory) response and it occurs due to the activation of memory cells which have been dormant following their differentiation during the primary immune response. These cells include antibody secreting plasma cells (which rapidly produce appropriate antibody) and T cell subsets which express T cell receptors that recognize the antigen and produce appropriate cytokines (Th1 or Th2 subsets).

Antibody-dependent cellular cytotoxicity (ADCC)

ADCC is a form of cytotoxicity in which an effector cell kills an antibody coated target cell. The effector cell carries receptors which recognize the FC region of the cell bound antibody. These reactions occur within minutes after the antigen combines with its appropriate antibody and is commonly stimulated by inhaled or ingested organisms, particularly helminth parasites. ADCC may cause significant host pathology (autoimmune pathology) but is known to have protective effects against some parasites, such as filarial nematodes in which ADCC is directed against the microfilariae in blood.

What makes parasites special pathogens?

Immunity to parasites is quite diverse, which reflects the diverse biology of the organisms. Studies in animal models have revealed that T lymphocytes and the cytokines they produce play a crucial role in determining the outcome of parasitic infection in terms of both protective immunity and immunopathology. Different parasitic infections in the context of different host genetic background can trigger polarized CD4+ Th cell subset responses. The set of cytokines produced by these different T helper cell subsets, in turn, can have opposing effects on the parasite, resulting in either control of infection or promotion of disease. Moreover, cytokines produced by one CD4+ subset can block either the production and/or activity of the cytokines produced by the other subsets. The establishment of this cross-regulation is important for parasite survival.

One of the most distinguishing features of most parasitic infections is their chronicity, reflecting the unusual adaptations these organisms have evolved for life inside of their hosts and for evasion of immune defences. The persistent antigenic stimulation resulting from chronic infection often leads to polarization of T cell subset populations and prominent immunoregulatory states. It is frequently argued that these immunoregulatory (often immunosuppressive) phenomena are induced deliberately by parasites to promote their own survival. A second important feature is the biological diversity of different parasites and their *in vivo* habitats which, in turn, lead to distinct forms of antigen presentation and T-cell activation. The number of different immunological scenarios is extensive and ranges from tissue-dwelling intracellular protozoa. For example, *Toxoplasma gondii*, which induce strong CD4+ Th1 and CD8+ responses, to large, gut-dwelling, multicellular helminths that elicit potent CD4+ Th2 responses. These diverse parasitic stimuli offer the immunologist an important comparative tool for understanding the cellular basis of differential T-cell activation.

Immune response to parasitic protozoa

Intracellular protozoa induce Th1 and CTL responses which produce IFN-γ, this may inhibit intracellular replication and activate innate cells such as macrophages which subsequently phagocytose the parasite-infected cells. Initial production of IFN-γ is probably reliant upon NK cells and tissue resident (intraepithelial) lymphocytes but the most significant source of IFN-γ production occurs from Th1 lymphocytes which have been differentiated by IL-12/IL-18 producing APCs. Host antibody production is also important during infections by parasitic protozoa since antibodies inhibit cellular invasion and function as opsonins, which increase the efficiency of phagocytosis (for a simplified model of immune response to intracellular parasites, see Fig. 3.3). Resistance to extracellular protozoa requires both cellular and humoral immune responses. Many studies have focused on the role of antibody classes during blood borne and mucosal extracellular protozoa infections and in some cases these studies have led to classic discoveries regarding immune evasion. However, T lymphocytes are essential not only because of their influence on the antibody response, but also due to the production of inflammatory cytokines which activate other effector cells.

Immune response to helminths

Parasitic helminths are large multicellular organisms which, with few exceptions, exist extracellularly. Consequently, antigen processing in helminth immune responses occurs primarily through the exogenous pathway, and although CD8+ T cells are induced in some infections, they have no established effector function. The major immunological 'hallmarks' of helminth infection are eosinophilia, elevated IgE, and in the case of certain parasites, mastocytosis. Importantly, each of these responses is stimulated by cytokines or cytokine combinations characteristic of Th2 cells: IgE by IL-4, eosinophilia by IL-5, and mastocytosis by IL-3, IL-4, and IL-I0. Much of the work on helminth immunology has focused on the questions of whether this Th2 response plays a functional role in immunity and how it is selectively induced. The best studied models are murine intestinal nematode infections (e.g. *Heligmosomoides polygyrus*, *Trichinella spiralis*, *Toxocara canis*) as well as rodent infections with the Schistosomes.

Self-cure

In many cases laboratory and farm animals expel nematode infections from their intestine, a phenomenon known as 'self-cure'. In the case of *Nippostrongylus brasiliensis* infection in rats, adult worms in the intestine cause a reduced intestinal contraction, which can also be shown by injecting E/S products into the intestinal lumen *in vitro*, and may serve as a biochemical holdfast, allowing the adult to attach to the intestine long enough to produce eggs. About 14 days post infection of rats with *N. brasiliensis*, self-cure occurs, expelling adults from the intestine, and in these immune rats there is antibody recognition of E/S products and when E/S products are injected into the intestinal lumen of these rats they have no effect on intestinal contraction. Innate immunity has for a long time been highlighted as a possible route by which self-cure can be achieved, with early studies suggesting that mast cell degranulation played an important role. However, in murine

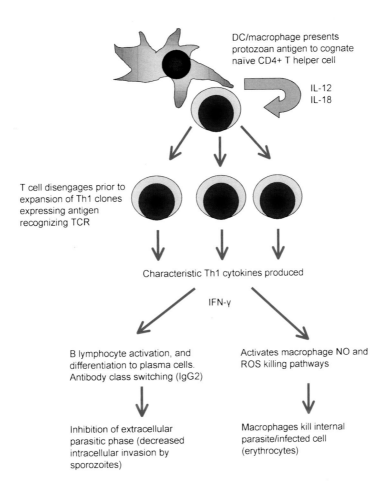

DC/macrophage presents
protozoan antigen to cognate
naïve CD4+ T helper cell

IL-12
IL-18

T cell disengages prior to
expansion of Th1 clones
expressing antigen
recognizing TCR

Characteristic Th1 cytokines produced

IFN-γ

B lymphocyte activation, and
differentiation to plasma cells.
Antibody class switching (IgG2)

Activates macrophage NO and
ROS killing pathways

Inhibition of extracellular
parasitic phase (decreased
intracellular invasion by
sporozoites)

Macrophages kill internal
parasite/infected cell
(erythrocytes)

Figure 3.3 The characteristic primary Th1 immune response against intracellular parasitic protozoa.

models devoid of mast cells, self-cure of *N. brasiliensis* infection still occurs. To date the mechanisms which drive self-cure are still not known but Th2 driven responses which may involve mast cells and goblet cells have been shown in some nematode/host infection models to be important.

Trichostrongyles infect sheep when L3 larvae are ingested from contaminated pasture. Infection induces 'self-cure' within a few weeks followed by strong protective immunity and studies in sheep have also indicated that Th2 responses are necessary to decrease adult gastrointestinal nematode survival and reduce faecal egg counts (FEC). For example when *Haemonchus contortus* (Barber's pole worm) infection was compared in resistant Gulf Coast native lambs and susceptible Suffolk lambs, significantly increased levels of IL-4 mRNA (in peripheral blood cells) and serum IgE were correlated with significant reduction of FEC in Gulf Coast sheep compared with Suffolk lambs. In pigs, self-cure has also been reported to correlate with elevated *Ascaris suum*-specific mucosal IgA and systemic IgG1 but not eosinophils or mucosal mast cells. This suggests that the 'self-cure' response may be associated with IgA and possibly Th2 cytokines (associated with IgG1 detection) rather than innate immune cells such

as eosinophils. However, other studies have reported *in vitro* mast cell degranulation in response to *A. suum* antigens and an increased expression of mast cell tryptase in the ileum, liver and bronchial-alveolar lavage fluid (BAL) *in vivo*, thus indicating an important immunological role for mast cells during *A. suum* infection of pigs.

Long-term adaptive response

The long-term survival of helminth parasites indicates their success in out-manoeuvring the immune system via achieving some form of balanced parasitism in which transmission is maintained and acute morbidity avoided. Helminths achieve this longevity despite the host immune response and their apparent inability to undergo antigenic variation. In some cases strong evidence exists for helminth-induced suppression of the host immune response. This probably increases worm survival but may also reduce the pathological affect of infection on the host tissues. Most animals become immune to parasitic worms and are capable of mounting very effective memory response (via T and B lymphocytes) upon secondary exposure to parasites. However, when cattle are exposed to *Ostertagia ostertagi* (brown stomach worm) immunity usually does not develop until after a year and even then sterile immunity (whereby no pathogens can live in the animal) never occurs. This is thought to be due to the induction of suppressor T lymphocyte subsets by APCs which present *O. ostertagi* antigens. These suppressor T cell subsets produce cytokines which inhibit both Th1 and Th2 activation and by doing so inhibit the host immune response.

Immune response to ectoparasites

There are many important ectoparasitic species affecting domestic animals. In many cases ectoparasites are important vectors of serious disease caused by parasitic protozoa (e.g. sandfly as a vector of *Leishmania*) or metazoan parasites such (e.g. Mosquito as a vector of *Dirofilaria*). However, heavy infestation by ectoparasites can seriously undermine the quality of an animal's life by causing intense irritation and in livestock this may manifest as reduced production and economic loss. The host immune response to ectoparasites can be very varied according to the parasite life cycle. To date there have been very few reported studies of the immune response to ectoparasites compared with the immune response to endoparasites, especially in veterinary species. Future studies will be needed to inform potential control strategies such as vaccination or hypersensitization treatments which are desirable given the amount of chemical treatments currently applied to pet animals and livestock, and which may have environmental impact or may induce resistance in future.

Parasite immune-mediated pathologies in host

The pathology associated with parasitic infection is often not only due to the direct activities of the parasite, but by the immunological and inflammatory responses of the host (Table 3.1). Parasitic pathogens commonly damage their host tissues via two main mechanisms; direct killing of host cells and killing of host cells via the aggressive host defences they provoke, the latter of which is most serious. Although host defences are designed to protect the host, they often do substantial damage to host cells as well as to parasites. At the site of parasitic replication, inflammatory and immune modulators are present at high concentration and provoke responses that damage healthy cells as well as parasite-infected cells. These responses are often destructive rather than protective for the host, and in some cases the longevity of the parasite may expose host tissues to these destructive responses for long periods of time.

Parasite vaccines

Although the animal and human body is remarkably adapted to controlling exposure to pathogenic parasites severe morbidity, mortality and economic losses may occur before this is achieved. The immune system can be augmented through either passive immunization, such as via transfer of antibodies (similar to the effect of passive transfer of antibody from Dam to neonate via colostrum and milk) or active immunization with parasite vaccine (which mimics the activation of the immune system during primary infection without causing pathology. Active vaccination, using avirulent parasite or parasite antigens, produces memory cells which can be rapidly activated if the animal is exposed to virulent parasite. Parasite vaccines are designed on a range of different antigen forms and preparations. These include the following:

- *Irradiated vaccines* use irradiated whole pathogen. Irradiation renders the parasite avirulent but maintains the integrity of many antigens. Dictol/Huskvac is an example of an irradiated vaccine used to control *Dictyocaulus viviparus* (cattle lungworm).
- *Somatic antigens* utilize internal parasite antigens which are released only when the parasite is killed and ground up. These are subunit vaccines which utilize much fewer antigens than irradiated vaccines.
- *Surface antigens* are subunit vaccines that utilize proteins from the parasite surface, e.g. the cuticle of nematodes.
- *Excretory/secretory antigens* are soluble proteins that are released by parasites (the excretory/secretory products of nematodes have also been trialled).
- *Stage-specific* vaccines consist of proteins that are developmentally regulated (stage specific).
- *Adjuvants* are substances (such as bacterial toxins) that induce non-specific immune responses – when administered in conjunction with a vaccine, adjuvants boost the immune response to the vaccine antigens.

Table 3.1 Types of immunopathological reactions and parasitic diseases

Anaphylactic: anaphylactic shock, e.g. sudden liberation of the parasite substances such as toxins into the body of the host, e.g. hydatid fluid

Cell-mediated: infiltration of the parasite-containing tissues with inflammatory cells such as eosinophils, epithelioid and giant cells, e.g. leishmaniosis, schistosomiasis, and trypanosomiasis

Cytotoxic: lysis of cell-bearing parasitic antigens, e.g. *Trypanosoma cruzi* infection

Granuloma formation: chronic inflammatory reaction characterized by mononuclear accumulation and macrophage activation, e.g. schistosomiasis

Immune complex: inflammation and tissue damage; deposition of small immune complexes in glomeruli, joints, skin vessels, and brain, e.g. angiostrongylosis, malaria, schistosomiasis, and trypanosomiasis

Perspectives

The constant battle for survival between parasites and their hosts has induced selective pressure which has given rise to some remarkable evolutionary characteristics of both the parasite and the host immune system. Not only is a better understanding of the associated immunology of parasitic disease essential to control these diseases by immunization, but also it continues to lead to important discoveries about the mechanisms employed by the immune system itself and also the biology of parasitic species.

Further reading

Andrade, Z. A. (2009). Schistosomiasis and liver fibrosis. Parasite Immunol. 31, 656–663.

Ashraf, M., Urban, J.F., Lee, T.D. and Lee, C.M. (1988). Characterization of isolated porcine intestinal mucosal mast cells following infection with Ascaris suum. Vet. Parasitol. 29, 143–158.

Dalton, J.P. and Mulcahy, G. (2001). Parasite vaccines – a reality? Vet. Parasitol. 98, 149–167.

Dawson, H.D., Beshah, E., Nishi, S., Solano-Aguilar, G., Morimoto, M., Zhao, A., Madden, K.B., Ledbetter, T.K., Dubey, J.P., Shea-Donohue, T., Lunney, J.K. and Urban, J.F. (2005). Localized multigene expression patterns support an evolving Th1/Th2-like paradigm in response to infections with Toxoplasma gondii and Ascaris suum. Infect. Immun. 73, 1116–1128.

Finkelman, F. D., Pearce, E. J., Urban, J. F., and Sher, A. (1991). Regulation and biological function of helminth induced cytokine responses. In Immunoparasitology Today, Ash, C., Gallagher R. eds (Elsevier Trends, Cambridge), pp. A62–A66.

Flynn, R.J., Mulcahy, G. and Elsheikha, H.M. (2010). Coordinating innate and adaptive immunity in Fasciola hepatica infection: implications for control. Vet. Parasitol. 169, 235–240.

Miller, H.R.P. and Jarrett, W.F.H. (1971). Immune reactions in mucous membranes. I. Intestinal mast cell response during helminth expulsion in the rat. Immunology 20, 277–288.

Miller, J.E. and Horohov, D.W. (2006). Immunological aspects of nematode parasite control in sheep. J. Anim. Sci. 84, E124–132.

Miquel, N., Roepstorff, A., Bailey, M. and Eriksen, L. (2005). Host immune reactions and worm kinetics during the expulsion of Ascaris suum in pigs. Parasite Immunol. 27, 79–88.

Mitchell, G. F. (1991). Co-evolution of parasites and adaptive immune responses. In Immunoparasitology Today, Ash, C., Gallagher R. eds (Elsevier Trends, Cambridge), pp. A2–A6.

Newton, S.E. and Munn, E.A. (1999). The development of vaccines against gastrointestinal nematode parasites, particularly Haemonchus contortus. Parasitol Today. 15, 116–122.

Shakya, K.P., Miller, J.E. and Horohov, D.W. (2009). A Th2 type of immune response is associated with increased resistance to Haemonchus contortus in naturally infected Gulf Coast Native lambs. Vet. Parasitol. 163, 57–66.

Uber, C.L., Roth, R.L. and Levy, D.L. (1980). Expulsion of Nippostrongylus brasiliensis by mice deficient in mast cells. Nature 287, 226–228.

Vallance, B.A., Galeazzi, F., Collins, S.M. and Snider, D.P. (1999). CD4 T cells and major histocompatibility complex class II expression influence worm expulsion and increased intestinal muscle contraction during Trichinella spiralis infection. Infect. Immun. 67, 6090–6097.

Section II
Diseases Associated with Helminths

Major Nematode Infections

Hany M. Elsheikha

4

Overview

Classification of nematodes has been traditionally based on the presence or absence of a posterior cuticular chemoreceptor called 'phasmid'. Nematode species with phasmid are known as phasmidea (Secernentea) and nematodes that lack phasmid are called aphasmidea (Adenophorea). It is important to realize that the parasite taxonomy is an evolving field and there is no a single scheme that is always acceptable. Class Nematoda includes many species which are important as agents of diseases in many animal species. This chapter focuses only on the most economically important nematode infections in livestock and companion animals. General taxonomy of nematodes considered in this chapter is given to the genus level (Table 4.1).

Angiostrongylosis

Aetiology

Canine angiostrongylosis is a snail-borne infection caused by the Metastrongylidae nematode *Angiostrongylus vasorum*. Adult worms live in the heart and pulmonary arteries of domestic dogs and wild canids causing severe respiratory and circulatory distress often resulting in the death of the animal. *A. vasorum* was also found in erratic sites, such as within pericardial sac, lumen of the bladder, kidney, and femoral artery often with fatal consequences in infected dogs.

Epidemiology and geographical distribution

The disease was originally reported in France in the early 19th century, although today, *A. vasorum* has a worldwide distribution in a wide range of hosts covering tropical, subtropical and temperate regions. In Europe it has a patchy distribution characterized by isolated endemic foci in France, Ireland, England and Denmark, with occasional cases outside endemic areas. The exact geographic range of *A. vasorum* in foxes or dogs is unknown as is how it is transported from one location to another.

Life cycle and pathogenesis

Angiostrongylus vasorum has an indirect life cycle (Fig. 4.1) which requires an intermediate gastropod (i.e. slugs and snails) and/or paratenic (e.g. amphibians, lizards, mice and rats) hosts for the development of first-stage larvae (L1) into the infective third-stage larvae (L3). Dogs become infected by ingesting the L3-infected intermediate or paratenic hosts. L3s penetrate the gastrointestinal wall and immature nematodes follow a lymphatic-hepatic-cardiopulmonary migratory route until they reach the right ventricle of the heart and/or pulmonary arteries, where they develop to sexual maturity and reproduce. Eggs laid by the female worms are transported to the pulmonary capillaries, where they hatch into L1. The L1s burrow through the capillaries and alveolar walls to the reach the airways. Irritation of airways leads to the larvae being coughed up, swallowed and subsequently passed in faeces. The intermediate or paratenic hosts become infected through ingestion of L1s. Pathological damages are attributed to the inflammatory response to eggs and migrating larvae.

Pathological findings

A thickened right ventricle, with pneumonia, breakdown in alveolar structure, presence of fibrous tissue, and inflammatory cell infiltration.

Clinical features

A wide range of clinical signs have been reported in dogs in association with *A. vasorum*. However, two clinical syndromes prevail: (1) respiratory disease and fibrosis caused by the inflammatory response to eggs and migrating larvae and (2) the haemorrhagic diatheses caused by coagulopathy. The most challenging clinical aspect of *A. vasorum* infection is to define the pathomechanisms leading to coagulopathies, as this is the most important factor causing mortalities.

Diagnosis

Detection of *A. vasorum* infection in dogs can be accomplished based on history, clinical signs and laboratory investigation. The latter includes (1) detection and morphological identification of L1 in faecal samples using the Baermann technique or faecal flotation; (2) cytological examination of samples collected from tracheal wash or bronchoalveolar lavage; (3) blood profile; (4) serological assays; and (5) PCR.

Table 4.1 Parasitic nematodes of veterinary importance

Order Suborder	Superfamily	Family	Genus
Rhabditida Strongylida*	Ancylostomatoidea	Ancylostomatidae	*Ancylostoma* *Bunostomum* *Uncinaria*
	Metastrongyloidea	Angiostrongylidae	*Aelurostrongylus* *Angiostrongylus*
		Crenosomatidae	*Crenosoma*
		Filaroididae	*Filaroides* *Oslerus*
		Metastrongylidae	*Metastrongylus*
		Protostrongylidae	*Muellerius* *Protostrongylus*
	Strongyloidea	Syngamidae	*Stephanurus*
		Chabertiidae	*Chabertia* *Oesophagostomum*
		Strongylidae	*Cyathostomum* *Strongylus* *Triodontophorus*
	Trichostrongyloidea	Dictyocaulidae	*Dictyocaulus*
		Trichostrongylidae	*Cooperia* *Haemonchus* *Hyostrongylus* *Nematodirus* *Ollulanus* *Ostertagia* *Teladorsagia* *Trichostrongylus*
Ascaridida	Ascaridoidea	Ascarididae	*Ascaris* *Parascaris* *Toxocara* *Toxascaris* *Baylisascaris*
Oxyurida	Oxyuroidea	Oxyuridae	*Oxyuris*
Rhabditida	Rhabditoidea	Strongyloididae	*Strongyloides*
Spirurida	Filarioidea	Onchocercidae	*Dirofilaria* *Dipetalonema* *Onchocerca*
	Habronematoidea	Habronematidae	*Draschia* *Habronema*
	Spiruroidea	Spirocercidae	*Spirocerca*
	Thelazioidea	Thelaziidae	*Thelazia*
Enoplida	Trichuroidea	Trichinellidae	*Trichinella*
		Trichuridae	*Capillaria* *Trichuris*
	Dioctophymatoidea	Dioctophymatidae	*Dioctophyma*

*Nematodes of the suborder Strongylida are known as bursate nematodes because of the presence of a copulatory bursa at the distal end of the male. The rest of these nematodes are non-bursate.

Treatment

The uses of fenbendazole, levamisole, ivermectin and milbemycin for the treatment of *A. vasorum* have been reported with variable degrees of success. Fenbendazole and imidacloprid/moxidectin were found to be effective against *A. vasorum* infection in naturally infected dogs.

Control

Various levels of control are possible to limit the spread of infection in dogs, from simple measures such as ensuring correct disposal of animal faeces, to prophylactic treatment. The most important step in control is to break the life cycle of the nematode, either by limiting the transmission to the intermediate/paratenic host, or from the intermediate to the definitive host.

Public health implications

There have been no reported cases of *A. vasorum* in humans; therefore it is assumed that humans are not at risk of contracting infection from dogs, foxes, molluscs or any other species. Humans can be infected with other *Angiostrongylus* spp., e.g. *A. cantonensis*.

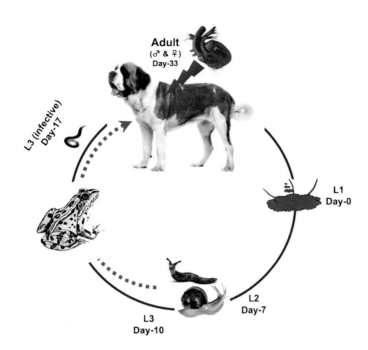

Figure 4.1 Life cycle of *Angiostrongylus vasorum*.

Ascariasis

Overview

Nematode worms from the ascarid family are well known parasites infecting a wide range of hosts. The species of veterinary interests include *Ascaris suum* (pigs), *Parascaris equorum* (horses), *Toxocara vitulorum* (buffalo and cattle), *Toxocara canis* (dogs), *Toxocara cati* (cats), and *Toxascaris leonina* (dogs and cats) (Table 4.2).

Ascarids are large nematodes with a predilection for the small intestine. They are lumen dwellers feeding on gut contents. Ascarids have a creamy white colour. Adult worms are characterized by the presence of three prominent lips (one dorsal and two ventro-lateral) surrounding the mouth opening, and rows of tiny denticles on the inner surface of each lip. Tail end of male is flexed ventrally, lacks a copulatory bursa but may have caudal papillae. Females are highly prolific, producing hundreds of thousands of eggs per day. Eggs have thick-shell and contain a single cell when passed in host faeces. Females are generally bigger than males.

The wide ranging prevalence, size, fecundity, and persistence in the environment make ascarids one of the most successful groups of parasites. Infections involving ascarids are most commonly observed in puppies, foals, and calves probably less than 6 months of age due to the development of acquired immunity by 18–24 months of age.

Ascarids have adapted well to their hosts, which is reflected by their development pattern within the host and the routes of infection. The life cycles of *Ascaris* spp. are direct, with a hepatotracheal migration within definitive hosts. Adult male and female worms live in the host's small intestine; unembryonated eggs are passed out in the faeces; development of the infective larvae usually occurs within 2 weeks under optimal conditions. Animal ingests embryonated eggs (containing L2); larvae are digested free of the egg in the gut of the host; larvae penetrate intestinal mucosa, pass through liver; carried in blood to lungs; breaks into alveoli; ascends respiratory tree; swallowed and develop to adult stages in intestine. There are some deviations from this general life cycle depending on the ascarid species. Ascarid life cycles in some species may involve transport hosts or additional routes of transmission.

High-intensity ascarid infections lead to poor growth and diarrhoea; sometimes obstructive jaundice, intestinal obstruction and respiratory signs. In toxocariasis, clinical signs are typically associated with the gastrointestinal tract: diarrhoea, emesis, stunted growth, abdominal discomfort, and, in severe cases, intestinal obstruction.

Diagnosis of ascarid is based on faecal flotation to demonstrate the distinctive ascarid-type dark brown eggs with thick mamillated wall (Fig. 4.2) in the faeces of animals with a patent infection. Marked eosinophilia may also be observed, although this is not exclusive to ascarid infection. Early stages of acute infection should be differentiated from enzootic pneumonia in pigs, chronic pneumonia in young foals, other forms of pneumonia in calves. Chronic infection should be differentiated from other causes of unthriftiness including malnutrition and chronic enteritis due to infections with *Salmonella* and *Brachyspira* spp.

Ascarid control is difficult because of the high fecundity and the resistance of eggs to environmental conditions. But, good parasite control measures especially in growing animals should be implemented. These include (1) keeping young stock away from sites where eggs are accumulated, (2) frequent removal of manure from stalls and pasture before the development of infective stages, (3) feeding animals off the ground in feeders that can be cleaned, and (4) prioritizing clean pastures for young animals and nursing mothers.

Table 4.2 Important ascarids covered in this section

Species	Primary host	Transmission
Toxocara vitulorum	Mainly cattle but also sheep and goats	Ingestion of eggs containing second-stage larvae; transmammary transmission
Ascaris suum	Pigs	Ingestion of eggs containing second-stage larvae
Parascaris equorum	Horses and donkeys	Ingestion of eggs containing second-stage larvae
Toxocara canis	Dogs	Ingestion of eggs containing second-stage larvae; ingestion of paratenic host (e.g. mice); prenatal transmission (transplacentally); transmammary transmission
Toxocara cati	Cats	Ingestion of eggs containing second-stage larvae; ingestion of paratenic host (e.g. mice); transmammary transmission
Toxascaris leonina	Dogs and cats	Ingestion of eggs containing second-stage larvae; ingestion of paratenic host (e.g. mice)
Baylisascaris procyonis*	Raccoons primarily, but occasionally in dogs	Ingestion of eggs containing second-stage larvae; ingestion of infected intermediate host

*Baylisascaris procyonis is an ascarid of raccoons that is occasionally found in dogs. It is implicated in serious neurological disease (larval migrans) in domestic animals and humans.

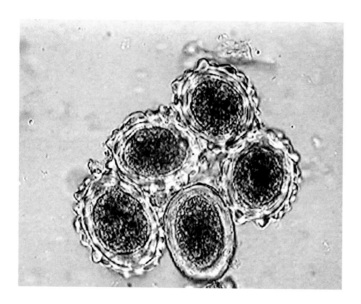

Figure 4.2 Ascarid-type eggs with the characteristic thick shell.

Humans are normal host for *Ascaris lumbricoides*. But some ascarids have a significant public health impact. For instance, human larval toxocariasis has been well documented, with several different syndromes described. Some of these manifestations can result in permanent ocular or neurological damage.

Ascariasis of pigs

Aetiology
Ascaris suum inhabits the small intestine of pigs, while its larvae can be found in the liver and lungs. *Ascaris suum* is the largest and commonest parasite encountered in pigs. Females measure from 25 to 40 cm, whereas males range from 15 to 25 cm and are thinner.

Epidemiology and geographical distribution
The common pig roundworm *A. suum* is a widely distributed parasite. A pig of any age can be infected.

Life cycle and pathogenesis
Life cycle is direct. Pigs are exposed to infection via ingestion of eggs containing second larval stage (L2) in contaminated feed and water. Earthworms may serve as paratenic hosts for *A. suum*. Pigs may also acquire eggs while suckling, when the eggs stick to the mammary glands. After ingestion of eggs, L2s hatch and migrate via liver to lung and then finally come back to mature in the small intestine. Migrating larvae can transfer bacteria to the lungs from the intestines causing bacterial pneumonia in young pigs. Prepatent period is 6–8 weeks.

Pathological findings
Grossly, large stout cylindrical worms, which in high-intensity infection can block the intestine (Fig. 4.3). Larval migration causes petechial haemorrhages in lungs and fibrotic spots on the liver known as 'milk spots'. This results in condemnations of the liver and economic losses. Microscopically, larvae are present in bronchioles and alveoli. The latter develop thickened walls and contain oedema fluid and cellular exudates in the lumens.

Clinical features
Reduced growth rate and poor feed conversion are seen. Adult worms are mildly pathogenic unless there are many. In this case the intestine and bile duct can be blocked leading to intussusception and death. Transient coughing may be seen caused by migrating larvae 1 week after infection.

Diagnosis
Diagnosis is based on clinical signs, worm egg count, and liver inspection. An ELISA test for serum antibody has been described.

Treatment
Broad-spectrum anthelmintics, e.g. ivermectin, doramectin, flubendazole, oxibendazole, pyrantel tartrate or levamisole, are effective.

Control
Control is difficult owing to the adhesive nature of the egg and its longevity on the ground. But, biosecurity measures and proper

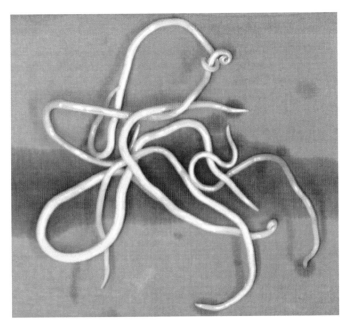

Figure 4.3 Adult *Ascaris suum* (ascarid of pigs).

sanitation are very important to complement the anthelmintic treatment.

Public health implications
Ascaris suum larvae may migrate in tissues of humans, but seldom become mature. Human cases have been reported in North America, Denmark and the UK.

Ascariasis of horses

Aetiology
Parascaris equorum infects horses and other equids.

Epidemiology and geographical distribution
Parascaris equorum occurs commonly in foals and has a cosmopolitan distribution.

Life cycle and pathogenesis
The life cycle is direct. Eggs are passed in manure and mature in the grass. While grazing, the horse swallows the eggs containing-larvae, which hatch and burrow into the walls of the intestine. From there, they are carried by the bloodstream into the liver and lungs. The horse coughs up the larvae and swallows them again. Larvae mature into egg-laying adults in the intestine. Damage is more widespread in foals, which have low resistance and may quickly accumulate massive worm infections. Large numbers of larvae breaking into the lungs cause haemorrhage. Migrating larvae can transfer bacteria to the lungs from the intestines have been occasionally associated with bouts of coughing and serous nasal discharge in foals.

Pathological findings
Mild eosinophilic pneumonia associated with the migration of larvae through the lungs.

Clinical features
Ascarids are dangerous to foals 6 months or younger. Severe infection in young horses can build up quickly and lead to liver and lung damage, poor growth, inappetence, rough hair coat and lethargy and even death. Acute infection is accompanied by severe enteritis, characterized by alternating constipation and foul-smelling diarrhoea. Lung damage in foals causes nasal discharge, coughing, fever, anorexia, and pneumonia from secondary infections. Adult horses rarely show clinical signs, as previous infections confer good resistance. In high-intensity infections, *P. equorum* can cause gut impactions and ruptures leading to a fatal peritonitis.

Diagnosis
Based on clinical signs and detection of characteristic eggs in faeces.

Treatment
Broad-spectrum anthelmintics, e.g. ivermectin, moxidectin, fenbendazole, mebendazole, oxibendazole or pyrantel embonate. Anthelmintic regimens tailored to the control of equine ascarid will also adequately control most other intestinal parasites of young horses except cestodes.

Control
Biosecurity measures, proper sanitation, and prophylactic deworming.

Public health implications
Unknown.

Ascariasis of cattle

Aetiology
Toxocara vitulorum is a parasitic ascarid of buffalo and cattle.

Epidemiology and geographical distribution
The parasite has a worldwide distribution, but found mostly in tropical and subtropical climates. *Toxocara vitulorum* is very uncommon in North America, but was reported recently in Florida.

Life cycle and pathogenesis
Calves become infected by ingesting third-stage larvae from an infected dam's milk, but not from ingesting eggs in the environment. Larvae ingested by calves develop into adults in 3–4 weeks, and then begin shedding eggs in the faeces. *Toxocara vitulorum* eggs do not hatch in the environment, but larvae in the eggs develop to the infective third-stage larvae. The infective eggs hatch in the host and the larvae penetrate the intestinal wall, and become hypobiotic in muscles. Patent toxocariasis is seen in young calves up to 6 months of age. In mature cattle, the larvae of *T. vitulorum* can undergo migration (visceral larva migrans) that inflicts inflammatory response to many organs, especially the liver and the intestine. Also, migration of the larvae through the lungs may cause the blood vessels of the lungs to haemorrhage.

Pathological findings

Gross changes in the intestine include enteritis, petechial haemorrhagic lesions, swelling and reduction in thickness of the intestinal wall. Changes in the liver include hepatitis and dark brown colour.

Clinical features

Low intensity infection is asymptomatic. Moderate infection is characterized by constipation and faeces mixed with blood and mucous. Severe infection can lead to frequent diarrhoea, unthriftiness, recumbency and death.

Diagnosis

Toxocara vitulorum can be diagnosed by clinical signs, examination of faeces for eggs and serological tests.

Treatment

Adult stage *T. vitulorum* can be effectively treated with piperazine, pyrantel, febantel, and oxfendazole. Treatment of beef calves less than 3 months of age with fenbendazole at 5 mg/kg is reasonably effective. Third-stage larvae of *T. vitulorum* in the intestine can be treated with pyrantel and levamisole.

Control

The administration of anthelmintics should be combined with other management procedures done early in the calves' lives to minimize infection. In general, preventive measures for other ascarids are also effective against *T. vitulorum*.

Public health implications

Unknown.

Ascariasis of dogs and cats

Ascarid infections of dogs and cats are cosmopolitan. Adult worms live in the small intestine of dogs (*Toxocara canis* and *Toxascaris leonina*) or cats (*Toxocara cati* and *Toxascaris leonina*) (Table 4.3). Fertilized female worms produce eggs that become infective approximately 3–4 weeks after being passed in the stools.

Pathology associated with ascarid infections in dogs and cats involves inflammatory and pathological alterations in the intestinal mucosa (caused by adults) and hepatopulmonary tissues (caused by migrating larvae).

Ascarids of companion animals have significant public health implications. For instance, humans can become infected with *T. canis* after ingestion of embryonated eggs present in soil contaminated with dog faeces. The larvae hatch from the ingested eggs, penetrate the small intestine and migrate to different tissues in the body inducing inflammatory responses. Migration of *T. canis* larvae leads to a syndrome known as visceral larva migrans (VLM). Symptoms of VLM include fever, hepatosplenomegaly, and respiratory distress such as wheezing, coughing, and episodic airflow obstruction. VLM can cause more serious outcomes if the larvae reach body tissues such as the brain or the eye. Cases of VLM from *T. leonina* have been reported; however, it seems to be of less importance than the risk from *T. canis*.

Canine hookworm infection

Aetiology

The name is derived from the mouth being subterminally positioned and anterior end is bent dorsally of the parasite. The mouth cavity of *Ancylostoma caninum* (in dogs) and *Ancylostoma tubaeforme* (in cats) has three pairs of sharp teeth at the ventral rim, while *Uncinaria stenocephala* (in dogs) lacks these teeth and the stoma is instead armed with rounded plates. *Ancylostoma caninum* females measuring 15–18 mm and males 9–12 mm. *Uncinaria stenocephala* females measure of 7–12 mm and males 4–5 mm in length.

Epidemiology and geographical distribution

Hookworms have a worldwide distribution. The development in the environment is highly temperature and humidity dependent and has been reported to be as short as 6–10 days. *Ancylostoma* is more prevalent in warmer climates; while *Uncinaria* is adapted well to the temperate climates and larvae are even able to survive over winter. Larvae in the environment are the principal source of infection. Main route into puppies is transmammary.

Life cycle and pathogenesis

The development of all hookworm species in the environment is similar. Hookworm eggs passed in dog or cats faeces contain a 4–16 cell morula. The larva hatches from the egg and become infective after two moults. Infection of the definitive host, the dog or cat, occurs in different ways depending on the species of hookworm and the age of the host animal. For *U. stenocephala*, infection occurs by means of the ingestion of larvae, while for *A. caninum*, infection with larvae may occur via the oral, percutaneous or transmammary routes. Hookworms are regarded as blood-sucking nematodes that feed on both blood and intestinal mucosa.

Pathological findings

Mucosal lesions with petechial bleeding caused by the feeding of the worms.

Clinical features

Low to medium worm intensities may lead to wasting and reduced growth in puppies. High worm intensities result in diarrhoea containing fresh blood from mucosal lesions, and are a cause of death in highly infected litters. Cutaneous infection with larvae may cause erythema at the penetration sites. The clinical signs that follow are dependent on the migration of the larvae within the body tissue. For example, when larvae reach the brain, ataxia may be seen.

Diagnosis

Diagnosis of hookworm infection can be based on faecal flotation. Eggs of *A. caninum* and *U. stenocephala* are soft-shelled nematode eggs, containing 4–16 cell morulae in fresh faeces. In general, *A. caninum* eggs are shorter and larger in width than *U. stenocephala*. The size is recorded at about 53–69 × 36–53 μm for *A. caninum* and 75–85 × 40–45 μm for *U. stenocephala*.

Table 4.3 Characteristic features of ascarids of dogs and cats

Toxocara canis

Host	Dogs
Signs	Low-intensity infection does not cause signs of disease. Young puppies are most likely to show clinical signs, and these will be worse if the puppy has a large number of worms or migrating larvae. Signs include coughing, nasal discharges, vomiting, diarrhoea, stunted growth rate, distended abdomen (pot-bellied appearance), or pale mucus membranes. Death is rare, but has been reported, and has been due to obstruction of the intestine or ulceration and perforation of the intestine wall
Life cycle	*Toxocara canis* have a complicated life cycle and can be transferred in four different ways:
	(i) **Ingestion of eggs.** After a dog eats the eggs, they hatch, and the larvae enter the wall of the small intestine. The larvae migrate through the circulatory system and either go to the respiratory system or other organs/tissues in the body. If they enter body tissues, they encyst especially in older dogs. In very young puppies, larvae move from the circulation to the respiratory system, are coughed up and swallowed. The larvae mature into adults. The adult worms lay eggs which pass out of the animal in the faeces. The eggs mature in the environment within 2 weeks
	(ii) **Ingestion of transport host.** If an animal ingests a transport host having encysted larvae, the migration is similar to that of ingesting infective eggs. Larvae are released from the transfer host when it is eaten and digested
	(iii) **Larvae through the uterus.** The dormant larvae in the tissues of pregnant bitch can migrate through the uterus and placenta and infect the fetal pup. This is called *in utero* transmission
	(iv) **Larvae through the milk.** Larvae can also enter the female's mammary tissues. The puppies can become infected through the milk while nursing. The swallowed larvae mature in the pup's intestine
Diagnosis	The eggs of *T. canis* are round in shape with a thick shell. The outer surface of this shell shows a characteristically rough surface. Eggs are not being shed into the faeces all the time, so false negative results are possible
Treatment	A wide assortment of drugs is available for use against *T. canis*. These include benzimidazoles (e.g. mebendazole), avermectins (e.g. milbemycin), pyrantel pamoate, or diethylcarbamazine. Because pregnant and nursing bitches are sources of infection they should be treated before and after whelping
Control	Periodic faecal examination and regular deworming. Reduce environmental contamination by maintaining good sanitation and hygienic disposal of dog faeces. In US, the CDC suggested deworming litter and bitch at 2, 4, 6, and 8 weeks of age

Table 4.3 continued

Toxocara cati

Host	Cats
Signs	occur mostly in young animals and consist of stunting, pot-belly, diarrhoea, poor coat and occasional deaths related to dehydration and weakness in high-intensity infections
Life cycle	Transmission occurs by three mechanisms:
	(i) **Direct ingestion of eggs.** When infective eggs are ingested, larvae undergo hepatic-tracheal migration as L2s → then are coughed up and swallowed and return to the gastrointestinal tract →enter the stomach wall for a time, return to the lumen → and mature into adult worms after three moults.
	(ii) **Via paratenic hosts.** Mice or rats ingest eggs and can serve as a paratenic host for *T. cati* in a manner similar to the other ascarids. Since migration occurs in paratenic hosts, no migration is seen in the cat. Direct development to adults occurs in the gut of cats. Cats can also become infected by eating other transport hosts such as earthworms and beetles.
	(iii) **Transmammary transmission.** Transmammary passage of larvae occurs in the colostrum and throughout the first 3 weeks of lactation. This mode of transmission is the most important source of infection in kittens. Unlike *T. canis*, *in utero* (transplacental/prenatal) infection does not occur with *T. cati*. The prepatent period for *T. cati* is about 8 weeks, which is longer than that of *T. canis* (4–5 weeks). Cats do not develop the immune response that dogs do
Diagnosis	Diagnosis is made by finding typical eggs or identifying adults. Weanling cats may not yet be shedding eggs. Adult *T. cati* is morphologically similar to *T. leonina*, which also occurs in cats, but may be differentiated by the broader 'arrowhead' cephalic alae and the 'bowed' head
Treatment	Similar to *T. canis*

Toxascaris leonina

Host	Dogs and cats
Signs	Similar to *T. canis*
Life cycle	Transmission occurs via two routes:
	(i) **Eggs, through ingestion of infective eggs.** The eggs hatch and the larvae mature within the small intestine. The adult female worm lays eggs which are passed in the faeces and mature in the environment.
	(ii) **Larvae, by ingestion of transport or intermediate host.** Mice and other rodents can act as intermediate or transport hosts of *T. leonina*. The rodent ingests the eggs, the eggs hatch, and the larvae migrate through the tissues of the rodent. If an animal eats the infected rodent, the larvae are released in the digestive system of the animal and develop into adults in the intestine. The prepatent period for *T. leonina* is about 11 weeks
Diagnosis	The egg surface of *T. leonina* is smooth. This characteristic is used to differentiate between *T. leonina* and *Toxocara* spp. Flotation methods are used to enrich eggs passed with the faeces
Treatment	Similar to *T. canis*

However, although the diagnosis of a hookworm egg is easily made, species determination requires good experience and/or PCR-based techniques. The latter are specifically used to determine the presence of low worm intensities and to permit accurate species identification. However, these are not available commercially.

Treatment

A wide range of anthelmintics are available such as fenbendazole, ivermectin, mebendazole, milbemycin oxime, pyrantel pamoate, or selamectin.

Control

Sanitary disposal of dog faeces and prophylactic deworming. Check the websites of Centers for Disease Control and Prevention (www.cdc.gov), Companion Animal Parasite Council (www.petsandparasites.org), and European Scientific Council for Companion Animal Parasites (www.esccap.org) for up-to-date recommendations.

Public health implications

Cutaneous larva migrans in man, also known as 'creeping eruption', is a dermatitis caused by migrating hookworm larvae. Infection occurs through skin contact with infective larvae and the most common sources of infection is soil contaminated with the faeces of infected dogs or cats. The clinical symptoms in humans are erythema at the sites of infection and intensive pruritus. Although a few cases of adult dog hookworms in the intestines of man have been reported, the risk of such infections does not appear widespread.

Capillariasis

Capillarid worms that have a veterinary significance are *Capillaria aerophila* (lung), *C. hepatica* (liver), and *C. plica* (kidney). *Capillaria* spp. have a worldwide distribution, but the actual prevalence is unknown.

Capillaria aerophila

The trichuroid nematode *C. aerophila* (also called *Eucoelus aerophilus*) is 2- to 4-cm-long nematode that infects the nasal cavity, trachea, bronchi and bronchioles of dogs and cats. Eggs are coughed up, swallowed and passed in faeces. The life cycle is direct, but earthworms may serve as transport paratenic hosts. Most infections are asymptomatic, but in severe infections coughing, nasal discharge, poor body condition, loss of weight, and dyspnoea can be seen. Diagnosis is confirmed by the presence of eggs (double operculated with asymmetrical plugs) in faeces or in airway cytology specimens, although shedding is intermittent. *Capillaria aerophila* eggs must be differentiated from morphologically similar eggs of *Trichuris vulpis* and *Eucoleus boehmi*. *Capillaria aerophila* eggs are smaller than *T. vulpis* eggs, and they have asymmetric plugs. Radiography may show a mild bronchial or interstitial pattern. Benzimidazoles such as fenbendazole are usually effective against respiratory parasites. Also, levamisole and selamectin can be used against *C. aerophila*.

Capillaria plica

Capillaria plica is a parasite that resides in the urinary bladder, ureters or rarely in the kidney pelvis of various wild carnivores. Hunting can be a risk factor for *C. plica* infection in dogs because fox populations represent a major source of infection for hunting dogs. The life cycle of this parasite is indirect and involves an earthworm as intermediate host; the ingestion of the intermediate host containing first-stage larvae is responsible for the infection of canids, definitive hosts. After two moults and a short dwelling period in the intestine, third-stage larvae reach the bladder, where they moult to adults and embed themselves deep into bladder mucosa (occasionally ureters and kidney pelvis). *Capillaria plica* in dogs has been considered to be of minor clinical significance. However, haematuria, dysuria, or even renal failure associated with glomerular amyloidosis may develop with or without periodic signs of clinical cystitis or secondary bacterial cystitis. Urinary sediment examination is the only diagnostic tool that permits the identification of *C. plica*. Since the excretion of *C. plica* eggs varies considerably from day to day, the sensibility of urinary sediment examination for diagnosing this infection is probably low and when this condition is suspected (or when it is necessary to confirm treatment efficacy) more than one examination of urine sediment should be performed. Urinalysis may also reveal mild proteinuria, microscopic haematuria and the presence of an increased number of transitional epithelial cells. Success in treating *C. plica* infection has been reported using benzimidazoles and levamisole. In dog shelters where *C. plica* is endemic several measures can be taken to avoid infection and reinfection from the environment such as limiting contact of dog with earthworms.

Capillaria hepatica

Capillaria hepatic occurs in rats. The specific diagnosis of *C. hepatica* infection is based on demonstrating the adult worms and/or eggs in liver tissue at biopsy or necropsy. Humans have been infected with this species.

Dioctophymosis (giant kidney worm infection in dogs)

Aetiology

Dioctophyma renale is the largest known parasitic nematode in domestic animals. Adult females can measure up to 100 cm long and 12 mm wide whereas males only reach 30 cm long and 6 mm wide. This parasite affects canines and mustelids.

Epidemiology and geographical distribution

The *Dioctophyma renale* is a worldwide occurring nematode. Infection appears more often in street dogs having less selective eating habits. Animals acquire infection via ingestion of raw fish/frogs or drinking water contaminated with the mud-worm infected by *D. renale* in its larval form.

Life cycle and pathogenesis

The life cycle of the worm is complex and includes intermediate, paratenic, definitive hosts. Eggs of *D. renale* are passed in the urine and ingested by the intermediate host, which are aquatic oligochaetes (mud-worms) where the nematode develops until the fourth larval stage. Oligochaetes are then eaten by paratenic hosts (fishes or frogs), where the infective larvae are encysted in tissues of these animals without further development. Definitive hosts (fish-eating carnivores) are infected by ingestion of contaminated oligochaetes or paratenic hosts. In these animals, the larva penetrates the duodenal wall, enters the abdominal cavity and migrates to the kidney, where it remains until the adult stage. The adult worm is commonly found in the renal pelvis. In dogs, the right kidney is more affected than the left one, due to its anatomic proximity to the duodenum.

Pathological findings

The main lesion is the progressive destruction of the renal parenchyma leaving only a thin capsule containing the worm and haemorrhagic exudates inside.

Clinical features

Most cases of canine dioctophymosis are asymptomatic. Death has been associated with urine retention and uraemia due to chronic renal insufficiency. When one kidney is affected, the signs of renal failure may not be evident, however haematuria can occur. If the parasite migrates to the peritoneal cavity, abdominal distension and peritonitis can be observed.

Diagnosis

The diagnosis is difficult due to the non-specificity of the clinical signs, especially in unilateral renal manifestation. Diagnosis can be achieved via detection of worm at necropsy, diagnostic imaging (radiography and ultrasound) may aid in localizing the presence of the parasite in the renal parenchyma. Urinalysis is conclusive, where the parasite eggs could be seen in the animal's urine. However, eggs will only appear in the urine sediment if a gravid parasite female is in the kidney causing the infection.

Treatment

There is no known therapy for animals infected with *D. renale*; but in cases of unilateral renal infection nephrectomy of the affected kidney can be done. In some cases it is necessary to perform an exploratory laparotomy or nephrotomy to remove the parasites.

Control

Limit contact of dogs with intermediate and transport hosts.

Public health implications

Dioctophyma renale cases have been described in humans.

Dirofilariasis (heartworm disease)

Aetiology

Heartworm (HW) is a parasitic disease caused by infection with the intravascular filarial nematode parasites of the Genus *Dirofilaria* that affects canine and less frequently feline hosts (Fig. 4.4). *Dirofilaria immitis* males measure 12–20 cm, and the females are 25–31 cm long. In general, *D. immits* is found primarily in the right ventricle and pulmonary arteries of the host and causes

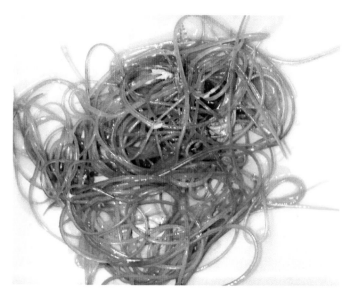

Figure 4.4 Adult *Dirofilaria immitis* collected from the heart of a dog with Heartworm disease.

respiratory and cardiac diseases. However, heartworms are not always restricted to the cardio-respiratory tract, and immune complex glomerulonephropathy has been also associated with HW.

Epidemiology and geographical distribution

Prevalence varies with geographic location, but widespread throughout North America and some European countries. Despite improved diagnostic tools, effective preventive and increased awareness, HW is considered highly endemic in many places in the United States. Recent research on the HW epidemiology showed that the disease prevalence is more likely to be affected by a climate change. The prevalence of HW is dependent on a number of factors, including the percentage of infected dogs, an environment conductive to mosquitoes and the density of susceptible dog populations.

Life cycle and pathogenesis

Dirofilaria immitis has a complex and indirect life cycle, with dog as definitive host and mosquito plays a crucial role as intermediate host (Fig. 4.5). Female adult worms release microfilaria (MFF) into the circulatory system where they can live for 2 years. MFF in circulation can be ingested by mosquitoes during feeding; develop to infective larval stage (L3) in the stomach of the mosquito and migrate to the salivary glands where they remain until the mosquito feeds and the L1s move down the mouth parts onto the skin and enter the bite wound into dog to migrate to heart. Microfilaria cannot develop in the dog of origin. They must pass through a mosquito to develop. Pre-patent period ranges from 6 to 7 months. Transplacental infection by microfilaria can occur, but no adults will develop from their entry into the dog.

Pathological findings

Adults live in the pulmonary arteries of dogs, leading to endothelial damage and myointimal proliferation. Pulmonary artery damage results in lobar arterial enlargement, tortuosity, and

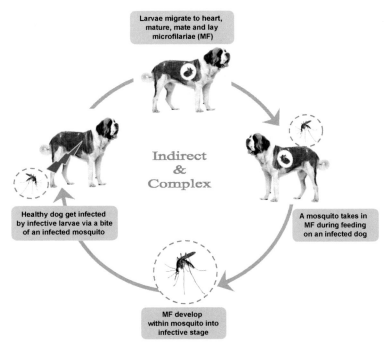

Figure 4.5 Life cycle of *Dirofilaria immitis*, the agent of heartworm disease.

Table 4.4 Clinical diagnostic features of stages of heartworm disease

Phase(s)		Major features
I	Mild to moderate	Chronic cough, decreased tolerance towards exercise, dyspnoea (difficult breathing), weight loss, pulmonary changes on thoracic radiography, packed cell volume (PCV) between 20 and 25
II	Moderate to severe	Cachexia, exercise intolerance, fainting (syncope), tachycardia, ascites indicates right-sided heart failure, hepatomegaly, pulmonary and cardiac changes on thoracic radiography, PCV < 20
III	Severe	Coughing up blood (haemoptysis) indicates severe pulmonary thromboembolism complications, congestive heart failure and vena cava syndrome occurs when vena cava is obstructed by adult worms, globinuria due to acute haemolytic shock

obstruction, causing pulmonary hypertension and thrombosis. Studies have shown that both dirofilarial antigens and those derived from its bacterial endosymbiont *Wolbachia*, interact with the host during canine and feline infections and participate in the development of the pathology and in the modulation of the host's immune response.

Clinical features

Severity of disease and damage to the dogs by HW are directly related to the number of adult worms, duration of infection, and host response. Infection with *D. immitis* causes multiple organ system dysfunctions, including pulmonary circulation, heart, liver and kidneys. Clinical signs range from being asymptomatic to heart failure. According to the severity of clinical signs, the diseases can be categorized into three phases (Table 4.4).

Diagnosis

Diagnosis of HW depends on obtaining an accurate patient history, recognition of clinical manifestations, and use of several diagnostic procedures. Given that each of the following diagnostic techniques has the shortcomings; their use in combination is required to optimize diagnostic accuracy.

- *Complete blood count*
  - anaemia: mild in phase II, severe in phase III
  - combined eosinophilia and basophilia is a sensitive indicator of HW disease
  - leucocytosis and thrombocytopenia are associated with thromboembolism.
- *Serum biochemical profile and urinalysis*
  - hyperglobulinaemia is an inconsistent finding
  - proteinuria is common in animals with severe and chronic infection and may be caused by immune-complex glomerulonephritis or amyloidosis
  - haemoglobinuria is caused by acute haemolytic crisis during vena cava syndrome.
- *Heartworm antigen tests* are specific, sensitive serological tests that identify adult female *D. immitis* antigen; widely available; standard tests for screening. Antigen tests take 7 months after infection to develop a positive status, therefore, are not used in testing pups less than 7 months.
- *Microfilaria identification tests* include the modified Knott's test, filter tests, and direct smear. Although rarely found because of the advent of monthly heartworm preventive agents, a blood

smear may reveal *D. immitis* microfilaria in a dog with HW disease.

- *Thoracic radiological examination* is performed not only as a diagnostic aid but also to predict stage of infection and extent of thromboembolism. Thoracic radiological examination also allows comparison between radiographs taken during treatment and recovery. Thoracic radiographic signs include:
  - enlargement of the main pulmonary artery
  - lobar arterial enlargement and tortuosity vary from absent (phase I) to severe (phase III)
  - parenchymal lung infiltrates of variable severity may extend into most or all of one or multiple lung lobes when thromboembolism occurs
  - allergic reaction to microfilaria induces diffuse, symmetrical, alveolar, and interstitial infiltrates.
- *Echocardiogram* may show right ventricular dilation and wall hypertrophy; parallel linear echodensities produced by the worms may be detected in the right ventricle, right atrium, and pulmonary artery.
- *Electrocardiogram (ECG)*, usually unremarkable, may reflect right ventricle hypertrophy in dogs with severe infection; heart rhythm disturbances rarely seen but may include atrial fibrillation especially in severe infection.
- *Angiography* is of little clinical importance.

Heartworm must be differentiated from (i) other causes of pulmonary hypertension and thrombosis, such as hyper-adreno-corticism, (ii) other causes of pulmonary disease include allergic lung disease, chronic obstructive pulmonary disease (COPD), neoplasia, parasitic lung disease, foreign body, pneumonia and (iii) other causes of ascites include dilated cardiomyopathy, hypoproteinaemia, hepatic disease, caudal caval or portal vein thromboembolism, neoplasia, pericardial effusion. Thoracic radiological examination and heartworm antigen tests should differentiate all these conditions from HW disease.

Dipetalonema reconditum males are 9–17 mm long, and the females are 20–32 mm long. *Dirofilaria repens* and *Dipetalonema reconditum* live in subcutaneous tissue, and are of limited veterinary importance, but cause lesions in cutaneous tissues due to microfilariae.

Treatment

The conventional approach is to kill all adult parasites first with an adulticide drug and then all circulating microfilariae with a microfilaricide. Some patients may need hospitalization during adulticide treatment, since severe post-treatment complications are likely. When adults die, the pulmonary arteries carry them to the lungs, where they eventually decay and are removed by the immune system. Although the adulticide drugs are designed to be slow-acting and prevent the accumulation of dead worms all at once in the animal's lungs, the load on the lungs is still immense and stressful to the treated animals. Restriction of activity is required for 4–6 weeks after adulticide administration especially for severe disease. Hospitalization and cage confinement for a week is recommended for dogs experiencing pulmonary

thromboembolic complications. Approximately 4 weeks following adulticide therapy, microfilaricide treatment should be initiated. This allows enough time for the dog to recover from any injuries associated with HW death. In dogs with severe disease and congestive heart failure, the latter should be treated until the dog becomes stable before administering adulticide. Also, stabilize pulmonary failure with antithrombotic agents (e.g. aspirin or heparin) and anti-inflammatory doses of corticosteroid; monitor the case using clinical and radiographic parameters. Dogs with vena cava syndrome require surgical removal of adult worms from right side of the heart and pulmonary artery via jugular vein by using fluoroscopy and a long, flexible alligator forceps. Recent research studies proposed the concept of 'tetracycline *Wolbachia* treatment of heartworms'. This hypothesis is believed to be attributable to clearance of *Wolbachia*, intracellular rickettsial-like organisms found within filarial tissues by Tetracycline treatment.

Control

Preventing HW is certainly safer and more economically efficient. HW disease is entirely preventable through medication and many products on the market are effective. Screening and chemoprophylaxis for HW are routine elements of the standard of care in veterinary practices designed especially to protect animals living in endemic/hyperendemic areas. New patients starting on prophylaxis for the first time must be tested for HW because most preventive drugs are not effective against adult heartworms. Thus, a dog with adult heartworms would still have infection even after being treated with preventive medicine. Antigen testing before starting preventive treatment in such cases is indicated to rule out possible adult infection, and if positive, consider adulticide treatment options. As long as patient is microfilaremic-negative prophylaxis treatment can be instigated.

Public health implications

Although canine heartworm has been known to exist in the Americas for more than 150 years (1847), the first human case was reported four decades later (1887). In general, cases of human infection are rare and heartworms represent no serious zoonotic potential. In some cases, heartworms were found to induce benign pulmonary nodules that can be radio-graphically confused with cancer. The adults do not develop in humans.

Heartworm disease in cats

Although the distribution of feline *D. immitis* infection parallels that in dogs, feline HW differs from canine HW in a number of characteristics.

- Cats are more resistant to heartworms than dogs.
- The cat does not serve well as a definitive host because of the low microfilaraemias.
- Aberrant migration of fourth-stage larvae (L4) occurs more frequently in cats than in dogs and ectopic heartworms have been found in the body cavities and central nervous systems of infected cats.
- There are fewer adults in feline infection (usually fewer than 6).

- The lifespan of the adults is only about half the length of that in dogs (2–3 years compared with 5–7 years).
- The average prepatent period is 7–8 months, 1–2 months longer than that in dogs.
- HW rarely reaches the adult stage in cats.
- HW infection in cats is often self-limiting (infected cats are frequently managed with supportive treatment).
- The overall prevalence in cats is between 5% and 10% of that in dogs in any given area.

Cats with mild signs may resolve the infection on their own. Microfilaricide treatment is usually unnecessary since cats have few circulating microfilariae. Surgical treatment, where adult worms are physically removed from the heart is indicated in cats that develop vena cava syndrome. Experts recommend taking preventive measures in areas where the prevalence of canine heartworm is high. A number of safe and effective macrocyclic lactone drugs are available for prophylaxis in cats. Monthly products like selamectin, ivermectin and milbemycin are considered safe and effective.

Habronemiasis

Aetiology
Cutaneous habronemiasis, also known as 'summer sores', is caused by a reaction to larvae of the equine stomach worms of the superfamily Spiruroidea, *Habronema muscae*, *H. majus* (syn. *H. microstoma*) and *Habronema megastoma* (syn. *Draschia megastoma*).

Epidemiology and geographical distribution
This condition occurs worldwide especially where the climate is warm and wet. The disease is common in spring and summer and less frequent in the winter. It is rare in the UK. The occurrence of lesions corresponds with the fly season, being caused by the aberrant intradermal presence of the larvae of stomach worms, *Habronema* spp.

Life cycle and pathogenesis
Adult worms live in the horses' stomach. Females pass eggs which develop and hatch to become first-stage larvae (L1) during transit through the intestinal tract and are passed out in faeces. The L1s are ingested by fly maggots. The house fly (*Musca domestica*) is an intermediate host for *H. muscae* and *H. megastoma*; the stable fly (*Stomoxys calcitrans*) is the intermediate host for *H. majus*. After maturation inside the fly vector, infective third-stage larvae (L3s) are deposited around a horse's mouth, nostrils, and conjunctiva or these are eaten in horse feed; the larvae are ingested; migrate to the digestive tract, and mature to adults in the stomach. Prepatent period is 6–8 weeks. The cutaneous form of habronemiasis occurs when L3s are deposited on wounds or other moist areas of the body and because these larvae cannot migrate they cause cutaneous lesions. Infective larvae rarely penetrate intact skin to cause lesions. The characteristic ulcerative granulomatous lesions of cutaneous habronemiasis are probably the result of a hypersensitivity reaction to parasite larvae. Evidence for the role of hypersensitivity reactions in the pathogenesis includes the seasonal recurrent nature of lesions, predilection of some horses to lesions, and response to systematic glucocorticoids as a sole treatment.

Pathological findings
Larvae may be found in skin scrapings, biopsies or discharges. Adult *H. megastoma* cause tumour-like lesions in stomach; other species cause catarrhal enteritis. Varying degrees of nodular to diffuse dermatitis, marked eosinophilia and mast cells, areas of coagulative necrosis that may contain nematode larvae, and granuloma formation around necrotic foci.

Clinical features
Cutaneous habronemiasis is characterized by large, rapidly proliferating reddish-brown granulomatous masses, and ulcerative lesions often observed in areas of uncovered wounds or on moist areas of the body (penis, urethral process of male horses, distal limbs, periocular lesions). These lesions are refractory to treatment and very pruritic. Adult *H. megastoma* cause intense irritation of the gastric submucosa, causing the formation of nodules that may affect digestion and, if they rupture, fatal peritonitis can develop.

Diagnosis
A tentative diagnosis can be often made on the history, clinical signs, and gross appearance of the lesions. *Gastric form:* eggs difficult to find in faeces. Gastroscopy can enable diagnosis. *Cutaneous form:* eosinophils, demonstration of larvae in biopsy using impression smear or scraping. Differential diagnosis should include bacterial granulomas, phycomycosis, zygomycosis, squamous cell carcinoma, sarcoid, and other skin neoplastic lesions.

Treatment
The objectives of treatment are to (i) reduce the size of the lesion, (ii) reduce the inflammation and (iii) prevent reinfection. Killing larvae in tissue can be achieved using macrocyclic lactones. Prednisolone orally has been effective for treatment of many horses. However, horses with large or refractory lesions may require surgery to debulk the lesions by conventional surgery or cryosurgery if the location of the lesions permits and before initiating medical therapy.

Control
Regular deworming of horses with ivermectin will kill adult stomach worms and minimize larval contamination of manure. Other measures include strict and regular removal of manure, prompt treatment of all skin wounds, and appropriate use of insecticides and fly repellents to control flies.

Public health implications
Not known.

Hyostrongylosis

Aetiology
The strongylid swine nematode *Hyostrongylus rubidus*, appears as small red streaks on the mucosa of stomach.

Epidemiology and geographical distribution
Transmission can occur in housed pigs but infection is mainly confined to outdoors animals.

Life cycle and pathogenesis
Hyostrongylus rubidus has a direct life cycle. Adult males and females reside in the stomach. Fertilized female produces strongyle-type egg in faeces. Larvae develop from L1 to L3 on pasture. Infection occurs via ingestion of pasture contaminated with L3s. Parasitic development is similar to that of *Ostertagia* spp. in ruminants where L3 larvae burrow into the gastric glands and moult from L4 to adults. Larvae can arrest in the gastric glands as L4. Inhibition of larvae in gastric mucosa is a common phenomenon in this infection and development of the inhibited stages with associated effects on the gastric mucosa occurs after farrowing. This resumption of development appears to be related to a hormonal basis, and attributed to lactation. Also, it may occur after therapy with an anthelmintic not effective against inhibited larvae. Pathogenesis depends on invasion of gastric glands with loss of parietal cell function. Protein leakage from the gastric lesions and increases in plasma pepsinogen can occur.

Pathological findings
Invasion of gastric glands by larvae can lead to inflammation; nodule formation and glandular cells may degenerate to mucus-forming type. Grossly, the gastric mucosa is thickened, catarrhal and has a cobble-stone or 'morocco leather' appearance. Microscopically, there is mucus metaplasia of parasitized and adjacent gastric glands. In chronic infections, submucosal lymphoid follicles may develop.

Clinical features
Generally asymptomatic, but heavy infections can produce gastritis. Adults suck blood, which can cause anaemia, inappetence and loss of weight, and may contribute to the 'thin sow syndrome'.

Diagnosis
Diagnosis is based on clinical signs of weight loss and finding strongyle eggs in the faecal sample, but the eggs can be confused with eggs of *Oesophagostomum* spp., which occur in pigs. Finding adult worms on necropsy and plasma pepsinogen levels are useful aids to diagnosis. *Hyostrongylus rubidus* must be differentiated from other causes of unthriftiness or emaciation such as swine dysentery, necrotic enteritis, coccidiosis, oesophagostomosis, and malnutrition.

Treatment
Doramectin, fenbendazole, flubendazole, oxibendazole, thiophanate or dichlorvos.

Control
Prophylactic treatment and good husbandry practices, such as rotating pastures.

Public health implications
Not known.

Ollulanus tricuspis infection

Aetiology
Ollulanus tricuspis is a small nematode of the stomach of cats and other mammals. It is characterized by its small size ≤ 1 cm, spiral coil of the head, and the presence of a well developed copulatory bursa in male and 3–4 short tooth-like structures (cusps) on the tail of female.

Epidemiology and geographical distribution
Ollulanus tricuspis has a worldwide distribution, but it mainly occurs in Europe, the Americas, Australia and the Middle East.

Life cycle and pathogenesis
The parasite has a direct life cycle. The females are viviparous, i.e. eggs hatch and larval development to L3 occurs inside the uterus of the female. The whole cycle can be completed endogenously in the same cat when infective L3s are released into the lumen of the stomach and develop into adults on the gastric mucosa in around 4–5 weeks. The L3s may be transmitted to another cat through the consumption of vomit containing L3s. Adult worms normally live under a layer of mucus in the stomach wall, but they may burrow into the gastric mucosa, leading to gastritis.

Pathological findings
Hypertrophic to fibrosing gastritis have been reported. Sometimes, no macroscopic lesions can be seen in the stomachs of infected cats.

Clinical features
Ollulanus tricuspis causes increased mucus production, anorexia, intermittent vomiting, emaciation, and haematemesis. However, severe chronic gastritis and occasional death have been reported in high-intensity infections in cats and other felids.

Diagnosis
Diagnosis is made by identification of larvae and adult worms in the vomit or stomach contents, or in scrapings collected by gastric lavage.

Treatment
Fenbendazole, levamisole or ivermectin can be effective.

Control
Good sanitation and prevention of contacts with infected cats.

Public health implications
Unknown.

Onchocerciasis

Aetiology

Onchocerciasis in equids is a filarial disease of the ligaments caused by *Onchocerca* spp. *Onchocerca cervicalis* affects the nuchal ligament whereas *O. reticulata* affect the suspensory ligament of the fetlock joint. Bovine onchocerciasis is caused by *O. armillata*, *O. gutturosa*, and *O. gibsoni*.

Epidemiology and geographical distribution

Observed throughout the world and its prevalence depends on the biology of the biting midge vector (*Culicoides* spp.).

Life cycle and pathogenesis

Adult worms live within the ligamentum nuchae, producing microfilariae which migrate in connective tissue to the upper dermis, especially the skin of the ventral midline and face where they are ingested by feeding *Culicoides*. Microfilariae migrate to the salivary glands of the fly and complete their life cycle when they are transferred to another host. Skin reactions are probably caused by hypersensitivity.

Pathological findings

Lesions are characterized by alopecia, scaliness, ulceration and pruritus, particularly along the ventral abdomen. Lesions may extend between the forelegs and hind legs to include the thigh, and in severe cases they may extend up the lower abdominal wall. The inner wall of the aorta may be corrugated, roughened, calcified, and swollen in case of *O. armillata* infection.

Clinical features

Although many horses are infected, the majority rarely show evidence of clinical disease. *Onchocerca cervicalis* causes fibrotic, caseous and calcified lesions in the ligamentum nuchae. The conditions known as 'poll evil' and 'fistulous withers' are no longer thought to be associated with this parasite. Microfilariae may sometimes be damaging. Those of *O. cervicalis* are occasionally observed in the cornea of horses. They can also induce hypersensitivity reactions in the skin of some individuals. Infections with *O. reticulata* may cause swelling of the suspensory ligament and a hot oedematous swelling of the posterior part of the cannon which persists for 3–4 weeks. After the swelling subsides, the suspensory ligament remains thickened. Affected animals are lame while the area is oedematous and swollen, but many recover when the swelling disappears.

In cattle, losses caused by adult filarial worms are slight although *O. gibsoni* infection causes unsightly lesions and rejection of beef carcasses from the high-quality meat trade. The nodules of *O. gibsoni* are usually freely movable and consist of fibrous tissue canalized by the long body of the worms.

Diagnosis

In onchocerciasis, microfilariae are not detectable in the bloodstream but may be found in skin biopsies. Some horses have lesions on the face, neck, or thorax. The lesions may be confused with those associated with horn fly feeding but these are more likely to include crusting and ulcerating dermatitis.

Treatment

Onchocerca microfilariae are eliminated by the macrocyclic lactones and systematic corticosteroids. The location site of the adult worms has a limited blood supply, which makes them difficult to eliminate. Continued microfilaria production by the adult parasites is responsible for recurrence of signs in the absence of regular administration of drugs.

Control

Fly control is the basis of any control programme.

Public health implications

Not known.

Oxyuriasis (equine pinworm infection)

Aetiology

Oxyuris equi (pinworm) nematode infection commonly occurs in the caecum, colon, and rectum of equids. The mature worm is white to slate grey in colour. The male is 1–2 cm long, but the female is much longer, up to 15 cm, and has a long sharply pointed tail.

Epidemiology and geographical distribution

The parasite is ubiquitous but of greater prevalence in areas of high rainfall. Eggs resist desiccation, may become airborne in dust and remain viable in stables for long periods.

Life cycle and pathogenesis

The life cycle is simple and direct. Fertilized female travels down the gut and crawls onto the perianal area, where she lays her eggs onto the perineal skin in a yellowish-grey gelatinous material around the anus. After completing egg lying, the females pass out of the anus and die. Frequently, eggs contain first-stage larvae when deposited. An embryo develops to an infective third-stage larva in about 3–5 days within the egg. Eggs may be licked off the skin and swallowed or they may eventually fall to the ground. Infection begins with ingestion of an embryonated egg containing an infective L3. The larvae hatch in the small intestine and invade the mucosal crypts of the caecum and colon. The prepatent period is approximately 5 months.

Pathological findings

Presence of eggs in yellow/grey streaks of gelatinous material on perineum.

Clinical features

The primary clinical sign of *O. equi* infection is intense pruritus of the tail head caused by drying and cracking of the egg masses in the anal region. The egg-laying behaviour of female *O. equi* provokes irritation of the perianal region, causing horses to rub and bite their tails. This can result in hair loss and physical damage to the tissues of the area. In severe infections, mild colic can result from inflammation of the caecum and colonic mucosa.

Diagnosis

Clinical signs are generally indicative. Detection of operculated eggs by the adhesive tape technique, slightly flattened on one side and with a mucoid plug at one pole, or by seeing adult worm in the faeces. The egg-laying behaviour of female *Oxyuris* means that eggs are rarely found in faeces taken from rectum.

Treatment

Treatment comprises the removal of egg masses, application of a mild disinfectant ointment to the perianal region and the administration of ivermectin, moxidectin, or any of the broad-spectrum benzimidazoles or pyrantels at the standard dose rate for horses.

Control

Sanitation and hygiene aimed at reducing the likelihood of reinfection. Frequent cleansing of the perineum will also limit spread.

Public health implications

Oxyuris equi has no zoonotic potential and does not infect other domestic animals. Humans serve as definitive hosts of *Entrobius vermicularis*, another oxyurid pinworm that is unique to primates.

Parasitic gastroenteritis

Overview

Gastrointestinal nematodes that infect ruminants are an important cause of disease and production loss. They contribute to a condition called parasitic gastroenteritis (PGE). PGE can be caused by many nematode species from spring to late autumn. The gastrointestinal nematodes of greatest importance in ruminants are members of the nematode of suborder Strongylida (the bursated nematodes) and most belong to the superfamily Trichostrongyloidea (Table 4.5).

Haemonchus contortus is the arguably the most important ruminant strongylid nematode worldwide. A second important abomasal nematode is *Teladorsagia circumcincta* (formerly *Ostertagia circumcincta*). *Nematodirus* spp. and *Trichostrongylus* spp. are further important genera that affect predominantly the small intestine of sheep particularly in Northern Europe although readily observed in New Zealand and Australia.

Other nematodes of different taxonomic orders also affect the gastrointistenal tract of small ruminants, such as *Bunostomum*, *Cooperia*, *Strongyloides* (small intestine), and *Chabertia*, *Oesophagostomum*, *Trichuris* (large intestine) are less common parasites. These nematodes vary in size from about 6 mm (*Trichostrongylus* spp.) to about 30 mm (*Haemonchus* spp.). Eggs of *Nematodirus*, *Capillaria*, *Trichuris* and *Strongyloides* are readily

Table 4.5 Nematodes of ruminants in UK

Predilection site	Species	Host*
Abomasum	*Haemonchus contortus*†	S, G, C
	Haemonchus placei†	C
	Ostertagia ostertagi	C
	Teladorsagia circumcincta	S, G
	Teladorsagia trifurcata	S, G
	Trichostrongylus axei	S, G, C
Small intestine	*Bunostomum trigonocephalum*	S, G
	Cooperia curticei	S
	Cooperia onchophora	S, C
	Cooperia pectinata	C
	Cooperia punctata	C
	Capillaria longipes	S
	Nematodirus battus	S, G, C
	Nematodirus filicollis	S
	Nematodirus helvetianus	C
	Nematodirus spathiger	S, G, C
	Strongyloides papillosus	S, G, C
	Trichostrongylus colubriformis	S, G, C
	Trichostrongylus longispicularis	S, G, C
	Trichostrongylus vitrinus	S, G
Large intestine	*Chabertia ovina*	S, G
	Oesophagostomum columbianum	S, G
	Oesophagostomum radiatum	C
	Oesophagostomum venulosum	S, G
	Trichuris ovis	S, G

*Traditionally considered host species: S, sheep; G, goats; C, cattle.
†May be same parasite.

distinguishable from each other. PGE has to be differentiated from other common causes of emaciation and diarrhoea in young animals such as: malnutrition, copper deficiency (in cattle), coccidiosis, Johne's disease, and chronic fascioliasis.

PGE occurs most often in young, non-immune animals, adult animals whose immunity has been compromised, or in small ruminants exposed to high levels of infection. The same life cycle generally applies to all the economically important stongylid parasites of ruminants. All have a direct, simple life cycle (Fig. 4.6). Adult female in the abomasum or intestine produces eggs that are excreted in the faeces. Development of the larval stages occurs in the faecal mass, which provides some protection from environmental conditions. A first-stage larva is formed that hatches out from the egg. Post hatching, larvae feed on bacteria and free-living protozoa and undergo 2 moults to reach the infective third larval stage (L3). L3 make their way out of the faecal material and onto the forage where they are ingested by ruminants. *Nematodirus* spp. are an exception to the general stongylid life cycle. The parasite has a long free-living period of its life cycle and eggs generally require a period of chilling followed by a mean day/night temperature of greater than 10 °C in order to develop to L3 and hatch. This strategy generally leads to a synchronized hatch into larvae in the spring. The concentrated exposure to L3 intensifies the pathogenic effects of this parasite. Once ingested by the host, the L3 larvae generally penetrate the mucosa in the site they normally inhabit (stomach, small intestine, large intestine), depending on the strongyle species and patent in a short period (14–49 days).

The geographic distribution of these parasites depends on their ability to adapt in the external environment. For example, *Haemonchus* generally requires warmth and moisture although recently outbreaks have been increasingly reported in Northern Europe; whereas others such as *Trichostrongylus*, *Teladorsagia*, and *Nematodirus* spp. will withstand drier, colder climates. The epidemiology of important species of gastrointestinal nematodes is strongly influenced by aspects of host–parasite interaction after infection occurs. Hypobiosis is the common example. In areas with cold winters, newly ingested larvae survive the winter months as arrested larvae inside the host. This means that as existing adults die they are not replaced. Also, eggs that are shed at the end of the grazing season are unlikely to develop or develop slowly, preventing further build up of L3 on pasture. In these areas with endemic hypobiosis, emergence and development of adult worms in late winter and early spring are followed by an increase in faecal egg counts. The rise in egg counts is magnified in periparturient sheep by a relaxation of immunity that increases survival and egg production in existing parasites and also increases susceptibility to further infection. The periparturient egg rise (PPR) can make an important contribution to L3 populations on pastures as young, susceptible animals begin grazing. In areas with mild weather, hypobiosis seems to be less important in the epidemiology of PGE.

Control is best accomplished by a combination of treatment and pasture management especially in wet and warm areas that promote survival of the larval stages. Treatment includes avermectins, milbemycins, benzimidazoles, probenzimidazoles; levamisole and morantel. Not all compounds are suitable for controlling hypobiotic larvae. Control methods differ widely according to climatic conditions, alternate grazing management options and the presence of anthelmintic resistance. The major aim is to maintain safe grazing by reducing pasture contamination. Integrated management schemes which reduce dependence on drug usage are preferred as anthelmintic resistance is a serious or emerging problem in many areas, particularly in sheep and goats.

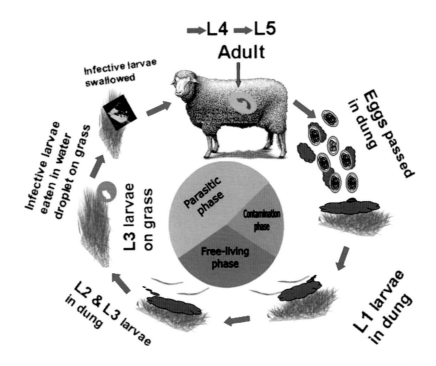

Figure 4.6 General life cycle of trichostrongylid nematodes.

Gastrointestinal nematodes that contribute to PGE will be discussed in more details with emphasis on the most economically important species.

Haemonchosis (barber pole worm infection)

Aetiology

Haemonchus contortus is a strongylate nematode of sheep and other ruminants. The name barber pole worm is derived from the macroscopically visible entwining of the blood-filled intestine and white egg filled uterus in the female worm. Male has a characteristic copulatory bursa (Fig. 4.7). Adults live in abomasum of ruminants. Female reach about 3 cm in length, making this species one of the largest of the strongylid nematodes of ruminants.

Epidemiology and geographical distribution

Geographic distribution includes UK – typically south/southeast, where climate is slightly warmer and dryer. Worldwide *H. contortus* is a very important parasite of sheep and goats in tropical/subtropical regions. In some cases resistant to all classes of current anthelmintics, which has made sheep farming in some regions non-sustainable. PPR or 'Spring Rise' is an important feature of *Haemonchus* infection. When adult animals are clinically affected by haemonchosis it is usually pregnant/lactating ewes, animals carrying a concurrent infection or animals under nutritional stress. The latter is particularly important in tropical regions where a chronic form of the disease can be observed. Drought conditions lead to poorer quality pastures and weight loss and animals that are less able to manage a continual loss of host resources caused by a small number of worms.

Life cycle and pathogenesis

Life cycle is direct. L3s shed their sheath in the rumen and moult to L4s within 48 hours. L4s use anterior piercing lancets to penetrate the lining of abomasum and to puncture blood vessels, leading to severe blood loss. It is estimated that on average each adult worm feeds for up to 12 minutes at a time and can remove 0.05 ml of blood either by ingestion or through seepage of the lesion. Each 'puncture wound' continue to haemorrhage for up to a further 7 min after the worm has stopped feeding. Adults develop in about

3 weeks of infection and begin to produce eggs. Unlike many other parasites of the gastrointestinal tract, *H. contortus* is not a primary cause of diarrhoea. Hence, its effects on a flock or herd are often insidious because routine observation of animals may not reveal the extent of infection and owners may not appreciate that disease is present until deaths occur. The feeding habit of the adult worms leads to a lowering in RBC count, plasma protein and haematocrit level. Infected hosts go through compensatory erythropoiesis while continually having to contend with loss in nutrient intake due to induced inappetence and decreasing iron and protein levels. This blood loss is what contributes mainly to the pathogenesis and clinical signs seen in haemonchosis. Another facet of the pathogenesis of haemonchosis is attributed to the damage of abomasal glands. Emergence of pre-adult worms from the abomasal glands triggers a hyperplastic reaction in neighbouring glands that causes larger nodular lesions, which if numerous may aggregate. The hyperplastic mucosal reaction may result in altered integrity/increased permeability of the epithelial sheet lining the inner mucosa of the abomasum, allowing for the leakage of protein into the lumen of the abomasum. In severe cases, this leads to hypoalbuminaemia, tissue oedema and weight loss. The gastric damage also involves the HCl-producing parietal cells, which become non-functional, and this leads to lack of production of HCl and increased abomasal pH to the alkaline side, which may rise to 6–7. The lack of gastric acidity produces the following effects. Firstly, incoming bacteria and ruminal protozoa are not killed and resident bacteria become overgrown. Second, pepsinogen is not converted to active pepsin as this is only initiated in an acidic environment; thus, no pepsin is available for protein digestion. This will be reflected by a diagnostic level of pepsinogen in the blood of infected animals.

Pathological findings

At necropsy, lesions include subcutaneous oedema of the intermandibular space, pale conjunctiva and oral membranes. Adult *Haemonchus* worms can be seen in the abomasal contents. The abomasum of infected sheep exhibits red haemorrhagic surface attributed to traumatic damage caused by feeding habit of the parasite.

Clinical features

Haemonchosis is a serious problem when lambs on pasture ingest large numbers of larvae. These parasites feed on blood and can cause severe anaemia. Diarrhoea, loss of body condition (weight gain in lambs) and wool thickness, and quality. In acute infections oedema and hypoproteinaemia, can be seen clinically as marked submandibular oedema 'Bottle jaw'. In chronic infections inappetence and weight loss are most readily observed.

Diagnosis

McMaster slides used to count and identify eggs. FAMACHA© system, and/or packed cell volume may be used to assess extent of anaemia in lambs infected with *Haemonchus*. During necropsy, adult female *H. contortus* (Fig. 4.8) and their unique barber pole appearance are not difficult to see in the abomasal contents.

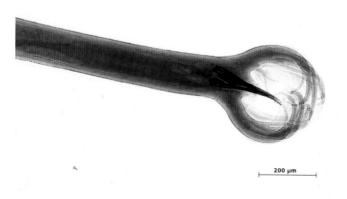

200 µm

Figure 4.7 Copulatory bursa of adult male *Haemonchus contortus*.

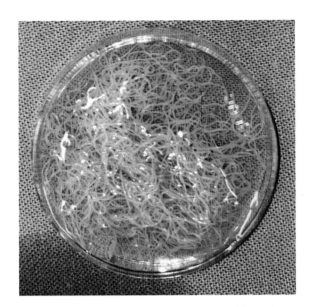

Figure 4.8 Adult *Haemonchus contortus* collected from abomasum of a sheep.

Treatment

Avermectins, milbemycins; benzimidazoles, probenzimidazoles; levamisole and morantel.

Control

Targeted deworming, sanitation and hygienic measures to prevent the spread of infection and pasture contamination.

Public health implications

Cases of human haemonchosis have been observed in Brazil and Australia.

Nematodirosis

Aetiology

Nematodirosis is common in temperate zones. It is of special significance to lambs in UK. *Nematodirus* spp. inhabit small intestine of ruminants (Fig. 4.5).

Epidemiology and geographical distribution

The disease spread from UK to Western Europe and USA, but its 'sudden' appearance in Scotland in early 1950s has never been explained. *Nematodirus* infection is usually associated with lambs (esp. recently weaned). Older animals are seldom affected but in recent years clinical cases have been reported. The major epidemiological feature of *N. battus* infection is the sudden appearance of infective larvae in spring following mass hatching of overwintered eggs. *N. battus* hatching can only occur from eggs excreted in previous year. However, some eggs deposited in spring can hatch in autumn of the same year causing contamination of pasture at this time. Due to the strict controlling factors, e.g. cold followed by day/night 10°C very large numbers can hatch at once in a restricted season (March-April) during which time the majority of deaths occurs. Climatic factors are important since a warm March would encourage an early hatch. Cool wet April/May will increase larval survival on pasture. Therefore, grazing lambs could be exposed to very high numbers of larvae. Weather conditions must therefore be taken into consideration and can be used to forecast problems.

Life cycle and pathogenesis

Nematodirus battus life cycle (Fig. 4.9) is a little different to common trichostrongyle life cycle. For example (1) preparasitic phase (L1–L3) occurs within egg shells. (2) larvae take months

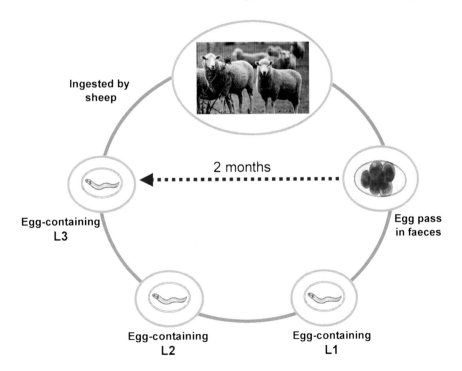

Figure 4.9 Life cycle of *Nematodirus battus* in sheep. This species does not have a common trichostrongyle Life cycle. Pre-parasitic phase is unique (L1–L3 occurs inside the egg).

to develop except *N. helvetianus*, which can develop and hatch in a few weeks. (3) eggs are extremely tough and resistant to freezing and drought, viable up to 2 years on pasture. (4) egg hatch is stimulated by cold period followed by a mean day/night temperature of ~ 10°C, but L3 are susceptible to climate and need to be ingested quickly. Therefore, this is usually the first nematode species to peak on pasture in spring. Nematodirosis is characterized by strong age-related immunity (immunity occurs after about 3 months of age), increased eosinophils and mast cells at site of infection, and villus shedding.

Pathological findings
The principal pathogenic damage is caused by larvae not adults. A large number simultaneously burrowing into the gut causes damage of villi and erosion of mucosa.

Clinical features
Acute onset in young lambs (6 weeks to 4 months). Ability of intestine to exchange fluids and nutrients is greatly reduced. This leads to rapid weight loss, watery diarrhoea, dehydration and sudden death.

Diagnosis
The primary laboratory test used for the diagnosis of all strongylid nematodes is a faecal flotation test for detection of the eggs of the nematodes. Because clinical signs appear during prepatent period faecal egg counts are of little value in diagnosis. However, *Nematodirus* eggs are very diagnostic. Strongylid nematodes shed eggs that are similar in morphology and cannot be easily differentiated. In faecal specimens they are all identified as strongylid or trichostrongylid eggs. To identify the genera of these nematodes, faecal culture and identification of L3 larvae are required. *Nematodirus* is the exception, where eggs are much larger than other strongylid species and contain distinctive dark cells. Remember the critical hatching requirements in this species. This is a condition which occurs in late spring, and disease usually first reported in May/June. Very often a vet will be called because of sudden death (onset and disease progression can be very fast). Also, consider grazing history, clinical signs and, if possible, necropsy.

Treatment
Ivermectin and levamisole are effective. Three treatments during May–June in years with predicted severe diseases, and two in other years.

Control
Alternative grazing with livestock which do not share parasites, having one species of animal following another one can be effective to break life cycle of the parasites. More than 2-year rotation is needed on previously infected pasture. Sheep following cows may also not work since calves have been known to carry *N. battus*. Sheep (Y1), cattle (Y2), conservation (Y3) if possible has been shown to be quite effective. When this alternative grazing is not available, control can be achieved by anthelmintics' prophylaxis. Ewes should be dosed prior to lambing.

Public health implications
Not known.

Ostertagiosis (brown stomach worm infection)

Aetiology
Ostertagia ostertagi in cattle and *Teladorsagia circumcincta* (formerly called *Ostertagia circumcincta*) in sheep are Strongylida (bursate) nematodes. Like *H. contortus*, *O. Ostertagi* is a parasite of the abomasum. However, unlike *H. contortus*, it does not feed on blood nor are the females prolific egg producers. Adults are slender and brown-coloured worms, 6–15 mm in length. Ostertagiosis is considered the most important helminthic disease in cattle in temperate climates.

Epidemiology and geographical distribution
Worldwide distribution, especially in moist and temperate regions of the world.

Life cycle and pathogenesis
Life cycle inside the host includes the following events: L3s exsheath in the fore-stomach. L3s migrate and moult to L4s inside the gastric glands. Immature adults emerge from the gastric glands (the main cause of pathology). Adults produce eggs and the cycle is complete. First immune response to *O. ostertagi* does not protect against re-infection with L3s (therefore repeated re-infection can occur). At certain times of the year, ingested larvae undergo arrested development or hypobiosis after a brief period of development. The damage in the abomasal wall (i.e. histological alterations) and associated complications (i.e. biochemical sequelae) that occur in haemonchosis are more of a problem in case of *Ostertagia* infection, and contribute to its main pathogenic effects. Hyperplastic epithelium becomes leakier, leading to protein loss into the abomasum and the characteristic protein-losing enteropathy. Accumulation of unabsorbable, osmotically active materials (undigested protein and bacteria) promotes the transfer of fluid from the extracellular spaces into the gut lumen, causing diarrhoea.

Ostertagiosis includes two important disease forms: type I and type II. Type I ostertagiosis occurs in calves (younger animals) turned out on pasture in April/May. This pasture has been grazed previous year (especially by calves). Thus, this disease results from the rapid acquisition of large numbers of L3 larvae that complete the development to the adult stages. Since L3 over winter large numbers may already be present as the calves are turned out. This is why rotation is important. Type II ostertagiosis occurs in animals which are old enough to have arrested larvae from previous grazing season, and associated with PPR or 'spring rise'. The synchronous development and maturation of inhibited larvae result in this clinical form of ostertagiosis.

Pathological findings
The abomasum of heavily infected cattle takes on the appearance of 'Morocco leather'. This cobblestone appearance is due to mucous cell hyperplasia and lymphoid nodules in the abomasal

submucosa elevating the overlying epithelium. Abomasitis characterized by an infiltration of chronic inflammatory cells, some eosinophils, a decrease in the number of parietal and chief cells, and hyperplasia of mucous cells in the abomasum.

Clinical features
Clinical signs result from the mechanical damage done to the abomasum. Diarrhoea, together with protein-losing enteropathy and loss of appetite, leads to rapid weight loss, hypoalbuminaemia and submandibular oedema ('bottle-jaw').

Diagnosis
McMaster slides used to analyse eggs. On necropsy, presence of brown nematodes, smaller than *H. contortus*, and more difficult to see without magnification. Condition of abomasum; cobblestone lesions in the abomasums caused by damage of the gastric glands. Elevated plasma level of pepsinogen. The abomasal contents are fluid, brown-green and fetid, as ingesta are partially putrefied because of the overgrowth of bacteria.

Treatment
More difficult to treat hypobiosis, but drugs such as ivermectin will kill the hypobiotic L4 larvae. In some cases very frequent drenching may be required around calving (type II). Frequent drenching may be required during the first grazing season, especially for animals raised on pasture on which calves grazed previous season.

Control
Sanitation and hygienic measures to prevent the spread of infection and pasture contamination. Common measures include lower stocking density. Rotate calves and adults, and rotate onto fresh pasture if possible.

Public health implications
Not known.

Trichostrongylosis

Aetiology
Nematodes in the genus *Trichostrongylus*, which inhabit alimentary tract of mammals (sheep, goats and cattle) and birds. Common species include *T. colubriformis* in small intestine, *Trichostrongylus axei* in abomasums, and *T. tenuis* in small intestine of birds. They are small, hair like worms that measure up to 0.7 mm long (difficult to see by naked eye). They have a small buccal capsule.

Epidemiology and geographical distribution
PGE due to trichostrongylosis has been seen in UK winter since warmer wetter winters have favoured increased L3 survival. Immune exclusion (exclusion of L3) and 'self-cure' (expulsion of adults in intestine) can occur.

Life cycle and pathogenesis
Life cycle is direct and non-migratory. Infection occurs via ingestion of free L3. Local and systematic changes associated with this parasite are similar to those inflicted by *Ostertagia* spp.

Pathological findings
Pathological lesions are mainly intestinal. Intestine is inflamed with hyperplasia and there may be blood spots. Mesenteric lymph nodes are enlarged.

Clinical features
Acute diarrhoea in young and chronic diarrhoea in older animals. A subclinical infection can reduce weight gains, wool growth, and milk production. The bottle jaw appearance can be seen. Reduced fecundity has been seen in *T. tenius*-parasitized birds.

Diagnosis
Faecal flotation test for detection of the strongyle-type eggs.

Treatment
Avermectins, milbemycins; benzimidazoles, probenzimidazoles; levamisole and morantel.

Control
General preventive programmes for parasitic gastroenteritis are also effective against *Trichostrongylus* spp.

Public health implications
Several species of *Trichostrongylus* have been known to infect humans, including *T. orientalis*, *T. colubriformis*, and *T. axei*.

Bunostomosis (hookworm infection)

Aetiology
Nematodes of the genus *Bunostomum* and related hookworms.

Epidemiology and geographical distribution
Worldwide, especially in warm, moist climates.

Life cycle and pathogenesis
Transmission is generally by skin penetration and is favoured by warm, humid conditions.

Pathological findings
Eggs and occult blood in faeces, anaemia, hypoproteinaemia. Red worms attached to mucosa of small intestine, nearby ingesta often blood-stained.

Clinical features
Anaemia, diarrhoea and anasarca.

Diagnosis
Necropsy to detect adult worms, and faecal flotation test for detection of the eggs.

Treatment
Most modern broad-spectrum ruminant anthelmintics are effective.

Control
General preventative programmes for parasitic gastroenteritis are also effective against hookworm.

Public health implications
Not known.

Chabertiasis

Aetiology
Chabertiasis of sheep, goat, and cattle is caused by *Chabertia ovina* (large-mouthed bowel worm), a worm 1–2 cm in length, which inhabits the colon and causes a clinical condition similar to that of oesophagostomosis. The adult worm has a characteristic, curved, bell-shaped buccal capsule which lacks teeth.

Epidemiology and geographical distribution
Chabertiasis is more common in sheep and goats than in cattle. It has a worldwide distribution, but it tends to be more common in temperate regions especially during winter months.

Life cycle and pathogenesis
The life cycle is direct and resembles that of other strongylids in the preparasitic phase. After ingestion by the final host, L3 larvae undergo a period of development in the wall of the small intestine before passing to the caecum and then to the colon. The prepatent period is approximately 6 weeks. Host immunity can reduce the fecundity of adult worms. Hypobiosis is also an important survival mechanism in the life cycle of this nematode with L4 being the hypobiotic stage in the mucosa of the small intestine or the caecum. In contrast to *Oesophagostomum*, the larvae do not cause any remarkable damage. Pathogenic effects are caused by the feeding adults that are attached to the mucosa and draw a plug of mucosa into the buccal capsule which is then digested. This results in area of mucosal ulceration and local haemorrhage with protein loss into the gut through these lesions.

Pathological findings
Thickening, oedema and petechiation of the wall of the colon, with intestinal contents tinged with blood. Adult worms with their characteristic large buccal cavities are confined to the first 25–30 cm of the colon, except in high-intensity infections.

Clinical features
Clinical manifestations are first seen about 3–4 weeks after infection. This coincides with the attachment of immature adults to the mucosa. Passing of soft blood flecked faeces with excess mucus. A protein-losing enteropathy, hypoalbuminaemia, weight loss. Death may occur in heavy infections.

Diagnosis
Faecal egg counts do not always correlate well with clinical signs as these may occur before the worms mature and hence, eggs will be absent from faeces. *Chabertia ovina* eggs are of the strongyle-type (i.e. eggs cannot be distinguished from the eggs of other trichostrongyles infecting the guts of ruminants). At necropsy the worms are readily identified from their location, size and characteristic shape of the buccal capsule.

Treatment
Most broad-spectrum anthelmintics are active against *Chabertia ovina*.

Control
General preventative programmes for parasitic gastroenteritis.

Public health implications
Not known.

Cooperiosis

Aetiology
Several species of the genus *Cooperia* occur in the small intestine of cattle. The adult worms measure 5–8 mm in length and males have a prominent bursa in relation to their size. Worms in all the species have a slightly bulbous appearance owing to the presence of the cephalic vesicle.

Epidemiology and geographical distribution
In temperate climates the epidemiology follow *Ostertagia* with winter hypobiosis. In subtropical areas the patterns of transmission follow those of *Haemonchus* with hypobiosis during the dry seasons.

Life cycle and pathogenesis
Their life cycle is essentially the same as that of other trichostrongylids. Arrested development is an important feature of the life cycle. The prepatent period is 12–15 days.

Pathological findings
Congestion, necrosis, and haemorrhages in the mucosa of the small intestine.

Clinical features
Cooperia are generally considered to be mild pathogens. They contribute secondary effects to the primary pathogens *Ostertagia* and *Haemonchus* in parasitic gastroenteritis. In heavy infections animals show profuse diarrhoea, anorexia, weight loss, poor productivity and emaciation, but no anaemia. These worms do not suck blood.

Diagnosis
The eggs usually can be differentiated from those of the common gastrointestinal nematodes by their parallel sides, but a larval culture of the faeces is necessary to definitively diagnose *Cooperia*

infection in the living animal. It is usually necessary to make scrapings of the mucosa to demonstrate *Cooperia* spp., which must be differentiated from other *Trichostrongylus* species via its coiled appearance.

Treatment
Most broad-spectrum anthelmintics are active against *Cooperia* spp.

Control
General preventative programmes for parasitic gastroenteritis.

Public health implications
Not known.

Oesophagostomosis

Aetiology
Oesophagostomosis is associated with infection with the bursate nematodes of genus *Oesophogostomum*, namely, *O. radiatum* (cattle), *O. dentatum* and *O. quadrispinulatum* (pigs), and *O. venulosum* and *O. columbianum* (sheep and goats). Adult worms have a characteristic cephalic inflation of the cuticle.

Epidemiology and geographical distribution
Oesophagostomum spp. have a worldwide distribution, but are common in wet temperate climates. Hypobiosis/Spring rise occurs to infect young animals.

Life cycle and pathogenesis
Life cycle is direct. Eggs develop to the infective larval stage in approximately one week. The preparasitic phase is typically strongylid, and infection is by ingestion of L3s. The larvae exsheath in the small intestine and burrow into the wall of the intestines where they remain for about 2 weeks and form nodules. They then re-enter the intestine to mature and lay eggs. The prepatent period is 30–45 days, depending on the species. *Oesophagostomum radiatum* induce strong protective immune response to low exposure; opposite to *O. ostertagi* where immune response takes a very long time to develop. The major damage arises from larvae penetrating the mucosa of the intestine.

Pathological findings
They are called 'nodular worms' because larvae developing in the colonic mucosa cause an inflammatory response leading to nodules in the wall of the large bowel which interfere with digestion and absorption. In high-intensity infections, the mucosa becomes inflamed and oedematous, with enlargement of regional lymph nodes.

Clinical features
Infection of sows is most important and high-intensity infections can lead to weight loss, reduced litter sizes, reduced litter weaning weights and oedema (pot belly). In lambs, *O. columbianum* is more pathogenic than *O. venulosum*, because the former

stimulates nodule formation. High-intensity infections can cause severe disease in young lambs (failure to thrive, scouring and weakness). *Oesophogostomum venulosum* can cause production loss but only in very high-intensity infection (usually no disease). In calves, severe disease can occur where adult worms can cause anorexia, anaemia, oedema, very dark diarrhoea, weight loss and death. In older cattle, strong protective immunity causes nodule formation. Nodules calcify and in very severe infections may cause intestinal intussusception, which may lead to stenosis (narrowing), ultimately the intestine is blocked or restricted.

Diagnosis
Diagnosis can be accomplished by faecal flotation for detection of strongyle-type egg and by detection of the worms at post-mortem examination. In acute infections clinical signs occur during the prepatent period and diarrhoea will occur without eggs being seen in faeces of infected animals. On necropsy, classic haemorrhagic nodules in cattle and fibrous nodules in pigs are caused by *O. radiatum*, and *O. dentatum*, respectively. In pigs, eggs can be confused with the eggs of *Hyostrongylus* and *Trichostrongylus* spp.

Treatment
Most commonly used anthelmintics, e.g. ivermectin and fenbendazole, are active against *Oesophogostomum* spp.

Control
General preventative programmes for parasitic gastroenteritis.

Public health implications
Not known.

Spirocercosis

Aetiology
The nematode *Spirocerca lupi* is primarily a parasite of dogs, although other carnivores may be affected.

Epidemiology and geographical distribution
Canine spirocercosis has a worldwide distribution, but is most prevalent in warm climate.

Life cycle and pathogenesis
The adult *S. lupi* is found in a nodular mass in the wall of the host's thoracic oesophagus. The female lays embryonated eggs that are transferred through a tract in the nodule and excreted in the host's faeces. Eggs are ingested by the intermediate host, coprophagus beetles, and develop to infective (L3) stage within 2 months. Carnivores are infected by ingestion of a beetle or a variety of paratenic hosts including birds, hedgehogs, lizards, mice and rabbits. In the carnivore host, the infective larvae penetrate the gastric mucosa, and migrate within the walls of the gastric arteries to the thoracic aorta. About 3 months post infection, the larvae leave the aorta and migrate to the oesophagus where they provoke the development of granulomas as they mature to adults over the next 3 months. The lesions caused by *S. lupi* are mainly due to

the migration and persistent presence of larvae and adults in the tissues.

Pathological findings

Oesophageal nodular masses and granulomas, and aortic scars and aneurysms are the most frequent lesions. Spondylitis and spondylosis of the caudal thoracic vertebrae are additional typical lesions. Neoplastic transformation of the granulomas to fibrosarcoma or osteosarcoma has been reported in dogs with spirocercosis. Less frequently, lesions may occur due to the aberrant migration of the worms. *S. lupi* worms and nodules have been reported in thoracic organs, the gastrointestinal tract, the urinary system, and the subcutaneous tissues.

Clinical features

The clinical signs depend on the location and severity of the lesions. Oesophageal lesions are associated with persistent vomiting and/or regurgitation followed by weakness and emaciation. Sudden death may be caused by rupture of an aortic aneurysm induced by migration of worms in the aortic wall.

Diagnosis

A definite diagnosis of spirocercosis is made by detection of characteristic eggs by faecal flotation. Thoracic radiographs of affected dogs show oesophageal granulomas as areas of increased density in the caudodorsal mediastinum and contrast oesophograms may outline granulomas. Oesophagoscopy and gastroscopy allow direct visualization of the nodules, which appear as broad-based protuberances with a distinctly nipple-like orifice.

Treatment

Several anthelmintics have been suggested for the treatment of canine spirocercosis. These include: diethylcarbamazine, disophenol, levamisole, albendazole, ivermectin and doramectin. Surgical excision of oesophageal granulomas and sarcomas is often not possible due to extensive or multiple lesions.

Control

Avoid contact with intermediate hosts.

Public health implications

A single case has been recorded.

Stephanurosis (swine kidney worm infection)

Aetiology

The kidney worm disease in pigs is associated with *Stephanurus dentatus*.

Epidemiology and geographical distribution

Mainly tropical and subtropical regions.

Life cycle and pathogenesis

The adult worms live in the kidneys and perirenal tissue and pass eggs into the urinary bladder. Earthworms can serve as an intermediate host. Pigs are infected by ingesting L3 larvae, or earthworms containing L3, by transmammary or transplacental transmission, or by L3 larvae penetrating the skin. Most of the damage is done by the migrating larvae to the liver and other organs.

Pathological findings

Liver lesions in the form of fibrotic tracks and fibrosis are caused by migrating larvae and immature adults.

Clinical features

Emaciation, failure to thrive and death. In rare cases, aberrant migrations of larvae to the spinal cord may cause a posterior paralysis.

Diagnosis

Diagnosis is usually made at necropsy where characteristic liver lesions and adult worms are seen in the perirenal areas; however, eggs can be identified in urine.

Treatment

Medicated early weaning is an effective programme whereby weaned pigs are separated from older pigs and medicated with broad-spectrum anthelmintics and antibiotics. *Boars* should be treated twice a year if in total confinement, otherwise, they should be treated every 3 months. *Gilts* should receive regular deworming at three month intervals until breeding if in confinement or every 6 weeks until breeding if in a contaminated environment. *Sows* should be treated with dewormers just prior to farrowing with a dewormer that kills migrating larvae. If sows are not maintained in farrowing crates, there should be a second treatment during early gestation to kill parasites they have acquired before they reach patency.

Control

Confinement does not eliminate parasites because of the extremely resistant eggs, so faecal flotation to check for parasites followed by strategic deworming with effective anthelmintics are necessary to ensure good productivity.

Public health implications

Not known.

Strongyloidiasis (thread worm infection)

Aetiology

Strongyloides ransomi in pigs, *S. westeri* in horses, and *S. papillosus* in sheep and cattle. All are parasites of the small intestine. They are thread-like and less than 1 cm in length.

Epidemiology and geographical distribution

Farm animals in many countries are exposed to infection with *Strongyloides*. Disease outbreaks occur in young pigs, foals, calves, and lambs but the overall economic importance of this parasite does not appear to be very significant.

Life cycle and pathogenesis
Only female worms are present in the intestine and so eggs are produced by parthenogenesis. The eggs are thin shelled and embryonated. The larvae that hatch out may develop into infective or non-parasitic forms. The latter become free-living males and females which live in decaying organic material and produce fertilized eggs that give rise to infective larvae. Transmission occurs when infective larvae enter the host either by ingestion or by skin penetration. In older animals they accumulate in subcutaneous tissues and migrate to the mammary gland when lactation starts. So, neonates can acquire infection during nursing via the milk. Infective larvae penetrating the skin of young animals travel via the blood to the lungs, where they break into alveoli, ascend the air passages to the pharynx and are then swallowed. They mature in the small intestine, where adult females lay eggs that do not require fertilization to develop. Eggs passed in faeces hatch to yield first-stage larvae, which develop in the manner, described as typical for roundworms, to become infective third-stage larvae. This life cycle is termed homogonic and includes a parasitic phase inside the host. However, the adult threadworms in the intestine can lay eggs that develop into a different kind of larvae. If warmth and humidity are conducive to survival of free-living forms, these larvae develop and moult into adult worms, which can live on pasture outside the host. This life cycle is termed heterogonic. Males and females of this type mate, producing fertilized eggs which eventually yield infective L3 larvae that are eaten by the host during grazing or actively penetrate host.

Pathological findings
Dermatitis, pulmonary haemorrhage and enteritis occur.

Clinical features
Diarrhoea in young animals is the most common clinical sign, but the penetration of massive numbers of larvae through the skin may also provoke dermatitis. Experimental infections in calves cause pallor and coughing, but cases of sudden death without previous signs have been ascribed to high-intensity infections with many migratory larvae. Sheep may develop lameness or be more subject to foot rot when subject to heavy infections. Dehydration, cachexia, foaming at mouth, anaemia and nervous signs have been reported in experimentally infected young goats. Pigs may show anorexia, listlessness and anaemia but diarrhoea is the principal clinical sign. Infection in pigs has been shown to reduce intestinal enzyme activity to increase intestinal plasma and blood loss and to reduce protein synthesis in the liver. In foals, high egg counts may be recorded in apparently healthy animals but may coincide with the onset of diarrhoea in other individuals.

Diagnosis
Baermann technique or flotation assay for the detection of the eggs and larvae in faeces (Fig. 4.10). Fresh faeces must be used because the eggs will hatch in older faeces.

Treatment
Most broad-spectrum anthelmintics are effective in eliminating this parasite. In foals, ivermectin is used at the standard equine dose but elevated doses of fenbendazole (50 mg/kg) and oxibendazole (15 mg/kg) are needed. The treatment of mares with ivermectin on the day of parturition doesn't prevent trans-mammary transmission but can reduce egg counts in the foals. Treatment of infected sows can be effective in removing arrested larvae from the subventral fat. Use of the ivermectin controlled-release bolus in lambs can prevent establishment of intestinal *Strongyloides* infections.

Control
Elimination of worms from warm, moist areas such as damp litters or beddings, which are suitable for parasite multiplication.

Public health implications
In general, this parasite is considered to have little zoonotic potential. However, human lesions of cutaneous larva migrans results from accidental exposure to infective larvae of *S. westeri* have been recorded.

Strongylosis (redworm infection)

Aetiology
The redworms (strongyles) are commonly seen in the large intestine of equids. Two nematode subfamilies: the Strongylinae (large strongyles) and Cyathostominae (≥40 species of small strongyles, small redworms, or cyathostomes). Strongylinae includes *Strongylus vulgaris*, *S. edentatus*, and *S. equinus*, which can migrate through the body, and *Triodontophorus* spp., and *Oesophagodontus robustus*, which do not. Strongyles vary in length from less than 12 mm (small strongyles) to 5 cm (large strongyles). But, some small strongyles, such as *Triodontophorus* spp., are nearly as large as *S. vulgaris*, the smallest of the large strongyles.

Epidemiology and geographical distribution
Worldwide distribution.

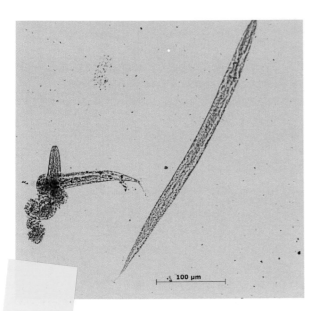

Fig. *Strongyloides* species larval stage.

Life cycle and pathogenesis

The life cycle is direct and infective larvae develop on pasture. Hypobiotic cyathostomin larvae can cause severe disease when they resume development in late winter and spring. Horses become infected by ingestion of infective larvae. In case of non-migratory strongyles, larvae enter the wall of the large bowl; remain in small subserous nodules for 2–4 months before breaking out into the intestinal lumen. Larvae of *S. edentatus* migrate via the portal vessels to the liver forming haemorrhagic tracts. Then, they migrate to the connective tissue under the peritoneum and form haemorrhagic nodules. Three months later, they return to the large bowl wall and again form haemorrhagic nodules, which rupture and release the worms into the lumen. *Strongylus equinus* also migrates via the liver to pancreas and peritoneal cavity but how they return to the intestine is unknown. *Strongylus vulgaris* is the most pathogenic of the large strongyles because of the prolonged (at least 4 months) and extensive migrations through the mesenteric arterial system and its branches before returning to mature in the large bowl. Larvae of *S. vulgaris* migrate via blood and form nodule in the cranial mesenteric artery. They return to intestine and form nodules in intestinal wall that rupture, releasing adults into intestinal lumen. *Strongylus vulgaris* larval migration within the blood vessels gives rise to non-strangulating intestinal infarction. Larval migration in all species induces peritonitis. Adult large strongyles are not blood feeders, but they cause blood loss from mucosal bites. Synchronous mass emergence into lumen of larvae arrested in development within intestinal mucosa causes typhlitis/colitis. High-intensity intestinal infection with large and small strongyle can alter intestinal motility, permeability and absorption.

Pathological findings

In general strongylosis a large numbers of adult worms are seen in caecum and colon; haemorrhagic inflammation of mucosa with multiple small ulcers, large and small nodules. In larval cyathostomiasis, mucosa is grossly inflamed with large numbers of larvae appearing as brown specks. In verminous arteritis the wall of cranial mesenteric artery is greatly thickened, with thrombi and larvae on internal surface. Ischaemia or necrosis of parts of intestinal wall is due to emboli. Migratory larvae are seen in various subserosal sites, and some cause nodules in the liver.

Clinical features

Larval stages rather than adults are responsible for the main pathogenic effects. General strongylosis: ill-thrift, weight loss, poor hair coat, and impaired performance. Verminous arteritis (caused by *S. vulgaris*): recurrent bouts of colic, diarrhoea, pyrexia, inappetence, depression. Larval cyathostomiasis: rapid weight loss, often with sudden onset diarrhoea. Prognosis is good for general strongylosis, fair for larval cyathostomiasis and poor for non-strangulating infarction.

Diagnosis

Judgement is made on the clinical history, presenting signs and laboratory findings [reduced haemoglobin, erythrocyte counts and packed cell volumes; leucocytosis; eosinophilia (with migrating larvae); hyperglobulinaemia; hypoalbuminaemia]; arteritis of cranial mesenteric artery sometimes palpable per rectum; immature worms sometimes in faeces in larval cyathostomiasis. At necropsy, the affected bowl is black, blood engorged and friable. Faecal examination for detection of strongyle eggs. All strongyles produce similar thin-walled eggs, each of which contains 4–16 brownish-coloured cells when deposited.

Treatment

Therapy may be targeted against immature and adult large and small strongyle worms in the intestinal lumen, against migrating *Strongylus* larvae, or against cyathostomin larvae in the intestinal lumen. General strongylosis: ivermectin, moxidectin; benzimidazoles; pyrantel. Migrating strongyles: ivermectin, moxidectin. In verminous arteritis (i.e. migrating *S. vulgaris* and *S. edentatus*) it may take some months after removal of the parasites for the lesion to resolve. Larval cyathostomiasis: fenbendazole, moxidectin.

Control

Twice-weekly removal of faeces from pastures; mixed or alternate grazing; routine dosing to prevent contamination of pasture with eggs. Larval cyathostomiasis: 5-day preventative fenbendazole treatment in early winter.

Public health implications

The large strongyles and cyathostomes nematodes have no zoonotic potential and cannot infect any animals other than equids.

Thelaziasis (eyeworm infection)

Aetiology

Thelaziasis, also known as eyeworm infection, is caused by nematodes of the genus *Thelazia* (Spirurida: Thelaziidae), which are transmitted by flies into the orbital cavities and surrounding tissues of many species of wild and domestic mammals. Out of 16 species of *Thelazia* described so far, *T. rhodesii* infect sheep, *T. skrjabini* infect cattle, and *T. californiensis* and *T. callipaeda* infect carnivores, cats, foxes, rabbits and wolves.

Epidemiology and geographical distribution

The disease is mainly seen in summer and autumn when the vector flies are active. It has been suggested that more than one species of diptera is involved in its transmission, i.e. *Musca domestica* (Muscidae family) and, experimentally, *Amiota variegata* (Drosophilidae family). Thelaziasis is usually more common in ruminants than horses and worms may be more abundant in beef than in dairy cattle.

Life cycle and pathogenesis

Thelazia larvae develop to infective stages in certain musci flies which act as an intermediate host. Adult worms live in the under the nictitating membrane and females release fi larvae (L1). When flies feed on the lachrymal secretio ingest L1 that go through two moults to the third-stage larvae (L3). Seasonality in the reproductive activity o *callipaeda* was demonstrated, probably coinciding with the activities of the vector(s).

Clinical features
Infection is often inapparent, but it may cause lacrimation, mucopurulent discharge, epiphora, conjunctivitis, keratitis and even corneal opacity and ulcers and photophobia. The infected animals can loose their vision.

Pathological findings
Conjunctivitis, keratitis, corneal ulceration, corneal oedema, abscess formation on the eyelids.

Diagnosis
Eyeworm is differentiated from infectious keratitis by observing the adult worm in the conjunctival sac or demonstrating first-stage larvae in eye washings.

Treatment
Treatment of thelaziasis is currently based on the mechanical removal of nematodes directly from the eyes of affected animals (after medication by local anaesthetic, e.g. proparacaine idrocloride hydrochloride), but this is an invasive option. Local instillation of antiparasitic drugs (i.e. organophosphates) and subcutaneous administration of ivermectin have also been described, and more recently ocular instillations of moxidectin have proved to be highly effective in the control of canine thelaziasis.

Control
The face flies and other *Musca* spp. are intermediate host for the parasite, and therefore fly control is essential for reducing infections.

Public health implications
Some *Thelazia* spp. (*T. californiensis* and *T. callipaeda*) cause human thelaziasis resulting in conjunctivitis, pain and excessive lacrimation. Humans are believed to be an accidental host, not the definitive host.

Trichinellosis (trichinosis)

Aetiology
Trichinellosis or trichinosis is associated with *Trichinclla spiralis*, tiny male and female adult worms (1.4–1.6 mm long). Infection of swine by this nematode parasite is of major economic importance to the swine industry and poses a serious health hazard to human beings.

Epidemiology and geographical distribution
Cosmopolitan distribution, but no evidence for its existence in the UK. Most often found on smaller farms with free ranging pigs. Rats can serve as a reservoir with pigs becoming infected by eating rats.

Life cycle and pathogenesis
The infective stage is L1 larva encysted in muscle; meat eaters become infected when they ingest meat with the encysted larvae; the larvae are digested out of the meat and undergo four moults in the small intestine to become adults; newborn (LI) larvae penetrate the intestine and spread throughout the body via the circulation and lymphatics; newborn larvae invade striated muscle; a nurse cell forms around the larva. Active muscles, such as tongue, masseter, diaphragm, and intercostal, laryngeal and extraocular muscles, are preferentially affected. The majority of the pathology is caused by the L1 when they penetrate muscle cells.

Pathological findings
Focal inflammation consisting of eosinophils, neutrophils, and lymphocytes occurs associated with invasion of the muscle by *Trichinella* larvae. After cyst formation, however, inflammation is minimal to absent. Over time encysted larvae can die and nurse cell becomes calcified.

Clinical features
No overt clinical disease is associated with *Trichinella* infection in swine. Pigs may show dyspnoea, periorbital oedema, slower growth and respiratory problems.

Diagnosis
Direct meat inspection for the detection of the characteristic encysted *Trichinella* larvae within muscle fibres (Fig. 4.11). Animals can be tested for the presence of anti-*Trichinella* antibodies in the serum or in the meat juice. Molecular diagnosis is used to genotype the recovered larvae to the species level.

Treatment
Once encysted in the muscle, *Trichinella* larvae are protected from host immune response and to anthelmintics therapy.

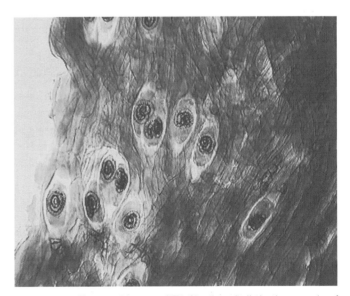

Figure 4.11 Encysted larvae of *Trichinella spiralis* in the muscle of a pig.

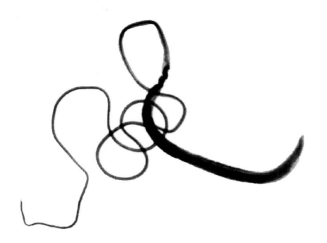

Figure 4.12 The whipworm, *Trichuris suis*. (Image kindly provided by Jerzy Behnke, University of Nottingham.)

Control

Control measures should target this parasitic infection in pigs and wildlife. Good sanitation with frequent manure removal along with separation of pigs from their faeces will decrease parasite burdens.

Public health implications

Humans can substitute as definitive host along with many other vertebrates. Encysted larval stage produces a characteristic facial swelling and oedema in affected people.

Trichuriasis (whipworm infection)

Aetiology

Whipworms are parasites of the caecum, and in high-intensity infections the colon, of many mammalian species. Adult worms (30–45 mm in length) are whip-like with thin anterior ends that wind through the mucosa (Fig. 4.12). Three species of whipworms are found in ruminants: *Trichuris ovis*, *T. discolor*, and *T. globulosa*, while *T. suis* occurs in pigs and *T. vulpis* in dogs. There is no evidence that *T. vulpis* is capable of infecting cats, which are uncommonly infected with *T. campanula*.

Epidemiology and geographical distribution

Whipworms are found worldwide and may be of considerable clinical significance disease. This occurs in sheep most commonly after hot, dry weather, which effectively cleanses the pasture of other nematode larvae but, the resistant *Trichuris* spp. eggs survive and are ingested when the sheep eat close to the ground to obtain grain given as drought feed.

Life cycle and pathogenesis

The life cycle is direct. Adult male and females live in colon; eggs are passed in the faeces. The eggs are very resistant to external environmental conditions and can survive for up to 6 years in environment, and for at least 2 years on pasture. Eggs embryonate in the environment in about 3 weeks. An infective larva develops inside the egg. In temperate climates, embryonation of *T. suis*

eggs may take more than 1 year. Infective stage is L1 larva within the egg which is ingested by the animal. Larvae are digested out of egg and penetrate the crypts of Lieberkuhn in colon and become intracellular for several days. Then, larvae develop from L1 to L2 to L3 to adults as they move from the base of the crypt to the superficial mucosa. Adult worms maintain their place in the colon by having their anterior end buried in the superficial mucosa.

Pathological findings

The faeces may contain blood-stained mucus and strips of necrotic mucosa. The nematodes lie with their thin anterior end superficially embedded in the wall of the caecum. The activities of the worms produce little tissue reaction *per se* but enable microorganisms in the gut microflora to become invasive. In high-intensity infections, a severe colitis and typhlitis occur, resulting in pseudonecrotic membranes and sloughing of colonic mucosa and leading to the death of young pigs.

Clinical features

Whipworms in farm livestock are usually considered to be relatively harmless. Light infections result in milder signs including diarrhoea, weight loss and a predisposition to bacterial infections of the colon including *Salmonella* and *Campylobacter*. High-intensity of infections can produce diarrhoea and dysentery and high mortality rate in recently weaned pigs. Severely affected animals are anorexic and rapidly lose weight. *Trichuris suis* is part of the complex of organisms that cause mucohaemorrhagic diarrhoea in young pigs.

Diagnosis

Diagnosis depends on detection in the faeces of the light brown oval eggs, which have a transparent plug at each end (Fig. 4.13). At necropsy, the adult worms which are 2–5 cm long are easily recognized by their whip-like appearance – the anterior two-thirds is much thinner than the handle-like posterior end.

Treatment

Most broad-spectrum anthelmintic compounds can be used, but not all are active against immature forms and repeat dosing may be necessary.

Control

Sanitation and proper hygienic measures.

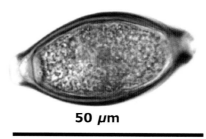

50 μm

Figure 4.13 Egg of *Trichuris* spp.

Public health implications

Trichuris trichura infects humans.

Verminous pneumonia (lung worm infection)

Overview

Lungworms are a group of parasitic nematodes that colonize the lower respiratory tract of livestock. They cause high morbidity, high mortality, and high economic costs throughout the world especially in temperate regions. The disease caused by lungworms has many local names, including verminous bronchitis, verminous pneumonia, parasitic bronchitis, hoose, fog fever, husk. Several factors known to affect the development and clinical manifestations of 'husk' include animal age, previous immunization or infection, presence of passively acquired antibodies, climatic condition, and anthelmintic treatment. Additional factors which may also play a role in clinical manifestations include the rate of intake of infectious larvae at exposure, host genetic and acquired factors, and the genotype and virulence of the worm.

It is evident that the circulation of lungworm infections throughout the world continues due to the lack of awareness, and inadequacy in the means of proper treatment and control. In the UK, an increase in husk cases has been reported especially in areas where vaccine use is low.

Clinically, the full spectrum of disease due to lungworm infection is now understood. Signs of lungworm infection range from moderate coughing with slightly increased respiratory rates to severe persistent coughing and respiratory distress and even failure. Moderate lungworm infections are common, elicit partial immunity, and do respond quickly to treatment. Severe lungworm infections can cause significant distress to the animal, reduced weight gains, reduced milk yields, unthriftiness, and death. Patent subclinical infections can also occur. Anthelmintics are commonly used as a prophylactic against lungworms and other nematode infections.

The term lungworm is generally used for a variety of different groups of nematodes, some of which use the lower air passages and the lung parenchyma as the final habitat. Others nematode species, such as ascarid larvae just migrate through the animals' lungs or respiratory tracts, causing various degrees of pathological damage according to the nature and intensity of the host–parasite interactions.

The major lungworms of livestock belong to one of two superfamilies, Trichostrongyloidea or Metastrongyloidea. However, not all the species in these superfamilies are lungworms. The lungworms in the superfamily Trichostrongyloidea include several species, which infect hoofed animals, including most common domestic species. Major features of worms belong to Trichostrongyloidea are their small size, hair-like shape, small mouth, small bursa in males and having direct life cycles. Common species include *Dictyocaulus viviparus* in cattle and deer, *D. arnfieldi* in donkeys and horses, *D. filaria* in sheep and goats. The lungworms in the superfamily Metastrongyloidea include species that infect a wider range of mammals. These species have indirect life cycles that involve intermediate hosts. Common species include

Protostrongylus rufescens in sheep and goats, *Muellerius capillaris* in sheep and goats, *Metastrongylus apri* in pigs.

Diseases caused by the three *Dictyocaulus* spp. are of most economic importance. The cattle lungworm *D. viviparus* is common in northwest Europe and is the cause of severe outbreaks of 'husk' or 'hoose' in young (and yearlings) grazing cattle. The lungworm of goats and sheep, *D. filaria*, is comparatively less pathogenic but does cause losses, especially in Mediterranean countries, although it is also recognized as a pathogen in Australia, North America, and Europe. *Dictyocaulus arnfieldi* can cause severe coughing in horses and, because patency is unusual in horses (but not in donkeys), differential diagnosis with disease due to other respiratory diseases can be difficult. *Muellerius capillaris* is prevalent worldwide and, while usually non-pathogenic in sheep, can cause severe signs in goats.

Bovine lungworms

Aetiology

Dictyocaulus viviparus is the only lungworm of cattle. Adults are slender, white nematodes; males are 3–8 cm long, and females are 3–10 cm long. They live in the lumen of bronchioles.

Epidemiology and geographical distribution

Distribution – seen mainly in temperate areas such as north-eastern USA and Europe. It requires moist, cool environment. Major outbreaks are seen from July to September, when non-immune calves have been on pasture 2–5 months and the parasites have had time to reproduce. *Pilobolus* fungi – facilitate the spread of lungworm larvae in a pasture. Larvae located on sporangiophore are shot several feet when sporangiophore explodes ejecting spores. Older animals are usually resistant, but they can act as carriers and spread the infection without showing any signs of the disease. Under favourable conditions *D. viviparus* larvae can over-winter on pasture. Bovine husk is a sporadic and unpredictable disease. This is because immunity develops more quickly than is the case with many other nematode infections.

Life cycle and pathogenesis

It has a direct life cycle, no intermediate host (Fig. 4.14). Infective stage is L3 larvae ingested with contaminated grass. The L3 larvae penetrate the gut, moult to L4 stage and enter lymphatics, migrate to lungs via circulation. L4 larvae moult to L5 (early adult stage) in the alveoli (may arrest at this stage). L5s migrate up through the bronchial tree as they mature. Adults are found in the bronchi and bronchioles. At ~21 days eggs containing L1 are shed by fertilized females, hatch almost immediately into L1s in the lungs, which pass up the bronchial tree, coughed up, swallowed and pass in faeces. On pasture, the L1 larvae moult into the third-stage infective form within less than a week (~5 days) in optimum environmental conditions.

Clinical features

Clinical signs range from bronchitis to severe consolidating pneumonia as eggs are inhaled to all areas of the lungs and inflammation commences. Acute pulmonary emphysema that is

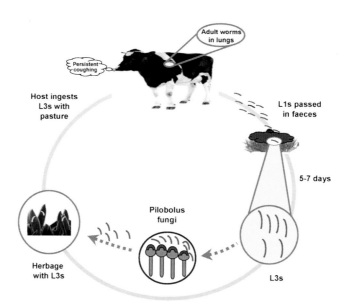

Figure 4.14 Life cycle of bovine lungworm, *Dictyocaulus viviparus*. First-stage larvae (L1), Third-stage larvae (L3).

associated with high-intensity infections of adult cattle previously exposed to this parasite in endemic areas.

Small ruminants lungworms
Lung worms in small ruminants (sheep and goat) are caused by three nematode species, namely *Dictyocaulus filariae*, *Protostrongylus rufescens* and *Muellerius capillaris*.

Dictyocaulus filariae
The most pathogenic species. It is similar to *D. viviparus* and is found in bronchi and bronchioles. It has a direct life cycle. Young animals are more susceptible. Affected animals exhibit respiratory signs: cough, dyspnoea, lethargy, weight loss, and catarrhal bronchitis. Goats differ from sheep by having diffuse interstitial rather than focal lesions.

Protostrongylus rufescens (red lungworms)
Long slender brown worms with moderate pathogenicity. Adult worms are found in the terminal bronchioles. It has an indirect life cycle, requires a snail or slug intermediate host. No age-related immunity; adults continue to be infected throughout life. Affected hosts show weight loss, loss of condition, respiratory signs and diarrhoea. Worms are found in granulomatous foci in the parenchyma and terminal bronchioles.

Muellerius capillaris (hair lungworms)
The most common but least pathogenic species. Small sized adults. Adult worms are found in the parenchyma of the lungs. It has an indirect life cycle, requires a snail or slug intermediate host.

Goats are most susceptible and can die from pneumonia. Worms are found in granulomatous foci in the parenchyma.

Equine lungworms
Lungworm infection of horses is associated with *Dictyocaulus arnfieldi*. The disease is usually recognized in late summer/autumn. It has a direct life cycle, no intermediate host. Horses become infected by ingesting larvae, which migrate to the lungs. In most horses, larval development becomes arrested and egg-laying adults do not arise. Adult parasites cause obstructive bronchitis, oedema and atelectasis. The microscopic lesion is eosinophilic bronchitis. Horses will have chronic cough (often paroxysmal in nature) which is non-responsive to antibiotics. Signs may be indistinguishable from COPD. Infection is often seen in horse grazing pasture with donkeys. Donkeys are natural hosts and may not show clinical signs. In these cases, horses may have low-level infections with no eggs seen in the faeces while donkeys will have patent infections (larvated eggs in faeces). Diagnosis suspected from historical information of grazing pastures contaminated by donkeys, clinical signs, and confirmed by presence of large numbers eosinophils and larvae in bronchoalveolar aspirate and detection of larvae in faeces using Baermann technique. However, faecal examination is usually negative since most infections are non-patent. Endoscopy may reveal larvae in the trachea or mainstem bronchi. The disease should be differentiated from coughing caused by *Parascaris equorum* larval migration.

Swine lungworms
Lungworm infection of pigs is associated with *Metastrongylus apri* and *M. edentatus*. Adults are found in bronchi and bronchioles.

The parasite has an indirect life cycle, requires earthworms as an intermediate host. Thus, this parasite occurs only where pigs have access to earthworm in an outside environment such as in feral swine and pastured swine. Young animals are more susceptible, adults appear to be immune. Clinical signs include bronchitis, pneumonia, persistent cough that may become paroxysmal, dyspnoea, lethargy and weight loss.

Diagnosis of lungworm infection

Ante-mortem diagnosis

- Diagnosis of lungworm infection in live animals is based on clinical signs, grazing history and knowledge of the patterns of the parasite epidemiology.
- Infection can be confirmed by the demonstration of L1 larvae in faeces and/or adult nematodes at necropsy of animals in the same herd or flock.
- L1 larvae can be recovered using faecal flotation and Baermann technique.
- Recovered larvae may be identified to species by their characteristic morphology as follows:
  - first-stage *D. viviparus* larva measures 310–390 μm by 19–25 μm and has a stout body and a conical tail
  - first-stage *D. filaria* larva measures 450–500 μm by 25 μm and has a blunt tail and a small knob at its anterior end
  - first-stage *M. capillaris* larva measures 300–320 μm by 14–15 μm and has a twice bent tail with a small dorsal spine at its base.
- Larvae are not shed in the faeces of animals in the prepatent or postpatent phases and usually not in the reinfection phenomenon. In these cases infection may be confirmed by the detection of immature stages in tracheal washes.
- Tracheal washes may also provide cytological evidence of eosinophilic inflammation consistent with parasitic bronchitis or pneumonia.
- Bronchoscopy and radiography may be also helpful.
- Different serological tests for *D. viviparus* infection have been described.
- Diagnosis can be made after failure of antibiotic therapy to ameliorate the condition especially in horses.

Table 4.6 Treatment options for lungworm infections by animal species

Parasite	Animal species	Treatment
Dictyocaulus viviparus, *D. filaria*	Cattle Sheep, goat	Ivermectin* Doramectin* Moxidectin* Eprinomectin* Fenbendazole† Albendazole† Levamisole
Dictyocaulus arnfieldi	Horse, donkey	Ivermectin Moxidectin
Metastrongylus apri	Pigs	Ivermectin Fenbendazole

*Macrocyclic lactones.
†Benzimidazoles.

Post-mortem diagnosis

- Post-mortem diagnosis can be made by the identification of lungworms and characteristic lung pathology at necropsy.
- Adult *D. viviparus*, found in the bronchi and trachea, are long, thin white worms with small buccal cavities. Males are 17–50 mm in length and females are 23–80 mm.
- Adult *D. filaria* can also be recovered from the bronchi and trachea at necropsy. Adult males are 25–80 mm long and have a short bursa, and adult females are 43–112 mm long with a conical, tapered tail.
- Adult *M. capillaris* are found in the lung parenchyma. Males measure 11–14 mm by 32–35 μm and have a posterior end coiled in 11–13 spirals. Adult females are 19–23 mm by 40–50 μm.

Treatment

Animals with slight cough and tachypnoea respond well to treatment, whereas those with dyspnoea, fever, anorexia, depression, and unthriftiness have a poor prognosis (either die or develop chronic form). Anthelmintic resistance is not yet considered to be a widespread problem of lungworms. The macrocyclic lactones and benzimidazoles are commonly used (Table 4.6) and are effective against larval and adult stages of the worm. However, decreased efficacy of using the macrocyclic lactone was recently observed in a study from Brazil. Levamisole is used in ruminants, but treatment may need to be repeated 2 weeks later as it is less effective against larvae during the early stages. Animals at pasture should be moved inside for treatment, and supportive therapy may be needed for complications that may occur. In severe cases non-steroidal anti-inflammatory drugs may also be helpful.

Control

Deworming

Lungworm infections in herds or flocks are controlled primarily by anthelmintics. Anthelmintic prophylaxis has become feasible with the advent of broad-spectrum, long-acting anthelmintics (macrocyclic lactones) and sustained-release intraruminal boluses containing oxfendazole or fenbendazole. Several strategic deworming programmes have been developed in Europe, which can effectively suppress developing established lungworm infection throughout the grazing season.

Vaccination

It is better to prevent than to treat established lungworm infection. Vaccination against husk is a vital component in the lungworm control strategy. The only lungworm vaccine available on the market in Europe is made up of irradiated infective larvae. The vaccine is effective and primes immune response against any exposure to infection. Two doses are given 4 weeks apart at least 2 weeks before animals can be turned out to allow the development of a protective level of immunity. If used properly, vaccination can prevent clinical disease, but some vaccinated animals may become mildly infected to the extent that larvae are excreted to perpetuate further infection.

Table 4.7 Major metastrongyloid nematode species associated with infections of the respiratory tract of dogs and cats

Parasite species	Host	Key features
Aelurostrongylus abstrusus	Cats	**Location:** alveolar ducts and terminal bronchioles
		Signs: nodule formation in lung, coughing, sneezing, dyspnoea, pneumonia
		Life cycle: Indirect with molluscs as intermediate host. Paratenic host occurs
		Diagnosis: (i) radiograph may show mixed bronchial, alveolar and interstitial patterns; (ii) detection of larvae in faeces or in tracheal wash samples; (iii) tracheal wash cytology may show eosinophils
		Treatment: benzimidazoles, levamisole, ivermectin
Crenosoma vulpis	Dogs	**Location:** trachea, bronchi and bronchioles
		Signs: coughing, sneezing, inappetence
		Life cycle: Indirect with molluscs as intermediate host. Paratenic host occurs
		Diagnosis: similar to *Aelurostrongylus abstrusus*
		Treatment: similar to *Aelurostrongylus abstrusus*
Filaroides (Andersonstrongylus) milksi and F. hirthi	Dogs	**Location:** terminal airways, bronchioles and alveoli
		Signs: usually asymptomatic, although coughing, dyspnoea may occur and miliary nodules may be seen at necropsy
		Life cycle: Direct and infection via ingestion of L1
		Diagnosis: (i) radiograph may show a diffuse interstitial or focal nodular pattern; (ii) detection of larvae or larvated eggs in faeces or in airway cytology specimens
		Treatment: benzimidazoles, ivermectin
Oslerus (Filaroides) osleri	Dogs	**Location:** within nodules on mucosa of distal trachea and tracheal bifurcation
		Signs: tracheobronchitis and nodule formation, exercise intolerance dyspnoea, or death
		Life cycle: Direct and infection via ingestion of L1
		Diagnosis: (i) bronchoscopy may show granulomatous nodules, containing worms in the trachea; (ii) detection of larvae in faeces or larvae and eggs in sputum. Be aware of the intermittent pattern of larval shedding; (iii) transtracheal wash for eosinophils
		Treatment: benzimidazoles, ivermectin or levamisole. Surgery is indicated to remove large nodules in case of severe airway obstruction

Management strategies

Effective control of husk should in addition to parasite management (e.g. chemotherapy and vaccination), provide other supplementary approaches. Sanitation and management practices are helpful for lungworm infection, because pasture herbage is the most common vehicle for transmission of infection. Some suggested measures include:

- Prevent overcrowding and avoid continuous use of the same pasture, particularly for young stock.
- Pastures that are known to be contaminated should not be restocked for at least 6 months.
- Avoid mixing sheep and goats on the same pasture.
- Horses should not be allowed to associate directly or otherwise with donkeys or mules, especially on pastures.
- Pigs should be housed indoors especially during high-risk seasons.
- Pre-turnout removal of adult worms and arrested larval stages from potential carrier yearlings or adult animals is necessary.
- Eliminate intermediate hosts to discontinue the life cycle, e.g. preventing access to infected earth worms in pigs.
- If animals are at grass, then it is necessary to treat the herd or flock and move onto a clean pasture that has not had the same animal species on before.

Public health implications

Lungworms described above are strict animal parasites and don't infect humans. However, there have been rare reports of human infections with the carnivore lung worm *Eucoleus aerophilus* in Morocco and Russia. The pig lungworm *Metastrongylus elongatus* has been reported in human three times; two of these involved the respiratory tract.

Lungworms of dogs and cats

Most of the bronchopulmonary parasites of dogs and cats are metastrongyloid nematodes, namely, *Oslerus (Filaroides) osleri*, *Filaroides hirthi*, *Andersonstrongylus (Filaroides) milksi*, *Crenosoma vulpis*, *Aelurostrongylus abstrusus* (Table 4.7). These nematodes can affect the lower and/or the upper part of respiratory tract of dogs and cats. Lungworm infections are relatively uncommon in domestic dogs and cats. Young animals are more susceptible.

Capillaria aerophila (Eucoleus aerophilus) is non-metastrongyloid nematode that affects respiratory tract of dogs and cats (see section on Capillariasis). *Angiostrongylus vasorum* and *D. immitis* reside within the pulmonary arteries and right atrium, respectively. They cause respiratory manifestations [see sections on Angiostrongylosis and Dirofilariasis (heartworm disease)]. Other nematodes can induce respiratory manifestations during the migratory phase of their life cycle, e.g. *T. canis, A. caninum,*

S. stercoralis. Migrating larvae induce some minor signs. During this phase no eggs are present in the faeces, but eosinophilia may be evident.

Acknowledgements

I would like to thank Ellis C. Greiner, Professor Emeritus at the College of Veterinary Medicine, University of Florida, Gainesville, Florida, USA, and Dr David J. Bartley from Moredun Research Institute, Scotland for their helpful advice and critical reading.

Further reading

Ashford, R.W. and Crewe, W. (2003). The Parasites of Homo Sapiens. An annotated checklist of the protozoa, helminths and arthropods for which we are home, 2nd Edn. London: Taylor & Francis.

Atkins, C.E., Atwell, R.A., Dillon, R., Genchi, C., Hayasaki, M., Holmes, R.A., Knight, D.H., Lukof, D.K., McCall, J.W. and Slocombe, J.O.D. (1996). Guidelines for the diagnosis, treatment and prevention of heartworm (*Dirofilaria immitis*) infection in cats. American Heartworm Society Bulletin 23, 1–7.

Bowman, D.D. and Atkins, C.E. (2009). Heartworm Biology, Treatment, and Control. Vet. Clin. North Am. Small Anim. Pract. 39, 1127–1158.

Brown, W., Paul, A., Venco, L., McCall, J.W. and Brunt, J. (1999). Roundtable discussion feline heartworm disease part 1. Feline Pract. 27, 6–9.

Chapman, P.S., Boag, A.K., Guitian, J. and Boswood, A. (2004). *Angiostrongylus vasorum* infection in 23 dogs (1999–2002). J. Small Anim. Pract. 45, 435–440.

Cury, M.C. and Lima, W.S. (1996). Aspectos clínicos de cães infectados experimentalmente com *Angiostrongylus vasorum* (Baillet, 1866) Kamensky, 1905. Arq. Bras. Med. Vet. Zootecnol. 48, 27–34.

Drudge, J.H. (1979). Clinical aspects of *Strongylus vulgaris* infection in the horse. Emphasis on diagnosis, chemotherapy, and prophylaxis. Vet. Clin. North Am. Large Anim. Pract. 1, 251–265.

Drudge, J.H. and Lyons, E.T. (1986). Large strongyles. Recent advances. Vet. Clin. North Am. Equine Pract. 2, 263–280.

Elsheikha, H.M. (2009). Growing economic backlash demands Lungworm awareness. Vet. Times 39, 12–14.

Garosi, L.S., Platt, S.R., McConnel, J.F., Wray, J.D. and Smith, K.C. (2005). Intracranial haemorrhage associated with *Angiostrongylus vasorum* infection in three dogs. J. Small Anim. Pract. 46, 93–99.

Gibbs, H.C. (1986). Hypobiosis and the periparturient rise in sheep. Vet. Clin. North Am. Food Anim. Pract. 2, 345–353.

Jacobs, D.E. (1986). Colour Atlas of equine Parasites. Bailliere, London.

Kaplan, R.M. (2002). Anthelmintic resistance in nematodes of horses. Vet. Res. 33, 491–507.

Koch, J. and Willesen, J.L. (2009). Canine pulmonary angiostrongylosis: An update. Vet. J. 179, 348–359.

Kramer, L., Grandi, G., Leoni, M., Passeri, B., McCall, J., Genchi, C., Mortarino, M. and Bazzocchi, C. (2008). *Wolbachia* and its influence on the pathology and immunology of *Dirofilaria immitis* infection. Vet. Parasitol. 158, 191–195.

Litster, A.L. and Atwell, R.B. (2008). Feline heartworm disease: a clinical review. J. Feline Med. Surg. 10, 137–144.

Maass, D.R., Harrison, G.B., Grant, W.N. and Shoemaker, C.B. (2007). Three surface antigens dominate the mucosal antibody response to gastrointestinal L3 stage strongylid nematodes in field immune sheep. Int. J. Parasitol. 37, 953–962.

Manfredi, M.T. (2006). Biology of gastrointestinal nematodes of ruminants. Parassitologia. 48, 397–401.

Manning, S.P. (2007). Ocular examination in the diagnosis of angiostrongylosis in dogs. Vet. Rec. 160, 625–627.

McKeand, J.B. (2000). Vaccine development and diagnostics of *Dictyocaulus viviparus*. Parasitology. 120, S17–23.

Morgan, E.R., Shaw, S.E., Brennan, S.F., De Wall, T.D., Jones, B.R. and Mulcahy, G. (2005). *Angiostrongylus vasorum*: a real heartbreaker. *Trends Parasitol.* 21, 49–51.

Morgan, E.R., Tomlinson, A., Hunter, S., Nichols, T., Roberts, E., Fox, M.T. and Taylor, M.A. (2008). *Angiostrongylus vasorum* and *Eucoleus aerophilus* in foxes (*Vulpes vulpes*) in Great Britain. Vet. Parasitol. 154, 48–57.

Oliveira-Júnior, S.D., Barçante, J.M., Barçante, T.A., Ribeiro, V.M. and Lima, W.S. (2004). Ectopic location of adult worms and first-stage larvae of *Angiostrongylus vasorum* in an infected dog. Vet. Parasitol. 121, 293–296.

Panuska, C. (2006). Lungworms of Ruminants. Vet. Clin. North Am. Food Anim. Pract. 22, 583–593.

Parsons, J.C. (1987). Ascarid infections of cats and dogs. Vet. Clin. North Am. Small Anim. Pract. 17, 1307–1339.

Ploeger, H.W. (2002). *Dictyocaulus viviparus*: re-emerging or never been away? Trends Parasitol. 18, 329–332.

Pozio, E. and Nöckler, K. (2009). Epidemiology, diagnosis, treatment, and control of trichinellosis. Clin. Microbiol. Rev. 22, 127–145.

Ribicich, M., Gamble, H.R., Rosa, A., Sommerfelt, I., Marquez, A., Mira, G., Cardillo, N., Cattaneo, M.L., Falzoni, E. and Franco, A. (2007). Clinical, haematological, biochemical and economic impacts of *Trichinella spiralis* infection in pigs. Vet. Parasitol. 147, 265–270.

Ryan, W. and Newcomb, K. (1995). Prevalence of feline heartworm disease – a global review, Proceedings of the Heartworm Symposium '95, Auburn, Alabama, American Heartworm Society, Batavia, Illinois.

Scott, I., Khalaf, S., Simcock, D.C., Knight, C.G., Reynolds, G.W., Pomroy, W.E. and Simpson, H.V. (2000). A sequential study of the pathology associated with the infection of sheep with adult and larval *Ostertagia circumcincta*. Vet. Parasitol. 89, 79–94.

Simcock, D.C., Scott, I., Przemeck, S.M. and Simpson, H.V. (2006). Abomasal contents of parasitised sheep contain an inhibitor of gastrin secretion *in vitro*. Res. Vet. Sci. 81, 225–230.

Simón, F., López-Belmonte, J., Marcos-Atxutegi, C., Morchón, R. and Martín-Pacho, J. R. (2005). What is happening outside North America regarding human dirofilariasis? Vet. Parasitol. 133, 181–189.

Simpson, H.V. (2000). Pathophysiology of abomasal parasitism: is the host or parasite responsible? Vet. J. 160, 177–191.

Smith, H.L. and Rajan, T.V. (2000). Tetracycline inhibits development of the infective-stage larvae of filarial nematodes *in vitro*. Exp. Parasitol. 95, 265–270.

Stromberg, B.E. and Gasbarre, L.C. (2006). Gastrointestinal Nematode Control Programs with an Emphasis on Cattle. Vet. Clin. North Am. Food Anim. Pract. 22, 543–565.

Tomlinson, A.J., Taylor, M. and Roberts, E. (2006). *Angiostrongylus vasorum* in canids. Vet. Rec. 159, 60.

Winter, M.D. (2002). *Nematodirus battus* 50 years on-A realistic vaccine candidate? Trends. Parasitol. 18, 298–301.

van Wyk, J.A. and Bath, G.F. (2002). The FAMACHA system for managing haemonchosis in sheep and goats by clinically identifying individual animals for treatment. Vet. Res. 33, 509–529.

Zajac, A.M. (2006). Gastrointestinal nematodes of small ruminants: life cycle, anthelmintics, and diagnosis. Vet. Clin. North Am. Food Anim. Pract. 22, 529–541.

Major Cestode Infections

5

Hany M. Elsheikha

Tapeworm infection: an overview

Cestoda is a class of parasitic flatworms (Platyhelminthes), commonly called tapeworms or cestodes. All tapeworms use vertebrates as a definitive host, and vertebrates or invertebrates (arthropods, crustaceans) as an intermediate host, depending on the species. The definitive host harbours the adult, sexual, or mature stages of parasite. Larval 'metacestode' development occurs in the intermediate host (IH), which will be eaten by definitive host. In the latter, larval stages attach to the gut mucosa and mature to adult tapeworms via a process called 'strobilation'. Most tapeworms are found in the small intestine of their host as adults or, as with *Thysanosoma* spp., have access to the intestine.

Strobilation

The cestode body is composed of three distinct regions, namely scolex, neck and strobila. The tapeworm's scolex ('head') is the hold fasting organ that anchors the worm to the intestinal wall of the definitive host. The scolex attaches to the neck, or proliferative region. From the neck, grows many proglottid segments which contain the reproductive organs of the worm. Strobilation (Fig. 5.1) is asexual process of forming segments in a tapeworm in which new proglottids are continuously formed in the neck just below the scolex (A). Along the length of the worm the proglottids increase in size and maturity, developing from premature (B) to mature carrying fully functional and active sexual organs (C), to the 'gravid' stage (D) in which essentially the entire proglottid is occupied with the uterus fully packed with eggs. The enlargement of segments as they mature results in the characteristic widening of the tapeworm body towards its distal end. Gravid proglottids break off from the end of the tapeworm and pass in the faeces. Eggs are released as the proglottids disintegrate, either within the animal body or on pasture in the faeces. In some species of tapeworms, intact proglottids are found in faeces. Neither the eggs nor the proglottids are infective for the host. To become infective metacestodes, eggs must first be ingested by IH and develop to the infective stage inside the IH *Hymenolepis nana* that infects mice, gerbils, hamsters, and humans (i.e. zoonotic) is an exception. Infection occurs via ingestion of eggs. This tapeworm can carry out both its adult stage and immature stage in the same host allowing infections to be build up even in the absence of an IH. The equivalent rat cestode, *Hymenolepis diminuta*, is not zoonotic; it needs an insect IH to complete its life cycle and so humans can only become infected by ingesting infected insects.

Metacestodes

The embryo that develops within the tapeworm egg is known as oncosphere or hexacanth (i.e. having three pairs of hooks). When ingested by the IH, it hatches and develops into an immature stage called a metacestode. Metacestodes vary greatly in structure among tapeworm species and depending on the type of the IH (Fig. 5.2). If the intermediate host is an invertebrate animal, embryos will migrate to the haemocoel and form cysticercoid metacestode inside the invertebrate body. Whereas if the IH is a vertebrate animal, the embryo will migrate into different tissues and develop to a generally fluid-filled cyst, the inner lining of which grows one or more immature scolices (heads) depending on the species of tapeworm. Infection of the definitive host occurs via ingestion of an IH containing a metacestode. Digestion releases the scolices, which mature in definitive host and become adult tapeworms.

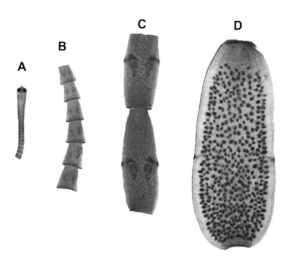

Figure 5.1 Stages of the cestode development.

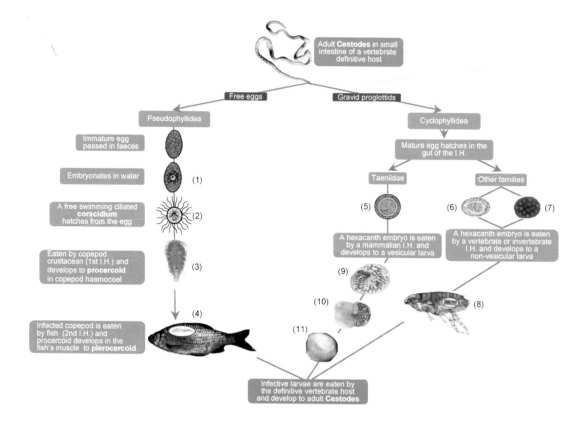

Figure 5.2 A summary of the general life cycles of parasitic tapeworms, Pseudophylidea and Cyclophyllidea. (1) Pseudophylidean egg; (2) free-living coracidium; (3) procercoid larva; (4) plerocercoid larva; (5) egg of family Taeniidae; (6, 7) eggs of other cyclophyllidean families; (8) cysticercoid larva; (9) cysticercus cyst; (10) coenurus cyst; and (11) hydatid cyst. IH, intermediate host.

Challenges with tapeworm infections

First, it is not known how tapeworm infection cycle through the year. Most nematode and trematode parasites reproduce on a seasonal basis, hence eggs are passed at a specific time of year when there is enough warmth for them to hatch, and forage plants for the hatching larvae to crawl onto, and so grazing animals can ingest them. It is unknown if this seasonal pattern occurs with cestodes. Second, current diagnostic test relies on seeing eggs in manure. If there is a period when tapeworms stop producing eggs, diagnostic test is useless during that time. In this respect, a DNA-based test is effective, since DNA is always leeching out of worms, whether they are juveniles or reproducing adults. Third, a tapeworm cannot be transmitted directly from one animal to another; it must undergo development in another host, so-called intermediate host.

Taxonomy of important tapeworms

The class Cestoda is divided based on the number of larval hooks into two subclasses: (1) subclass Cestodaria in which the larval stages have 10 hooks and are thus described as decacanth, and (2) subclass Eucestoda, whose larvae have six hooks (hexacanth). Eucestoda includes species that have a public health importance and/or clinical relevance in veterinary medicine. These species are found in two orders, Pseudophyllidea and Cyclophyllidea, recognized by their different life cycles and morphological attributes.

General taxonomy of cestodes considered in this chapter is given to the genus level (Fig. 5.3).

Adult tapeworm infection

Equine cestodes

Aetiology

Equines can be host to three tapeworm species of the anoplocephalid family, namely *Anoplocephala perfoliata*, *Anoplocephala magna*, *Paranoplocephala* (*Anoplocephaloides*) *mammillana*. All the three species are similar in that the scolex is devoid of rostellum, hooks, or hooklets, and suckers are unarmed. In addition, *A. perfoliata* has unique lappets/flaps on the scolex just below each sucker (Fig. 5.4). Anoplocephalid are flat, broad, triangular and relatively short compared with tapeworms found in other animal species. They live at a junction between the small and large intestine (i.e. the ileocaecal junction).

Epidemiology and geographical distribution

Anoplocephala perfoliata is the most prevalent and most frequently associated with clinical disease and has a worldwide distribution. Grazing horses are at risk of infection, due to the existence of oribatid mites, the intermediate host that passes tapeworms to horses.

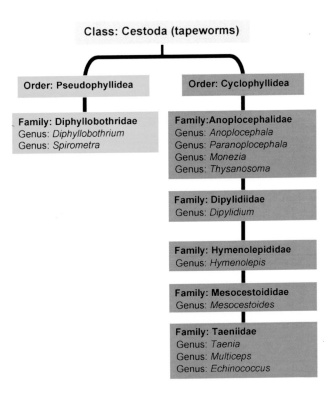

Class: Cestoda (tapeworms)

Order: Pseudophyllidea

Family: Diphyllobothridae
Genus: *Diphyllobothrium*
Genus: *Spirometra*

Order: Cyclophyllidea

Family: Anoplocephalidae
Genus: *Anoplocephala*
Genus: *Paranoplocephala*
Genus: *Monezia*
Genus: *Thysanosoma*

Family: Dipylidiidae
Genus: *Dipylidium*

Family: Hymenolepididae
Genus: *Hymenolepis*

Family: Mesocestoididae
Genus: *Mesocestoides*

Family: Taeniidae
Genus: *Taenia*
Genus: *Multiceps*
Genus: *Echinococcus*

Figure 5.3 General taxonomy of cetsodes of veterinary medical importance.

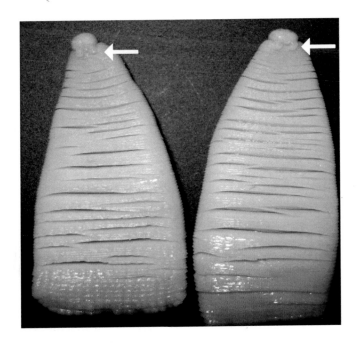

Figure 5.4 Adult *Anoplocephala perfoliata* tapeworm of horses. Lappets (arrows) are evident just below each sucker. (Image reproduced by kind permission, John W. McGarry, University of Liverpool.)

Life cycle and pathogenesis

The life cycles of all equine tapeworms are similar in that the infective eggs (containing hexacanth larvae with six hooks), are ingested by free-living oribatid mite on pastures. In the mite, a small larval form, the tadpole-like cysticercoid, develops to the infective stage within 2–4 months. Transmission occurs by ingestion of infected pasture mites. Once ingested by the horse, the larval stage is released from the mite and develops into an adult tapeworm in 6–10 weeks. The mechanical damage caused by the suckers on the scolex of the tapeworms at the site of attachment and parasite antigens play a role in the pathogenic process. Lesions caused by the inflammatory changes at the site of parasite attachment and changes in bowl wall diameter at the ileocecal junction may be a potential cause of colic and intussusception. Tapeworms compete with the host for nutrients, hinder normal gut motility, and excrete some toxic wastes into the host' bowl.

Pathological findings

Extensive inflammation and ulceration of various depths from the superficial mucosa to the muscularis mucosa and submucosa at the site of attachment near the ileocecal junction. Mild prolapse of the terminal ileum into the lumen of the ileocecal junction. Presence of yellow diphtheritic membrane and gross oedema of the mucosa. A granulomatous lesions project from the mucosa at the ileocecal junction.

Clinical features

Most of infections are asymptomatic. But, horses with tapeworms might have diminished performance, increased susceptibility to other disease conditions. In heavy infection may cause failure to thrive and, increased risk of cecal perforation, cecal torsion, spasmodic colic and ileal impaction, ileocecal intussusception and less frequently anaemia.

Diagnosis

A presumptive diagnosis can be made by finding proglottids in the faeces, or findings characteristic eggs (Fig. 5.5) on direct smears or faecal flotation. The eggs often have a peculiar shape, varying from almost round to somewhat square or D-shape, with an outer vitelline membrane and a thick, dark, albuminous middle shell. The innermost membrane consists of a chitinous pyriform apparatus. The pyriform apparatus contains the hexacanth embryo characteristics of cyclophyllidean cestode eggs. Serological tests (e.g. ELISA) can be used. Also, whole worms may be seen at necropsy and can be collected in 5% formaldehyde or 70% ethanol for examination. These worms are found in clusters at or near the ileocecal junction. Tapeworm infections in horses should be differentiated from other causes of unthriftiness and colic.

Treatment

All approved anthelmintics are more than 95% effective against tapeworms. Dewormers containing broad-spectrum anthelmintic (e.g. ivermectin or moxidectin) plus praziquantel with the cestocidal activity are used with a high degree with success in the USA. Also, pyrantel pamoate 13.2 mg/kg oral (USA) or pyrantel embonate 38 mg/kg oral (Europe) has showed good efficacy. Because of the nature of the life cycle that involves a free-living invertebrate intermediate host, animals can be reinfected after treatment, which might give rise to the incorrect impression that treatment was ineffective. Ileocecal intussusception can be very serious, and requires surgical interference to save the horse.

Control

Control is difficult and necessitates control of the intermediate hosts. Measures should aim at reducing both the numbers of eggs passed into the environment in faeces and the exposure of animals to cysticercoid-containing mites. Rotation of pastures also has been suggested as a means of prevention. Ploughing and reseeding pastures have been suggested to reduce the number of oribatid mites. Newly purchased animals should be isolated and treated prophylactically with an appropriate cestocidal drug before entering the grazing area.

Public health implications

Equine cestodes are not zoonotic.

Ruminant cestodes

Aetiology

Cestodes in cattle and sheep belong to the anoplocephalid family, including *Moniezia expansa* and *Moniezia benedini*. The scolex is devoid of rostellum, hooks, or hooklets, and suckers are unarmed. *Monezia* spp. can reach lengths of 4 m (Fig. 5.6). *Thysanosoma actinioides* occurs in sheep and measures 25–30 cm long. Its proglottids are 5–6 times wider than long and have a conspicuous fringe on their posterior surface, hence called 'fringed tapeworm'. *T. actinioides*, besides inhabiting the small intestine, often invades bile duct and pancreatic duct and causes many livers to be condemned.

Epidemiology and geographical distribution

The majority of anoplocephalid species have a cosmopolitan distribution.

Life cycle and pathogenesis

The life cycle of *Moniezia* spp. is the same as that of the *Anoplocephala* spp. found in horses, and they use similar free-living mites. The cycle of *T. actinioides* is not known. The egg of the common sheep tapeworm (*M. expansa*) is ingested by oribatid mites, in which the metacestode develops. The life cycle is completed when sheep eat infected mites containing cysticercoid larva. The mechanical damage caused by the suckers on the scolex of the

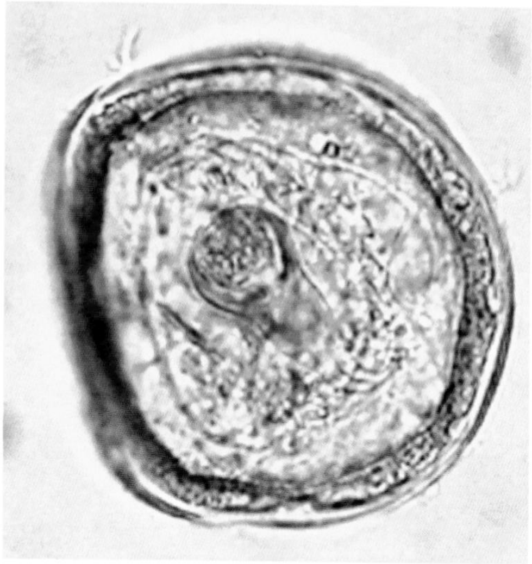

Figure 5.5 *Anoplocephala perfoliata* egg measures about 65–85 μm. Note the pear shaped structure called 'pyriform apparatus' around the oncosphere in the centre of the egg. (Image reproduced by kind permission, John W. McGarry, University of Liverpool.)

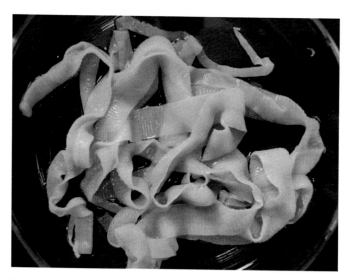

Figure 5.6 Adult *Monezia expansa* of sheep. (Image reproduced by kind permission, John W. McGarry, University of Liverpool.)

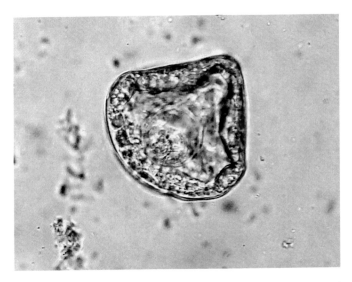

Figure 5.7 *Monezia expansa* egg showing the 'pyriform apparatus' and measure approximately 56–67 μm. (Image reproduced by kind permission, John W. McGarry, University of Liverpool.)

tapeworms at the site of attachment and parasite antigens play a role in the pathogenic process. Tapeworms compete with the host for nutrients, hinder normal gut motility, and excrete some toxic wastes into the host' bowl.

Pathological findings
Ulceration and mild inflammation of intestinal mucosa at the site of attachment may be seen on necropsy.

Clinical features
Little pathogenicity, most of infections are asymptomatic. In heavy infection may cause failure to thrive and less frequently anaemia.

Diagnosis
A presumptive diagnosis can be made by finding proglottids or eggs in the faeces on direct smears or faecal flotation. Anoplocephalid eggs are round to triangular in shape, with an outer vitelline membrane and a thick, dark, albuminous middle shell (Fig. 5.7). The innermost membrane consists of a chitinous pyriform apparatus. Also, diagnosis can be made at necropsy. Ruminants' tapeworm infections should be differentiated from other causes of unthriftiness and colic.

Treatment
Treatment options include albendazole, fenbendazole, mebendazole, oxfendazole and praziquantel. Because of the free-living nature of the invertebrate intermediate host, animals can be reinfected after treatment, which might give rise to the false assumption that treatment was ineffective.

Control
The same measures used to control equine tapeworms.

Public health implications
Cestodes of ruminants are not zoonotic. A single case of *Monezia* infection was reported in a human in Egypt.

Cestodes of dogs and cats

Aetiology
Dogs and cats can be host to parasites belong to the two major groups of Cestodes, namely cyclophyllideans (true cestodes) and pseudophyllideans (pseudocestodes); however, true cestodes are more commonly encountered (Table 5.1).

There are several species of genus *Taenia* that can infect dogs and one species that infect cats (Table 5.2). Prepatent period varies according to the species but it is generally ranges from 6 to 10 weeks. Depending on species mature worm can reach up to 5 m in length.

Epidemiology and geographical distribution
The species of tapeworms found in dogs and cats depends on their geographic location and the amount of free-ranging activity the animals can have. Hence, hunting dogs or cats at higher risk of infections, and puppies or kittens are less likely to be carrying tapeworms as infection is acquired via eating prey. *E. garnulosus* is

Table 5.1 Common cestodes in dogs and cats

Parasite species	Dog or cat	Intermediate Host[a]	Infective stage
Cyclophyllidean cestodes			
Dipylidium caninum	Both	Fleas, lice	Cysticercoid
Taenia spp. (see Table 5.2)	Both	Rabbit and ruminants (definitive host – dogs); rodents (definitive host – cats)	Cysticercus
Mesocestoides spp.	Both	Non-fish vertebrates	Tetrathyridium
Echinococcus granulosus, *E. multilocularis*	Both	Ruminants (definitive host – dogs); rodents (definitive host – fox, dogs, coyotes, cats)	Hydatid cyst; alveolar echinococcosis
Pseudophyllidean cestodes			
Spirometra spp.	Both	Non-fish vertebrates (amphibians, reptiles)	Plerocercoid
Diphyllobothrium latum	Both	Fish	Plerocercoid

[a]Final intermediate host from which the dogs and cats acquire infection because some cestodes have complex life cycles that require multiple intermediate hosts, e.g. *D. latum* (broad tapeworm) requires copepods as 1st IH and fish as 2nd IH. Also, *Spirometra* spp. requires crustacean as first IH and non-fish vertebrate as second IH.

Table 5.2 Common *Taenia* spp. reported in dogs and cats

Taenia spp.	Definitive host	Intermediate host	Larval stage and site
T. pisiformis	Dogs and wild canids	Rabbit	*Cysticercus pisiformis*: liver/body cavities
T. hydatigena	Dogs and wild canids	Ruminants (cattle, sheep, deer, elk and moose)	*Cysticercus tenuicollis*: liver/abdominal cavity
T. multiceps	Dogs and wild canids	Sheep and cattle	*Coenurus cerebralis*: CNS
T. ovis	Dogs and wild canids	Ruminants (cattle, sheep, deer, elk, and moose)	*Cysticercus ovis*: muscles
T. serialis	Dogs and wild canids	Rabbit	Coenurus serialis: connective tissues
T. krabbei	Dogs and wild canids	Reindeer	*Cysticercus tarandi*: muscles/abdominal cavity
T. taeniaeformis	Cats	Mice, rats, and other small rodents	*Strobilocercus fasciolaris*: liver

found in limited areas in the UK, including Wales and the Hebridean islands. All cestodes of dogs and cats have an intermediate host (IH) in which the larval stage develops (Tables 5.1 and 5.2).

Life cycle and pathogenesis

Members of true cestodes that infect pets shed egg-laden proglottids in their faeces. When the appropriate IH ingests these eggs, larval cysts develop. Dogs and cats are infected when they ingest the IH that contains these larval cysts. These animals may then begin shedding proglottids of *D. caninum* or *Mesocestoides* spp. as soon as 2–3 weeks after infection. For *Taenia* and *Echinococcus* spp., the prepatent period may be as long as 1–2 months. In contrast, adult pseudophyllidean cestodes, such as *Spirometra* spp. or *D. latum*, discharge individual operculated eggs through a median genital pore in the segment. These eggs hatch upon contact with water and develop in a copepod first IH and a vertebrate second IH before being ingested by a cat or dog definitive host and developing into an adult tapeworm. Dogs and cats may begin shedding pseudophyllidean tapeworm eggs as soon as 10 days after infection. Infections will only occur when dogs and cats ingest larvae in prey species or in undercooked animal tissue in an area where infection is cycling in nature.

Pathological findings

Ulceration and mild inflammation of intestinal mucosa at the site of attachment may be seen on necropsy.

Clinical features

Disease in dogs and cats due to infection with adult cyclophyllidean cestodes is rare. Most of tapeworm infections are asymptomatic. However, heavy infection may occasionally cause disease, intestinal disturbance, failure to thrive and anaemia. Also, passage of proglottids may be associated with perianal irritation. Motile segments on the animal's coat can be seen.

Diagnosis

Diagnosis of *Taenia* spp. and *D. caninum* infections is normally made by finding the proglottids (body segments), or chain of proglottids, around the host's anal region or on its furs. Although the eggs will float, they are usually not released to mix with the faeces. When freshly shed, *D. caninum* proglottids have rounded edges with a cucumber seed-shape (Fig. 5.8), whereas those of

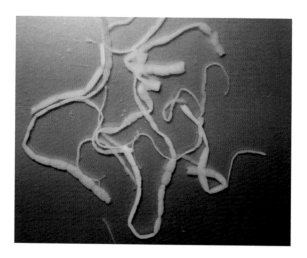

Figure 5.8 Adult *Dipylidium caninum* showing the cucumber-seed appearance of its segments. Adult worms may reach up to 50 cm in length. (Image reproduced by kind permission, John W. McGarry, University of Liverpool.)

Taenia spp. are more rectangular with sharp corners (Fig. 5.9). Often, *D. caninum* or *Taenia* spp. infection is diagnosed based on a client's observation of proglottids, which can be motile when fresh or appear like grains of rice (or sesame seeds) when desiccated on or around the pet. *Taenia* spp. have one genital opening per proglottid, whereas *D. caninum* has two, one on either side. Further identification of *Taenia* spp. beyond the genus designation can be achieved via morphological characterization of the internal structures. *E. granulosus* eggs frequently mix with the faeces (unlike *Taenia* spp.), but the eggs are typical *Taenia*-type eggs, possessing thick, striated shells (Fig. 5.10). *D. caninum* eggs, if seen in faeces, occur in packets contained within a thin-walled membrane (Fig. 5.11).

Treatment

Several treatments are available for the treatment of tapeworm infections in dogs and cats, e.g. praziquantel, epsiprantel, or fenbendazole. Praziquantel and epsiprantel are considered the treatments of choice because they are highly effective against *D. caninum*, the most common tapeworm of dogs and cats, as well as *Taenia* spp. and *Echinococcus* spp. Only praziquantel is labelled as effective against *Echinococcus* spp.

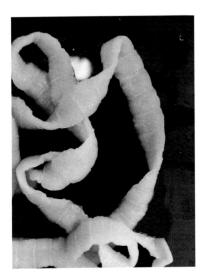

Figure 5.9 Adult worms of *Taenia* spp. (Image reproduced by kind permission, John W. McGarry, University of Liverpool.)

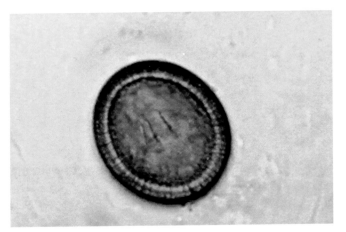

Figure 5.10 *Echinococcus* egg is indistinguishable from *Taenia* spp. egg. (Image reproduced by kind permission, John W. McGarry, University of Liverpool.)

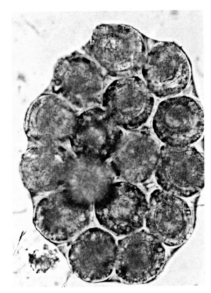

Figure 5.11 *Dipylidium caninum* egg cluster. Each egg cluster contains up to 20 eggs and within each is an oncosphere bearing 3 pairs of hooks. (Image reproduced by kind permission, John W. McGarry, University of Liverpool.)

Control

Always remember that maintenance of the cestode life cycle depends on pets gaining access to infected prey. Thus, treatment of tapeworms in dogs and cats must be combined with appropriate control measures and husbandry modifications, such as effective flea control and prevention of ingestion of prey species; in the absence of these changes, reinfection is likely to occur. Control depends on the tapeworm species. For example, the presence of *D. caninum* necessitates control of fleas and lice. In other tapeworm species dogs and cats should not have access to the flesh or viscera of the infected intermediate host. Preventing predation and scavenging activity by keeping cats indoors and dogs confined to a leash or in a fenced yard will limit the opportunity for pets to acquire infection with *Taenia*, *Echinococcus*, or *Spirometra* or *D. latum* through ingestion of intermediate hosts. Because both flea infestations and scavenging behaviours are difficult to prevent totally, routine monthly deworming of dogs and cats with a broadly cestocidal compound may be indicated, particularly for dogs and cats in areas endemic for *Echinococcus* spp. *E. multilocularis* is not indigenous to the UK. Because of its serious zoonotic potential the praziquantel requirement of the Pet Travel Scheme (PETS) was instigated to treat dogs and cats prior to entry to the UK to keep this zoonotic cestode out of the UK.

Public health implications

See section on Public health implications.

Larval tapeworm (metacestode) infection

Certain tapeworms use domestic animals as intermediate hosts. Metacestodes in domestic animals appear as fluid-filled cysts that occupy special locations in the animal's body depending on the species involved. Cattle may harbour *Cysticercus bovis* 'measly beef', the metacestode of *Taenia saginata* (the beef tapeworm of humans) in their muscles including heart, tongue, masseters, diaphragm, intercostal, and other skeletal muscles of fore and hind limb. *C. bovis* may undergo degenerative changes or even classification. Infections in cattle are usually asymptomatic. Heavy experimental infections can lead to myositis, myocarditis, and signs of muscular stiffness or weakness. *Taenia solium* (the pork tapeworm of humans) occurs in pigs as *C. cellulosae* (pork measles). *Cysticerus bovis* (cattle), *C. ovis* (sheep), *C. dromederii* (camel) and *C. cellulosae* (swine) have also economic significance resulting from condemnation or down grading of infected carcases.

Other metacestodes can lead to severe disease conditions in the affected animals. Coenurosis ('gid' or 'sturdy') is a disease of the brain and spinal cord caused by *Coenurus cerebralis*, the intermediate stage of *Taenia multiceps* which inhabits the intestine of dogs, cats and wild carnivores. The clinical disease occurs in sheep and rarely in cattle. *C. cerebralis* causes cortical meningitis and encephalitis. Affected sheep holds its head to one side and turns in circles. There may be blindness, paralysis of limbs and pressure atrophy of the brain and bones of the skull adjacent to the cyst. *Cysticercus tenuicollis* (Fig. 5.12) infection is caused by the larval stage of tapeworm *Taenia hydatigena* which is found in dogs and cats. *C. tenuicollis* causes no overt clinical signs but during passage

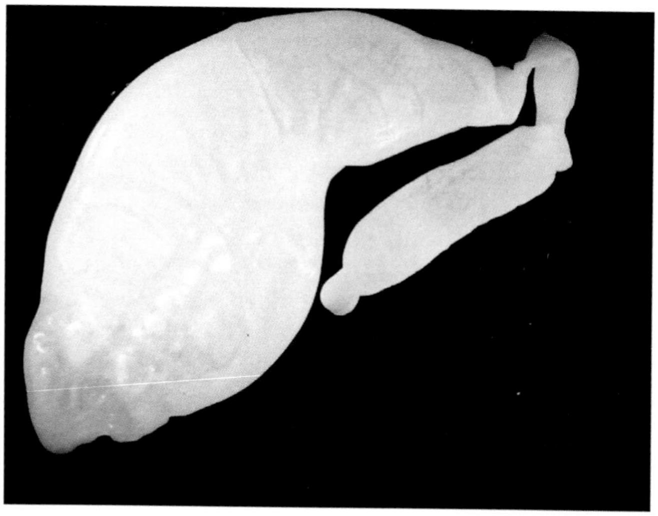

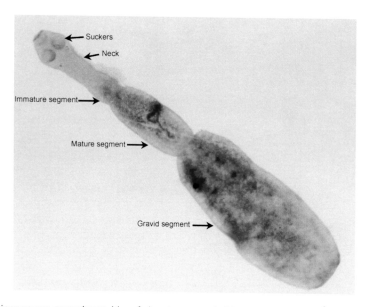

Figure 5.12 *Cysticercus tenuicollis*, larval stage of *Taenia hydatigena*. (Image reproduced by kind permission, John W. McGarry, University of Liverpool.)

of the onchospheres in the liver they induce hepatic lesions in the form of haemorrhagic tracts. Migrating onchospheres may be accompanied by anaerobic microorganisms, which may cause small necrotic hepatic foci resulting in liver damage. Acute disease occurs only with the presence of large numbers of cysticerci, and is characterized by depression and weakness. Chronic stage is usually asymptomatic. No treatment is available to cysticerci infection in farm animals and control is challenging because it requires treating infection in the definitive host (dogs) and preventing contact with dogs.

Dogs, cats and other carnivores are the definitive hosts of *Echinococcus granulosus* (Fig. 5.13). This adult tapeworm is of little concern to the dog, but its metacestode, known as a hydatid cyst, can grow in almost any mammal including humans when these

hosts ingest the eggs of *E. granulosus*. The embryos inside the eggs will hatch and the embryos migrate to the blood stream, which carries them to various organs and develop into hydatid cysts (Fig. 5.14). These can achieve a considerable size of 5–10 cm or more in diameter, which may damage animals by putting pressure on neighbouring organs, particularly liver and lungs, impairing their function. Animals with hydatid cysts are a perpetual reservoir of metacestodes that are infective – if they contain hydatid sand (Fig. 5.15) – for dogs, which in turn may infect humans. Hydatid cyst must be differentiated from cysts of *C. tenuicollis*, *C. cellulosae*, and calcified TB lesions.

Public health implications

Humans are normal definitive host for a wide range of adult cestodes that inhabit small intestine (Table 5.3).

Even though adult tapeworm infection in humans is not life-threatening, humans can be infected by a wide range of metacestodes, which cause adverse health consequences. Metacestodes that can be found in humans include; *Cysticercus cellulosae* (in various muscles especially those of the eye), *Coenurus cerebralis* (in brain and spinal cord), hydatid cyst (in liver, lung, brain, and other organs). Hydatid cyst infection (echinococcosis or hydatidosis) can be cystic (caused by *E. granulosus*) or alveolar (caused by *E. multilocularis*). Sparganosis is caused by accidental ingestion or drinking of the cyclops infected with procercoid stage of *Diphyllobothrium mansoni* where the procercoid larvae penetrate the intestine and migrate to the subcutaneous and musculature and develop into sparganum (= plerocercoid) in different organs. *Spirometra* spp. are also zoonotic; humans who accidentally ingest *Spirometra* species-infected copepods in water or spargana in the tissue of an infected second IH can develop sparganosis. In general, care must be taken when handling materials that might be infected with eggs or metacestodes of tapeworms as many of these are infective to humans.

Figure 5.13 Adult stained *Echinococcus granulosus* (dwarf dog tapeworm). Mature worm measures 5–6 mm in length with the terminal (3rd gravid) segment comprising nearly half the length of the worm. (Image reproduced by kind permission, John W. McGarry, University of Liverpool.)

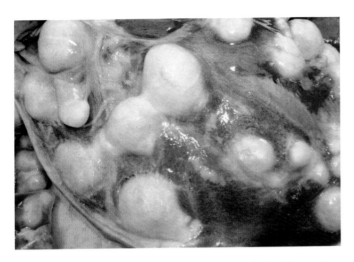

Figure 5.14 Typical echinococcal hydatid cysts in the tissue of an intermediate host. Fertile cyst contains many protoscoleces, but infertile cyst is devoid of protoscoleces. (Image reproduced by kind permission, John W. McGarry, University of Liverpool.)

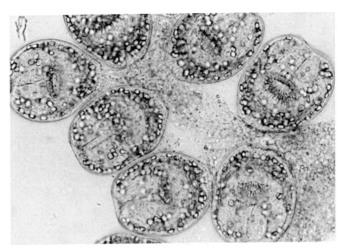

Figure 5.15 Protoscoleces (known as hydatid sand) recovered from the hydatid fluid. Each protoscolex is a potential tapeworm in the final host. (Image reproduced by kind permission, John W. McGarry, University of Liverpool.)

Table 5.3 Basic features of adult tapeworms affecting humans

Tapeworm	Intermediate host	Infective stage	Mode of infection
Taenia saginata	Cattle	Cysticercus bovis	Ingestion of undercooked infected beef
Taenia solium	Pigs	Cysticercus cellulosae	Ingestion of undercooked infected pig meat
Hymenolepis nana	Human and fleas	Eggs or cysticercoid	Auto-infection, ingestion of eggs, or ingestion of infected fleas
Hymenolepis diminuta	Rat fleas	Cysticercoid	Ingestion of infected flea or its larval stage
Dipylidium caninum	Dog fleas	Cysticercoid	Ingestion of infected fleas or its larval stage
Diphyllobothrium latum	Fresh water fish	Plerocercoid	Eating undercooked fish

Acknowledgements

I like to thank Professor John W. McGarry from University of Liverpool for helpful advice and permission to use certain images.

Further reading

Bucknell, D.G., Gasser, R.B. and Beveridge, I. (1995). The prevalence and epidemiology of gastrointestinal parasites of horses in Victoria, Australia. Int. J. Parasitol. *25*, 711–724.

Carabin, H., Budke, C.M., Cowan, L.D., Willingham, A.L. and Torgerson, P.R. (2005). Methods for assessing the burden of parasitic zoonoses: Echinococcosis and cysticercosis. Trends Parasitol. *21*, 327–333.

Conboy, G. (2009). Cestodes of dogs and cats in North America. Vet. Clin. North Am. Small Anim. Pract. *39*, 1075–1090.

Craig, P.S., McManus, D.P., Lightowlers, M.W., Chabalgoity, J.A., Garcia, H.H., *et al.* (2007). Prevention and control of cystic echinococcosis. Lancet Infect. Dis. *7*, 385–394.

Elshazly, A.M., Azab, M.S., Elbeshbishi, S.N. and Elsheikha, H.M. (2009). Hepatic hydatid disease: four case reports. Cases J. *2*, 58.

Fetcher, A. (1983). Liver diseases of sheep and goats. Vet. Clin. North. Am. Food Anim. Pract. *5*, 525.

Garcia, H.H., Moro, P.L. and Schantz, P.M. (2007). Zoonotic helminth infections of humans: echinococcosis, cysticercosis and fascioliasis. Curr. Opin. Infect. Dis. *20*, 489–494.

Gasser, R.B., Williamson, R.M. and Beveridge, I. (2005). *Anoplocephala perfoliata* of horses—significant scope for further research, improved diagnosis and control. Parasitology. *131*, 1–13.

Georgi, J.R. (1987). Tapeworms. Vet. Clin. North Am. Small Anim. Pract. *17*, 1285–1305.

Ghazaei, C. (2007). Evaluation therapeutic effects of antihelmintic agents albendazole, fenbendazole and praziquantel against coenurosis in sheep. Small Ruminant Res. *71*, 48–51.

Moro, P. and Schantz, P.M. (2009). Echinococcosis: a review. Int. J. Infect. Dis. *13*, 125–133.

Scala, A. and Varcasia, A. (2006). Updates on morphobiology, epidemiology and molecular characterization of coenurosis in sheep. Parassitologia. *48*, 61–63.

Major Fluke Infections

6

Philip J. Skuce

Dicrocoeliasis

Aetiology
Dicrocoeliasis is caused by *Dicrocoelium dendriticum*, which is also known as 'lancet fluke' or 'small liver fluke'. It can infect sheep, goats, cattle, deer, rabbits and occasionally horses and pigs (Fig. 6.1).

Epidemiology and geographical distribution
Dicrocoeliasis is a widespread problem worldwide in grazing livestock. The epidemiology of *Dicrocoelium* depends upon the environment and on the presence of its intermediate and definitive hosts.

Life cycle and pathogenesis
Ingested metacercariae hatch in the small intestine and the immature fluke migrate up the bile ducts to the liver, hence there is no migratory phase within the liver. The life cycle differs from other fluke in that there are two intermediate hosts, namely land snails and brown ants. Miracidia are already embryonated within the eggs when shed in faeces, these hatch and are ingested by suitable snails. Cercariae are released as slime balls, which are subsequently eaten by ants. These are, in turn, ingested by grazing animals. The chances of this happening are greatly enhanced by the parasite within the ant's brain altering host behaviour, such that infected ants migrate to the tips of grass swards. The transmission of *D. dendriticum* is, therefore, more terrestrial and not dependent on access to water, unlike *F. hepatica*.

Pathological findings
Because there is no migratory phase within the liver, infected livers can be relatively normal. However, in heavy infestations, there can be extensive focal liver damage accompanied by distension of the bile ducts (Fig. 6.2).

Clinical features
Often subclinical, but in heavy infestations anaemia, oedema, emaciation have been reported.

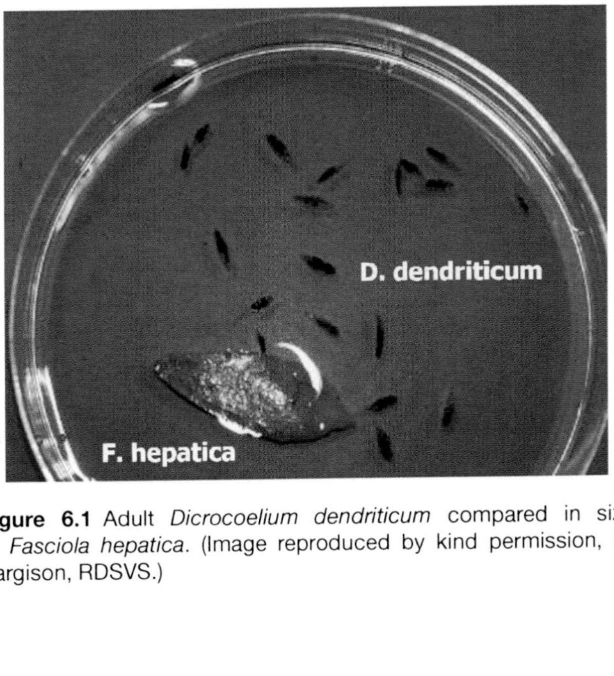

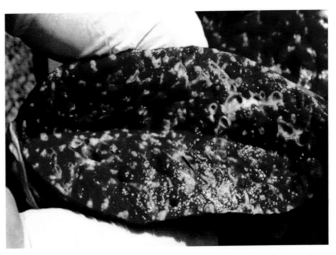

Figure 6.1 Adult *Dicrocoelium dendriticum* compared in size to *Fasciola hepatica*. (Image reproduced by kind permission, N. Sargison, RDSVS.)

Figure 6.2 Liver damage caused by severe *Dicrocoelium dendriticum* infection. (Image reproduced by kind permission, N. Sargison, RDSVS.)

Diagnosis

Diagnosis is based on the presence of *D. dendriticum* eggs in faeces or flukes in the bile ducts.

Treatment

Difficult to treat because many fasciolicides show little/no activity against *D. dendriticum* at normal dose rates. Netobimin, albendazole and fenbendazole show good activity, but at very high dose rates.

Control

Control compromised by the persistent nature of the eggs and the presence of multiple intermediate and reservoir hosts in the environment.

Public health implications

Dicrocoelium spp. do pose a zoonotic risk but are very uncommon in humans; most cases are likely to be non-symptomatic.

Fascioliasis

Aetiology

Liver fluke disease (fascioliasis) is caused by the parasitic flatworm, *Fasciola hepatica*. The parasite itself is leaf-shaped, approximately 2–5 cm in length as an adult (Fig. 6.3) and causes severe liver damage with associated production losses, in sheep and cattle. Whilst primarily a parasite of livestock, *F. hepatica* has a broad host range and can also infect goats, deer, rabbits and man. The disease has traditionally been associated with the wetter, milder parts of Europe, and also with parts of S. America where it is also a risk to humans. Tropical fascioliasis is caused by the

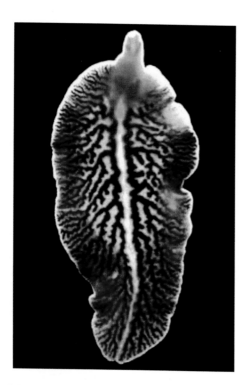

Figure 6.3 Adult liver fluke. (Image reproduced by kind permission, S. Stammers)

closely-related species, *F. gigantica*, and is a significant constraint on livestock production in large parts of Asia and Africa.

Epidemiology and geographical distribution

The epidemiology of liver fluke disease is intimately associated with the epidemiology of its snail intermediate host. In the northern hemisphere, snails infected in spring will typically shed cercariae on pasture in the late summer to early autumn. Most livestock are at risk of ingesting viable cysts at this time but can also pick up infection in the late winter/early spring by ingesting cysts that may have survived over winter. The epidemiology of the disease is also influenced by the grazing habit of the livestock. High rates of infection would normally be associated with mild winters and warm/wet summers but can also be seen in drier periods as animals are forced to seek out more lush pasture, which will increase exposure to infected snails.

Life cycle and pathogenesis

The fluke has a complicated two-host life cycle (Fig. 6.4), involving a mammalian definitive host (in which the adults live) and a snail intermediate host (in which the larval stages develop and multiply). The adult flukes live in the bile ducts of sheep and cattle where they shed large numbers of eggs. These pass out onto pasture in the host's faeces. A single adult fluke can shed up to 50,000 eggs per day and even in a light infection, up to 500,000 eggs can be deposited on pasture from a single sheep. At temperatures above approximately 10°C, a larval stage known as the miracidium will develop inside the egg, a process which takes approximately 2–4 weeks. The miracidia are free-swimming and, upon hatching, have approximately 3 hours in which to locate and penetrate a suitable snail intermediate host. In the UK and northern Europe, this is a particular species of small mud snail, *Galba truncatula*, which is approximately 5–6 mm in length and can be found in water courses, wheel tracks, hoof marks, etc., on poorly drained land. Following penetration of the snail, the parasite develops through a series of further larval stages within the snail's tissues and emerges some 6–8 weeks later as the infectious cercarial stage. Fluke numbers are hugely amplified at this point because for each miracidium infecting a snail, hundreds if not thousands of cercariae are produced. These are also free-swimming but quickly lose their tails to become the infective metacercarial cyst stage adhering to blades of vegetation or herbage. Under optimum conditions, the infectious cysts can survive for approximately a year on pasture but are susceptible to drying-out and prolonged freezing. The life cycle is completed when metacercarial cysts are ingested by grazing livestock. The cysts will hatch in the intestine in response to acid conditions and bile, to release immature fluke, which then penetrate the gut wall and pass into the body cavity where they locate the liver. The young fluke migrate through the liver tissue, causing severe liver damage, and after approximately 8–10 weeks, reach the bile ducts where they mature into egg-laying adult parasites to start the cycle again. It is possible to see immature fluke in the liver tissue and adult fluke in the bile ducts of the same animal at the same time. The threat to livestock is further increased by the presence of wildlife reservoir hosts, including deer, hares and rabbits which maintain

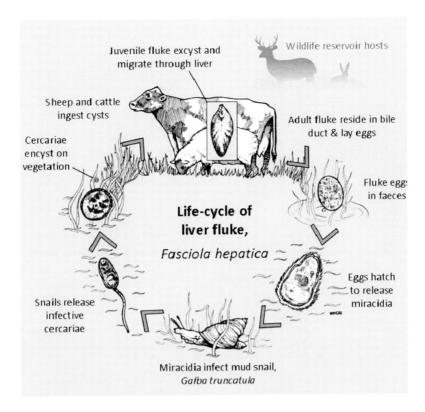

Figure 6.4 Liver fluke life cycle. (Image reproduced by kind permission from the Moredun Research Institute ©).

the life cycle even when there are no livestock present or when livestock have been successfully treated for fluke.

Pathological findings

Acute and subacute fascioliasis result from liver damage associated with the migrating juvenile flukes. Upon post-mortem examination, the liver may be enlarged and pale in colour and, typically, possess numerous haemorrhagic fluke tracts (Fig. 6.5). In severe cases, animals can be extremely anaemic as a result of haemorrhagic blood loss (Fig. 6.6). Chronic fascioliasis results from reduced liver function combined with the anaemia caused by the blood-feeding adult flukes. Upon post-mortem, varying degrees of fibrosis are seen in the liver parenchyma and the bile ducts are often distended and hyperplastic (Fig. 6.7). In chronically infected cattle, the bile ducts can become extensively calcified, a condition known as 'pipestem fibrosis' (Fig. 6.8).

Clinical features

Liver fluke disease is often classified into three clinical forms, with varying degrees of severity. These are dependent on the timing, level and duration of ingestion of metacercarial cysts.

Acute fluke disease

This is more often seen in sheep than in cattle and occurs when animals ingest massive numbers of infective metacercariae over a short period of time from herbage in the autumn/early winter. The simultaneous migration of large numbers of immature fluke through the liver causes severe pathological damage and haemorrhage and frequently results in sudden deaths in autumn/early

winter, often following handling as the liver can be fragile. Deaths typically occur before the immature fluke have developed into egg-laying adults so there will be no fluke eggs in the faeces. Other sheep in the flock will often be anaemic with the inside mucosa of eyelids pale (Fig. 6.9) and the abdomen swollen. Acute fluke infection can predispose animals to clostridial necrotic hepatitis or 'black disease', but this is less commonly seen nowadays with the advent of effective clostridial vaccines.

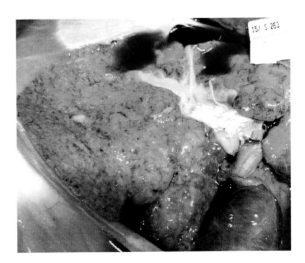

Figure 6.5 Acute fluke damage in an ovine liver. Note pale colour and haemorrhagic fluke tracts. (Image reproduced by kind permission, R. Reichel, VLA © 2010 Crown copyright)

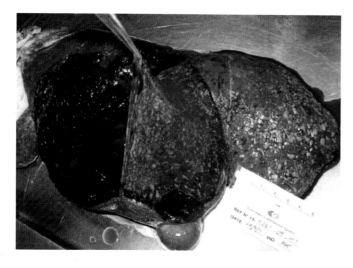

Figure 6.6 Acute fluke damage in an ovine liver. Note mottled necrotic regions and extensive haemorrhage. (Image reproduced by kind permission, R. Reichel, VLA © 2010 Crown copyright)

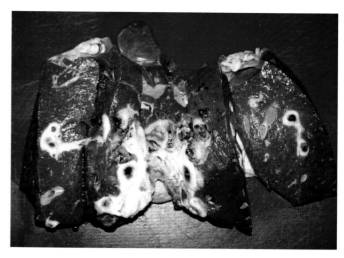

Figure 6.8 Classic 'pipestem fibrosis' in a chronically infected bovine liver. (Image reproduced by kind permission, N. Sargison, RDSVS.)

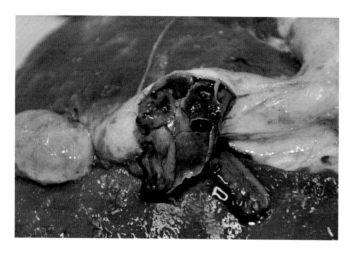

Figure 6.7 Adult fluke emerging from distended hyperplastic bile ducts in a chronically infected ovine liver. (Image reproduced by kind permission from the Moredun Research Institute ©)

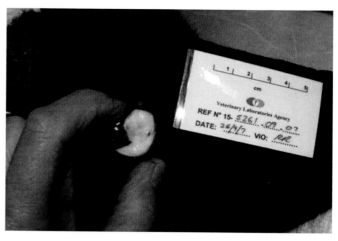

Figure 6.9 Severe anaemia in a chronically infected ewe. (Image reproduced by kind permission, R. Reichel, VLA. © 2010 Crown copyright)

Subacute fluke disease

In this form of fascioliasis, infection is acquired over a more prolonged period, there is damage to the liver tissue and also the presence of adult flukes in the bile ducts. Infected animals tend to show rapid weight loss and poor body condition during mid and late winter. Deaths often occur later in the year than for acute fascioliasis, typically around late November-February.

Chronic fluke disease

This is the most common and widespread form of fluke disease in both sheep and cattle and can be associated with either 'summer' (after the main peak of shedding) or 'winter' infection of snails. Disease is, therefore, often seen in late winter/spring or early-summer. It is associated with a prolonged intake of low to moderate numbers of metacercariae from herbage and results in a progressive loss of body condition associated with the accumulation of adult flukes in the bile ducts of the liver. Anaemia is

often severe in undernourished sheep and they may also exhibit submandibular oedema ('bottle jaw'), an accumulation of fluid caused by low blood protein (or hypoalbuminaemia) (Fig. 6.10). Deaths are uncommon in well nourished sheep but chronic fascioliasis is often exacerbated by poor nutrition.

Diagnosis

Confirmation of disease is usually through post-mortem examination of livers. In the live animal, the presence of the classic gold-coloured, operculate fluke eggs in sheep/cattle faeces is taken as evidence of a fluke infection. However, egg counting is only indicative of a patent or adult infection (immature fluke do not lay eggs). Moreover, fluke egg counting is not an accurate indication of actual fluke burden, because egg-laying adult fluke reside in the bile ducts, so eggs only appear sporadically in the faeces. Blood enzyme profiles, looking specifically for liver/bile duct damage, may be of use in chronically infected animals. Also, a number of fluke-specific ELISA tests are commercially available.

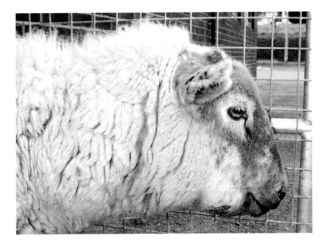

Figure 6.10 'Bottle jaw' in a chronically infected ewe. (Image reproduced by kind permission, R. Reichel, VLA © 2010 Crown copyright.)

These detect anti-fluke antibodies in blood and/or milk and indicate that an animal has been exposed to fluke infection. These are useful as survey tools; however, their diagnostic potential is questionable because anti-fluke antibodies can persist well after an animal has been successfully treated for fluke. More recently, an ELISA test capable of detecting minute traces of antigens released by the fluke into the host's faeces (i.e. coproantigens), has become available. This has the potential to discriminate between current and previous infection and, because the readout from the test is essentially quantitative, may also provide an indication of the efficacy of treatment. Acute fascioliasis should be differentiated from haemonchosis, infectious hepatitis, eperythrozoonosis, anthrax, and enterotoxaemia. Chronic fascioliasis should be differentiated from nutritional deficiencies of copper, cobalt, Johne's disease, and other internal parasitisms, including parasitic gastroenteritis (particularly haemonchosis in sheep and ostertagiasis in cattle).

Treatment

Control of liver fluke infections in livestock relies heavily on the strategic use of flukicidal drugs. There is a wide selection of such products on the market. All are capable of killing the adult fluke in the bile ducts but vary in their ability to kill the juvenile fluke in the liver (Fig. 6.11). They are usually formulated as single product flukicides but are also available as combination fluke and worm drenches. More recently, pour-on products have been developed for use in cattle. The emergence of parasite populations that are resistant to products used for their control is an inevitable consequence of repeated treatment and selection pressure. Where resistance or lack of efficacy in fluke has been reported to date, it has concerned triclabendazole, the active ingredient in a number of leading flukicides and the drug of choice to treat acute fluke outbreaks. Triclabendazole-resistant fluke have been reported in the west of Scotland and southwest Wales. The extent of triclabendazole resistance in the UK is currently unknown but probably low at this time.

Control

On some farms it may be possible to drain localized wet areas, particularly in the early spring, to reduce the snail populations. Molluscicidal treatment of snails, whilst common practice in the past, is now deemed environmentally unacceptable. Fencing off localized snail habitats may be practical in some circumstances, especially during high-risk periods. Avoiding grazing the wettest areas in autumn/winter will reduce the intake of metacercariae and lessen the incidence of disease. Avoidance or drainage of snail habitats; strategic anthelmintic dosing programmes.

Public health implications

Whilst being primarily a parasite of livestock, *F. hepatica* is also a major parasite of public health importance. As many as 17 million

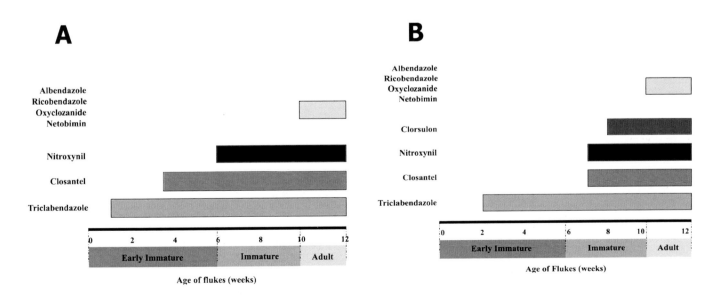

Figure 6.11 Spectrum of activity of major fasciolicides in (A) sheep and (B) cattle. (Image reproduced by kind permission from the Moredun Research Institute ©).

people are thought to be infected with fluke in over 40 different countries, mostly in the Middle East, South-East Asia and South America. Endemic fascioliasis in humans requires the combined presence of the snail intermediate host, domestic grazing livestock, appropriate climatic conditions and the suitable dietary habits of at risk human subjects. Humans become infected by ingesting metacercarial cysts on aquatic vegetation, such as watercress and water chestnuts. Pathogenesis depends on the number of cysts ingested and is similar to that reported in other animals.

Paramphistomosis

Aetiology

Rumen fluke disease (paramphistomosis) is caused by *Paramphistomum cervi*, *P.* microbothrioides and related flukes. Paramphistomes in their early stage are located in the small intestine and abomasum, from where they move to the rumen to finally establish as adults.

Epidemiology and geographical distribution

Paramphistomum spp. have a worldwide distribution and are considered to be important parasites of a number of ruminant species, particularly in tropical and subtropical areas. Geographical distribution, seasonality, and disease risk are determined by the occurrence of intermediate molluscan hosts (planorbid and bulinid snails). *Paramphistomum* infection requires the coexistence of favourable temperature and humidity and the presence of intermediate hosts. Paramphistomosis has been described in low and easily flooded lands, rice growing areas and natural grass pastures with slow running water, as well as in areas of lakes and marshlands. Snails reproduce during the warm and rainy months, when their number increases and they become easily infected with *Paramphistomum* miracidia.

Life cycle and pathogenesis

Within the intermediate host, the external phase in the life cycle of *Paramphistomum* spp. is similar to that of *F. hepatica*. Within the definitive host, when the metacercariae are ingested and reach the anterior part of the small intestine, the immature flukes are shed and remain attached to the intestinal wall, feeding on cellular detritus. Once they have developed sufficiently, they migrate towards the rumen, where the parasites will reach the adult stage, remaining there and living on ruminal fluid.

Pathological findings

The adult parasites in the rumen appear to cause relatively little pathology, unless in heavy infections. The major pathological effects are seen in the intestinal phase of the infection, where the immature fluke become attached to the ileum and duodenum, causing severe erosion of the duodenal mucosa. Large numbers of small, flesh-coloured flukes can be seen attached to the ruminal mucosa (Fig. 6.12).

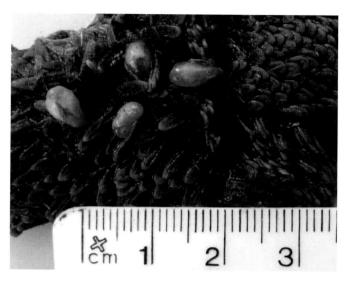

Figure 6.12 Paramphistomes on the surface of a bovine rumen. (Image reproduced by kind permission H. Carty, SAC VIS.)

Clinical features

Enteritis, fetid diarrhoea, anaemia, protein loss, which generates a generalized oedema (hydrothorax, hydropericardium, ascites, lung oedema).

Diagnosis

Demonstration of immature flukes in faeces. Faecal sedimentation to detect eggs. Eggs are similar in shape to those of *F. hepatica* but slightly larger, and transparent in aspect. Paramphistomosis should be differentiated from nutritional deficiency of copper, infection with intestinal roundworms, infectious enteritides, usually accompanied by fever, Johne's disease in adult animals, but this is a much more chronic disease, and poisonings, including many weeds, inorganic arsenic and lead.

Treatment

Oxyclozanide.

Control

Avoidance or drainage of snail habitats; anthelmintic treatments to prevent contamination of pastures with eggs.

Public health implications

None known, it would appear that the adults cannot develop in non-ruminant hosts.

Acknowledgements

The author would like to thank the following for helpful advice and permission to use certain images: Mr Sinclair Stammers, scientific photographer; Dr Neil Sargison (Royal Dick School of Veterinary Studies, RDSVS); Dr George Mitchell and Ms Rita Deuchande (Scottish Agricultural College Veterinary Investigations Service, SAC VIS); Mr Rudolf Reichel (Veterinary Laboratories Agency, VLA) and Professor Bob Hanna, Agrifood and Biosciences Institute Northern Ireland, AFBINI).

Further reading

Chen, M.G. and Mott, K.E. (1990). Progress in assessment of morbidity due to *Fasciola hepatica* infection: a review of recent literature. Trop. Dis. Bull. *87*, R1-R38.

Hopkins, D.R. (1992). Homing in on helminths. Am. J. Trop. Med. Hyg. *46*, 603–609.

Mas-Coma, S., Bargues, M.D. and Esteban, J.G. (1998). Human Fasciolosis. In Dalton, J.P., ed. (CABI Publishing, Oxon, UK), pp. 411–434.

Mezo, M., Gonzalez-Warleta, M., Carro, C. and Ubeira, F.M. (2004). An ultrasensitive capture ELISA for detection of *Fasciola hepatica* coproantigens in sheep and cattle using a new monoclonal antibody (MM3). J. Parasitol. *90*, 845–852.

Sargison, N.D. (2008). Sheep Flock Health – a Planned Approach. Blackwell Publishing. Chapter 2, pp. 197–205.

Skuce, P.J. (2009). Liver fluke in Sheep and cattle. Moredun Foundation News Sheet, Vol. 5, No. 4.

Spithill, T.W., Smooker, P.M. and Copeman, D.B. (1999). *Fasciola gigantica*: epidemiology, control, immunology and molecular biology. In Fasciolosis, Dalton, J.P., ed. (CABI Publishing, Oxon, UK), pp. 465–525.

Taylor, M.A., Coop, R.L. and Wall, R.L. (2007). Veterinary Parasitology, 3rd edn (Blackwell Publishing, Oxford, UK), pp. 208–210.

Diseases Associated with Protozoa

Diseases Caused by Protozoa

7

Naveed A. Khan and Hany M. Elsheikha

Acanthamoeba granulomatous encephalitis

Aetiology

Acanthamoeba granulomatous encephalitis is caused by opportunistic free-living amoeba, *Acanthamoeba* spp.

Epidemiology and geographical distribution

This is a rare disease that is generally limited to hosts with a weakened immune system. It has been reported in the majority of vertebrates, worldwide. The exposure of hosts (especially in the presence of skin lesions) to standing water, soil, mud, or swimming in contaminated water, i.e. lakes, untreated pools may attribute to this fatal infection.

Life cycle and pathogenesis

Acanthamoeba has two stages in its life cycle: a vegetative trophozoite stage, which under harsh conditions transforms into a dormant cyst stage (Fig. 7.1). Trophozoites are about 15–35 μm, contain a single nucleus, feed on bacteria, and reproduce by binary fission. Cysts are double-walled, approximately 8–15 μm, and are highly resistant to physical, chemical and radiological conditions.

Acanthamoeba enter into the lungs via the nasal route. Next, they traverse the lungs into the bloodstream, followed by haematogenous spread. Finally, *Acanthamoeba* cross the blood–brain barrier and enter into the central nervous system (CNS) to produce disease. It is noteworthy that *Acanthamoeba* may bypass the lower respiratory tract and directly enter into the bloodstream via skin lesions. The pathophysiological complications involving the CNS most likely include induction of pro-inflammatory responses, invasion of the blood–brain barrier and neuronal damage leading to the brain dysfunction. The affected organs other than the CNS may include subcutaneous tissue, skin, liver, lungs, kidneys, pancreas, prostate, lymph nodes and bones.

Pathological findings

Post-mortem examination often shows severe oedema and haemorrhagic necrosis and the presence of cysts in tissues.

Clinical features

Neurological manifestations vary, and may include fever, behavioural changes, hemiparesis, agitation, cranial nerve palsies and increased intracranial pressure, finally leading to seizures, coma and death.

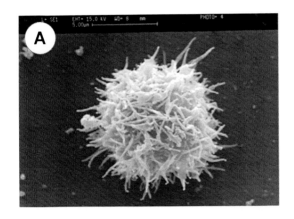
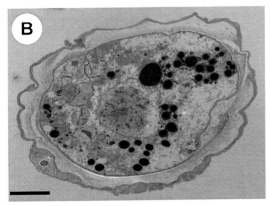

Figure 7.1 (A) Scanning electron micrograph depicting *Acanthamoeba* trophozoite. Scale bar = 5 μm. (B) Scanning electron micrograph depicting *Acanthamoeba* cyst. Scale bar = 2 μm.

Diagnosis

The diagnosis can be made by demonstrating organisms (cysts) in infected tissues. The brain image analyses using computed tomography or magnetic resonance imaging scan may show multifocal areas of signal intensities or lesions indicating brain abscesses or tumours suggestive of the CNS defects. The cerebrospinal fluid findings reveal pleocytosis with lymphocytic predominance with elevated polymorphonuclear leucocytes, increased protein concentrations, decreased glucose concentrations, minimal cloudiness and possible presence of amoebae. The high levels of *Acanthamoeba*-specific antibodies (> 1:200) in serum using indirect immunofluorescence assays may provide a useful and straightforward method to suspect this infection. It is helpful to inoculate a portion of the CSF and/or brain biopsy for amoebae culturing. The clinical specimens can be inoculated onto non-nutrient agar plate seeded with Gram-negative bacteria. *Acanthamoeba* feeds on bacteria as food source and depending on the number of amoebae in the specimen, trophozoites can be observed within a few days. PCR-based methods have been developed for the clinical diagnosis of amoebae infections and provide rapid diagnosis from the clinical specimens. In addition, matrix-assisted laser desorption–ionization time of flight MS (MALDI-TOF-MS) may be of potential value in the rapid identification of *Acanthamoeba* in the clinical specimens.

Treatment

There is no recommended treatment and the majority of cases are identified at the post-mortem stage. If diagnosed early, a combination of ketoconazole, fluconazole, sulfadiazine, pentamidine, amphotericin B, azithromycin, or itraconazole may be effective. Alkylphosphocholine compounds, such as hexadecylphosphocholine have shown promise.

Control

Exposure of animals to standing water, lake water, freshwater may contribute to this infection. In the presence of skin lesions, avoid contact with muddy water or organic-rich soil.

Public health implications

There is no information on *Acanthamoeba* granulomatous encephalitis as a zoonotic disease. Accidental intake of amoebae cysts orally is not the route of infection. The exposure of hosts to contaminated soil and water (especially in the presence of skin lesions) may attribute to this fatal infection in humans and animals. Humans and animals become infected from common environmental sources.

Amoebiasis

Aetiology

Amoebiasis (amoebic dysentery and amoebic liver abscesses) is caused by protozoan pathogen, *Entamoeba histolytica*.

Epidemiology and geographical distribution

Amoebiasis is caused by the ingestion of infective cysts in contaminated water. Infection is transmitted by faecal–oral route; cysts shed from infected animals. It has been reported in dogs, cats, pigs, rats and primates with a worldwide distribution.

Life cycle and pathogenesis

The life cycle of *E. histolytica* alternates between the cyst and the trophozoite forms. Cysts are the infectious stage of the parasite. The cysts are hardy and can survive harsh environmental conditions. Infection begins when a new host ingests cysts in contaminated food, water, fomites or by the faecal–oral route. Trophozoites emerge from the cysts and divide asexually by binary fission. Pathogenic amoebae invade the mucosa causing ulceration and dysentery. Amoebae may disseminate to other organs where large abscesses may form. Amoebae secrete proteases which facilitate their invasion of tissues. Amoebae transform into cyst which are passed in faeces to continue the cycle.

Pathological findings

Flask-shaped ulcers can be observed in the mucosa of the large intestine. Abscess formation in liver, lungs and brain.

Clinical features

Clinical signs include diarrhoea or dysentery.

Diagnosis

Entamoeba histolytica can be diagnosed in faeces by the direct smear technique (phase microscopy or fluorescent antibody detection). Trophozoites and cysts are best demonstrated by iodine, trichrome or iron haematoxylin staining or it can be cultured. Trophozoites are approximately 12–30 µm, while cysts are 10–12 µm and contain four nuclei. Parasite reproduces asexually by binary fission and form cysts for transmission. PCR-based assays as well as serology-based assays have been developed for rapid diagnosis.

Treatment

Treatment requires combined use of metronidazole and diiodohydroxyquin.

Control

Clean water supplies together with improved hygiene and ensuring correct disposal of faeces should limit this infection.

Public health implications

Entamoeba histolytica can produce severe diarrhoea or dysentery in humans which can result in disseminated infection.

Babesiosis

Aetiology

Babesiosis is a malaria-like parasitic disease caused by protozoan, *Babesia* spp.

Epidemiology and geographical distribution

Babesiosis occurs in a variety of animals including cattle, sheep and goats, horses, and dogs with a worldwide distribution.

Life cycle and pathogenesis

Transmission is by blood-sucking ticks, *Ixodes* spp. Sporozoites are inoculated into the host by the feeding tick. These organisms invade erythrocytes (Fig. 7.2), where they multiply. The destruction of erythrocytes releases parasite which invade more erythrocytes resulting in a rapidly increasing parasitaemia. This results in an acute syndrome characterized by haemolytic anaemia and injury to multiple organs. *Babesia* spp. produce acute disease by two main mechanisms: haemolysis and circulatory disturbances. A chronic stage is associated with anaemia and weight loss, and a carrier state. The next stage in the life cycle is infection of the vector tick by these blood stages.

Pathological findings

Post-mortem examination shows carcass as pale and jaundiced while the blood appears thin and watery.

Clinical features

Anaemia, haemoglobinuria, jaundice, fever, loss of appetite, pregnant animals often abort, and high fatality rate.

Diagnosis

The history and clinical sign together with vector presence in the environment should be of diagnostic value. The presence of parasites in blood during a febrile attack can provide confirmation. The morphology of the parasites in stained thin blood smears is variable, but typically they appear as ring forms that may be round, oval or amoeboid, with a small nucleus and conspicuous vacuole, usually with chromatin extending round the margins except when the parasite is degenerating, when it has a punctuate appearance. The demonstration of high levels of *Babesia*-specific antibodies in serum using indirect immunofluorescence assays may provide a useful and straightforward diagnostic tool. PCR-based methods employed on blood samples have been developed for the clinical diagnosis of Babesiosis infections and provide rapid diagnosis.

Treatment

Early diagnosis together with administration of appropriate drugs (diminazene and imidocarb) is generally effective, while combined therapy with atovaquone and azithromycin eliminates parasites and prevents recrudescence.

Control

Vector (tick) control should limit the spread of infection. Live vaccines are available as prophylactic measures.

Public health implications

There are several species of *Babesia* that can infect humans, but *B. microti* (a rodent-borne piroplasm) and *B. divergens* (the bovine piroplasma) are the most prevalent etiological agents of human babesiosis in the United States and Europe, respectively.

Balamuthia amoebic encephalitis

Aetiology

First diagnosed in a mandrill baboon, *Balamuthia* amoebic encephalitis is a rare disease caused by opportunistic free-living amoeba, *Balamuthia mandrillaris*.

Epidemiology and geographical distribution

Balamuthia has been shown to produce infection in the majority of vertebrates, worldwide. The exposure of hosts (especially in the presence of skin lesions) to standing water, soil, mud, swimming in contaminated water, i.e. lakes, untreated pools may attribute to this fatal infection.

Life cycle and pathogenesis

Balamuthia mandrillaris has two stages in its life cycle, a vegetative trophozoite stage and a dormant cyst stage (Fig. 7.3). Trophozoites are about 30–60 µm, generally contain a single nucleus, feed on other eukaryotic cells, reproduce by binary fission and form cysts under harsh conditions. Cysts are triple-walled, approximately 10–30 µm, highly resistant to physical, chemical and radiological conditions. *Balamuthia* enter into the lungs via the nasal route. Next, they traverse the lungs into the bloodstream, followed by haematogenous spread and cross the blood–brain barrier to enter into the CNS to produce disease. *Balamuthia* may bypass the lower respiratory tract and directly enter into the bloodstream via skin lesions. The pathophysiological complications involving the CNS most likely include induction of pro-inflammatory responses, invasion of the blood–brain barrier and neuronal damage leading to the brain dysfunction. The cutaneous and respiratory infections can lasts for months, but the involvement of the CNS can result in fatal consequences within days or weeks.

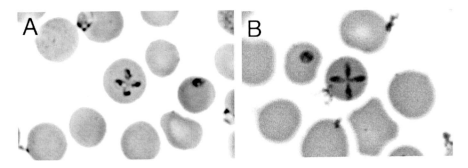

Figure 7.2 Maltese cross forms in gerbil (*Meriones unguiculatus*) erythrocytes: (A) *Babesian microti*, (B) *Babesia divergens*. (Credit: Jeremy S. Gray and Louis M. Weiss, University College Dublin.)

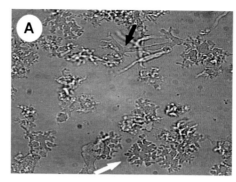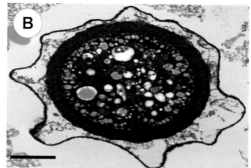

Figure 7.3 (A) *Balamuthia mandrillaris* trophozoites under a phase-contrast microscope. Arrows indicate pseudopodial extensions. Magnification ×450. (B) Transmission electron micrographs depicting *Balamuthia mandrillaris* cyst. Scale bar = 2 μm.

The affected organs other than the CNS may include subcutaneous tissue, skin, liver, lungs, kidneys, pancreas, prostate, lymph nodes and bones.

Pathological findings

Post-mortem examination often shows severe oedema and haemorrhagic necrosis and the presence of cysts in tissues.

Clinical features

Neurological manifestations vary, and may include fever, behavioural changes, hemiparesis, agitation, cranial nerve palsies and increased intracranial pressure, finally leading to seizures and coma.

Diagnosis

The brain image analyses using computed tomography or magnetic resonance imaging scans of the head may reveal single or multiple space occupying lesions indicating brain abscess or tumours suggestive of the CNS defects. The cerebrospinal fluid (CSF) obtained by lumbar puncture rarely show the presence of *Balamuthia* and may resemble that of aseptic meningitis. The cerebrospinal fluid findings, while not confirmatory, but are of value showing pleocytosis with lymphocytic predominance with elevated polymorphonuclear leucocytes, normal or slightly low glucose level, increased levels of proteins (> 1000 mg/dl), and minimal cloudiness. Cysts are observed in the brain tissue and exhibit three layers. The demonstration of high levels of *Balamuthia*-specific antibodies in serum using indirect immunofluorescence assays may provide a useful and straightforward method to diagnose this infection. It is helpful to inoculate a portion of the CSF and/or brain biopsy for amoebae culturing. For *Balamuthia*, the clinical specimens can be inoculated onto mammalian cell monolayers. *Balamuthia* feeds on eukaryotic cells as food source and depending on the number of amoebae in the specimen, trophozoites can be observed within a few days. PCR-based methods have been developed for the clinical diagnosis of amoebae infections and provide rapid diagnosis from the clinical specimens. In addition, matrix-assisted laser desorption–ionization time of flight MS (MALDI-TOF-MS) may be of potential value in the rapid identification of *Balamuthia* in the clinical specimens.

Treatment

No recommended treatment and it usually proves fatal. Early diagnosis followed by administration of a combination of 5-fluorocytosine (flucytosine), fluconazole, sulfadiazine, clarithromycin, trifluoperazine, and pentamidine isethionate may improve prognosis. Despite the limited success, the prognosis remains extremely poor.

Control

In the presence of skin lesions, avoid contact with organic-rich soil and/or muddy water.

Public health implications

There is no information on *Balamuthia* amoebic encephalitis as a zoonotic disease. The exposure of hosts to contaminated soil and water (especially in the presence of skin lesions) may attribute to this fatal infection in humans and animals.

Balantidiasis (also known as balantidiosis)

Aetiology

Balantidiasis is an intestinal infection, caused by ciliated protozoan pathogen, *Balantidium coli* (Fig. 7.4).

Epidemiology and geographical distribution

Balantidium coli is the only ciliate that is pathogenic. This is a rare disease that is generally limited to hosts with a weakened immune system. *Balantidium* has been shown to produce infection in vertebrates including horses, pigs, and non-human primates with a worldwide distribution.

Life cycle and pathogenesis

The life cycle consists of both the trophozoite and cyst forms. The trophozoite is quite large, oval, and covered with short cilia; it measures approximately 50–100 μm in length and 40–70 μm in width. There are two nuclei within the trophozoite, one very large bean-shaped macronucleus and the smaller round micronucleus.

The organisms normally live in the large intestine. The cyst is formed as the trophozoite moves down the intestine. Nuclear division does not occur in the cyst; therefore, only two nuclei are present, the macronucleus and the micronucleus. The cysts measure from 50 to 70 μm in diameter. The infection fundamentally affects the colon and causes variable clinic pictures, from asymptomatic to serious dysenteric forms. Parasite may invade tissues other than intestine. Proteases have been suggested as important factors that may be associated with the pathogenicity of *B. coli*.

Pathological findings
Intestinal haemorrhage, perforation, ulcerative colitis. For extraintestinal infections, tissues reveal inflammation, ulceration, necrosis, and the presence of parasites.

Clinical features
Chronic infection present non-bloody diarrhoea, while fulminating balantidiasis result in passing mucoid, bloody stools with weight loss as well as intestinal haemorrhage and perforation with life-threatening consequences.

Diagnosis
Routine stool examinations, particularly wet preparation examinations of fresh and concentrated material, will demonstrate cysts. These organisms do not stain well (too large and thick) on the permanent stained smear (trichrome, iron-hematoxylin) and can be confused with faecal debris (including helminth eggs), hence the use of wet smears (from direct mounts or concentrate sediment) is recommended.

Treatment
Tetracycline is the drug of choice, although it is considered investigational for this infection. Iodoquinol or metronidazole may be used as alternatives.

Control
Hygiene while handling pigs and other infected animals. Affected animals should be isolated and treated.

Public health implications
A major risk factor for humans is close contact with pigs. Crowding in dwellings can facilitate the spread of infection. Others at risk are workers in abattoirs where pig intestines are handled. Farmers working with pig faeces are at risk of contracting the infection. Given the numbers of simians carrying these organisms zookeepers can be at risk as well as veterinarians and veterinary students working with sick hogs are at risk of infection.

Besnoitiosis

Aetiology
Besnoitiosis is a disease of the skin, subcutis, blood vessels, mucous membranes, and other tissues, caused by *Besnoitia* spp.

Epidemiology and geographical distribution
Infection has been reported in a variety of animals, in particular, cattle, goats, horses, and opossums with a worldwide distribution.

Life cycle and pathogenesis
Besnoitia spp. are protozoa that form cysts in the infected host tissues. It has a life cycle that requires intermediate host (where asexual reproduction occurs) and definitive host (where sexual reproduction occurs). Life cycle of *Besnoitia* is similar to that of *Toxoplasma gondii*. Definitive hosts (cats for majority of species) become infected by ingesting tissues containing cysts through cannibalism, and schizonts and gamonts are formed in the intestinal mucosa. Oocysts are shed in faeces. Intermediate hosts become infected by ingesting food or water contaminated with oocysts excreted by definitive host (such as cats). After infection, organisms emerge from oocyst and disseminate within the host and can invade different cell types, cross biological barriers and can cause severe pathology depending largely on the host immunological status and the parasite virulence. The parasite develops in connective tissue, and cysts may become macroscopic and can affect various tissues.

Pathological findings
Cysts in dermis, subcutaneous, and other fascia.

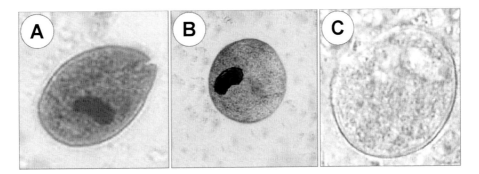

Figure 7.4 *Balantidium coli*. Saline/iodine wet mount, (A) *B. coli* trophozoite, note the large bean-shaped macronucleus and the cilia ('fuzz') around the periphery; (B) *B. coli* cyst, note the more rounded shape, cilia are more difficult to see, and the presence of the macronucleus. (C) Saline wet mount without iodine; note that the organism characteristics are somewhat difficult to see. However, the macronucleus is still visible. (Credit: Lynne S. Garcia, LSG and Associates.)

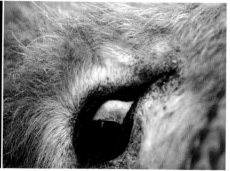

Figure 7.5 *Besnoitia bennetti* cysts in the mucous membrane of the upper lip and sclera of a miniature donkey.

Clinical features

Anasarca, alopecia, hyperpigmentation and scleroderma, and infertility. Pin-point nodules (cysts) on the scleral conjunctiva and mucosal surfaces (Fig. 7.5).

Diagnosis

Diagnosis can also be made by demonstrating organisms (crescent-shaped bradyzoites) in skin scrapings, biopsy, or conjunctival scrapings. An ELISA test for bovine besnoitiosis is now available.

Treatment

Besnoitiosis is non-pathogenic in cats, and no treatment is necessary. No recommended treatment for the tissue cyst. Early diagnosis together with administration of antimony and sulfanilamide complex can prevent cyst development, while oxytetracycline have shown promise as an early therapeutic intervention.

Control

Hygiene measures include avoiding contact with carnivores. In some countries, cattle are immunized with a live, tissue-culture-adapted vaccine. Affected animals should be isolated and treated symptomatically. Reduction of biting insects and ticks may also reduce transmission.

Public health implications

There have been no reported cases of besnoitiosis in humans; therefore it is assumed that humans are not at risk of contracting infection from infected animals.

Blastocystosis

Aetiology

Blastocystosis is an infection of the gastrointestinal tract caused by highly prevalent protozoan pathogen, *Blastocystis* spp.

Epidemiology and geographical distribution

This is a rare disease that is generally limited to hosts with a weakened immune system. *Blastocystis* is a waterborne commensal, recognized as a protozoan that inhabits human and animal intestinal tracts with a world-wide distribution. Prevalence of infection is highest in areas of poor sanitation. The parasite has been reported in annelids, arthropods, amphibians, reptiles, birds (notably with domestic chickens) and mammals.

Life cycle and pathogenesis

The life cycle of this protozoan parasite begins with ingestion of resistant faecal cysts that develop into vacuolar forms (Fig. 7.6). The latter replicate by binary fission. Some of these forms mature into cysts that are shed in the faeces and continue transmission via the faecal–oral route. Parasite proteases, predominantly of the cysteine type, have been shown to be important for virulence.

Pathological findings

The pathology associated of blastocystosis may be limited but may include inflammation of the intestinal mucosa and invasion of the superficial layers together with damage to the intestinal wall.

Clinical features

The organism has been found in a high percentage of clinically healthy animals; its pathogenic role in dogs or cats is uncertain. With a weaker immune system, the clinical consequences of *Blastocystis* infection are mainly diarrhoea and abdominal pain as well as non-specific gastrointestinal symptoms such as nausea, weight loss, bloating, lassitude, and dizziness.

Diagnosis

The diagnosis can be made by demonstrating organisms in faeces but requires familiarity with the morphological features. Internal structures of the organism can be visualized by electron microscopy. As is the case with light microscopy, a thin rim of cytoplasm surrounds a large central vacuole. The most commonly observed forms in *in vitro* culture are the vacuolar form, and less commonly seen forms are the amoeboid, cystic, multivacuolar and avacuolar forms. The vacuolar form is spherical and may vary widely in size, ranging from 2 to 200 µm within a single culture, with diameters averaging 4–15 µm, while the cyst forma are as small as 2–15 µm. The mode of division is binary fission. PCR-based assays have been developed for rapid diagnosis.

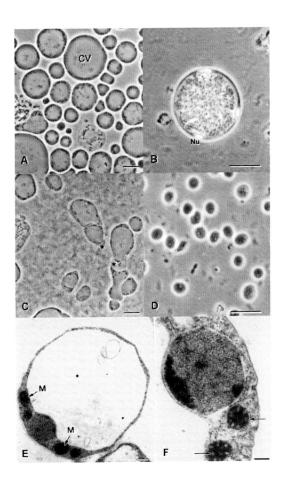

Figure 7.6 Morphological forms of *Blastocystis* by phase-contrast (A–D) and transmission electron (E, F) microscopy. (A) vacuolar forms from *in vitro* axenic culture, displaying extensive size variation; (B) granular form with distinct granular inclusions within central vacuole; (C) amoeboid forms from colonies grown in soft agar with pseudopod-like cytoplasmic extensions (*); (D) ovoid faecal cysts; note small size and refractile appearance; (E) transmission electron micrograph of vacuolar form revealing large central vacuole resulting in a thin band of peripheral cytoplasm. The nucleus is flanked with electron dense mitochondria-like organelles (MLOs); (F) at higher magnification, the nucleus reveals features typical of *Blastocystis* with course nucleoplasm and peripheral chromatin mass. The MLOs possess distinct saccate cristae (arrows). CV, central vacuole; Nu, nucleus; M, MLO. A–D: bar = 10 µm; E and F: bar = 0.5 µm. (Credit: Kevin S.W. Tan, National University of Singapore.)

Treatment

Although the pathogenicity of *Blastocystis* is somewhat controversial, treatment is applied only when cause of diarrhoea is apparent. Metronidazole for 10 days has been used to treat affected hosts, although relapses may be observed, presumably as a result of re-infection. Nitazoxanide has also been used.

Control

Clean water supplies together with improved hygiene by ensuring correct disposal of animal faeces should limit this infection. Introducing measures to ensure passive transfer of colostral antibodies should minimize infection pressure.

Public health implications

Pigs, rodents and domestic birds represent huge reservoirs of the parasite for zoonotic transmission. Though *Blastocystis* may also be a commensal, it is associated with signs of diarrhoea and cutaneous rashes in immunocompromised people.

Coccidiosis

Aetiology

Coccidiosis is a parasitic disease of the intestinal tract of animals. It is caused by a variety of protozoan pathogens, two of which (genus *Eimeria* and genus *Isospora*) are described here while others are covered elsewhere in this chapter.

Epidemiology and geographical distribution

The severity of the infection depends on environmental conditions (warmth, moisture), stocking intensity, age, and previous exposure. It occurs most commonly in crowded conditions both in barns and on pasture, especially in calves, lambs and chicken, with a worldwide distribution.

Life cycle and pathogenesis

Infection is transmitted by the faecal–oral route; oocysts shed from infected animals. Oocysts of the *Eimeria* spp. sporulate in the environment and reach the infective stage in the same manner as do *Isospora* spp. (Fig. 7.7). *Eimeria* spp., however, develop four sporocysts, each of which contains two sporozoites, for a total of eight infective forms per oocyst. Young calves, lambs, piglets, kids and foals are affected. Immunity develops after infection; clinical disease occurs rarely in adult cattle. Infection rate is high, while clinical disease is much less common. High morbidity with low case fatality rate is reported.

Pathological findings

Infection causes ileitis, caecitis and colitis.

Clinical features

Diarrhoea, dysentery, tenesmus, appetite normal appetite or inappetence, mild abdominal pain in lambs, nervous signs in calves with coccidiosis in cold climates, loss of body weight, anaemia in some cases but not common. Epidemics occur in calves and lambs, especially feedlot animals. Diarrhoea without blood in faeces of piglets. Diarrhoea with a large amount of blood in foals.

Diagnosis

Demonstration of oocysts in faeces; and merozoites in intestinal tissues is of high diagnostic value. However, wet preparation examination of fresh material either as the direct smear or as concentrated material is recommended rather than the permanent stained smear. PCR-based assays have been developed for clinical diagnosis.

Treatment

For *Eimeria* spp., treatment includes sulfonamides compounds, while toltrazuril is recommended for *Isospora* infection.

Control

It is recommended to control population density to minimize number of oocysts ingested while immunity develops. In addition, prevention of contamination of feed and water, and the use of dry bedding are important control strategies.

Public health implications

Zoonotic potential is unknown for *Eimeria* spp. while *Isospora* spp. are known to produce clinical symptoms including diarrhoea, which may last for long periods (months to years), weight loss, abdominal colic, and fever; diarrhoea is the main symptom. Bowel movements (usually 6–10 per day) are watery to soft, foamy, and offensive smelling, suggesting a malabsorption process. Infection can be severe in people with weaker immune system. Effective eradication of *Isospora* infection in humans has been achieved with co-trimoxazole, trimethoprim-sulfamethoxazole, pyrimethamine–sulfadiazine, primaquine phosphate–nitrofurantoin, and primaquine phosphate–chloroquine phosphate; while the drug of choice is trimethoprim–sulfamethoxazole.

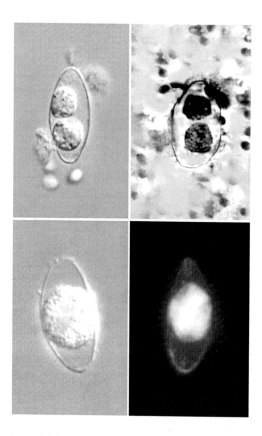

Figure 7.7 Top panel: *Isospora belli.* Oocysts containing two sporoblasts; these oocysts are normally seen in patients with more normal stools and are not infective when passed. Left: Wet mount from stool sedimentation concentration. Right: Stained with modified acid-fast stain. Bottom panel: Oocysts containing a single sporoblast; stained using optical brightening agent stain (Calcofluor white). (Credit: Lynne S. Garcia, LSG and Associates.)

Cryptosporidiosis

Aetiology
Cryptosporidiosis is a diarrhoeal disease caused by protozoan parasites of the genus *Cryptosporidium*.

Epidemiology and geographical distribution
Infection is predominant in ruminant neonates and may cause diarrhoea, especially if there is concurrent infection with other enteropathogens, nutritional, or environmental stress. Infection has been reported in the majority of mammals, worldwide.

Life cycle and pathogenesis
Infection begins with the ingestion of an oocyst by the host through contaminated water. Sporozoites (which are haploid) emerge from the ingested oocyst via excystation in the gut and invade host epithelial cells (Fig. 7.8). Replication typically takes place in the small intestine, or in the colon. The trophozoite grows, and through a process called merogony, and produces several merozoites within a single meront (maturing trophozoite). Merozoites develop into the sexual stages of the parasite: microgamonts or macrogamonts which fuse to produce a zygote. Zygotes develop into oocysts that are environmentally resistant form and are released in the faeces and transmission continues via the faecal–oral route.

Pathological findings
Abnormality of the small intestinal mucosa with crypt hyperplasia, resulting in flattening of the mucosa and the appearance of atrophy of villi (villous atrophy).

Clinical features
Malabsorption-type diarrhoea similar to that seen with rotavirus infection. The diarrhoea is usually liquid and yellow. Affected animals are often active, alert, and nursing. Diarrhoea can vary from mild and self-limiting to severe, especially with mixed infections, which are quite common.

Diagnosis
Acid-fast staining of air-dried faecal smears is a quick and easy method of diagnosis. Oocysts are roughly spherical and range from 4 to 8 μm in length or width. Length/width ratios range from 1.0 to 1.2 depending upon species. Within the oocyst, sporozoites may be visible, along with a structure that is referred to as the residual body. Although oocysts are considered to be the infective stage of the parasite, it is the individual zoite that bears the apical complex and invades a host cell. Demonstration of lesions and organism by immunofluorescent assay confirms diagnosis. In addition, PCR-based assays have been developed for rapid diagnosis.

Treatment
Halofuginone and paromomycin are known to be effective.

Control
Clean water supplies together with improved hygiene by ensuring correct disposal of animal faeces should limit this infection. Introducing measures to ensure passive transfer of colostral antibodies should minimize infection pressure.

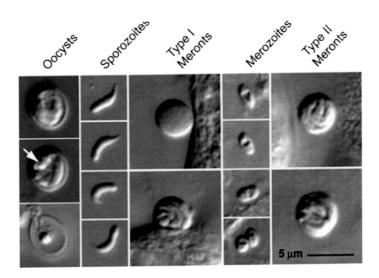

Figure 7.8 *Cryptosporidium parvum* asexual life cycle. The top oocyst contains four sporozoites surrounded by the oocyst wall. The residual body can be seen in the middle oocyst (arrow). The bottom oocyst has excysted – only an empty shell with an open suture and the residual body remains. Excysted sporozoites then develop into type I meronts. The meront in the top has not yet undergone cellularization, while portions of the eight merozoites can be seen within the mature meront in the bottom image. Upon emergence, merozoites invade nearby cells and frequently form clusters of two or more merozoites (as seen in the bottom image). type II meronts may form from type I merozoites and contain only four developing merozoites. The sexual stages (not pictured) are then thought to develop from type II merozoites. The meronts and merozoites were from *in vitro* cultures at 24 hours post infection with HCT-8 cells as hosts. (Credit: Stanley Dean Rider Jr. and Guan Zhu, Texas A and M University.)

Public health implications

This is a highly zoonotic pathogen that can produce severe diarrhoea, especially in individuals with a weaker immune system.

Cyclosporiasis

Aetiology

Cyclosporiasis is a diarrhoeal disease caused by *Cyclospora* spp. that has characteristics similar to other coccidia.

Epidemiology and geographical distribution

It has been reported in dogs, poultry, primates and reptiles with a worldwide distribution; however its role in producing infection in animals is incompletely understood.

Life cycle and pathogenesis

The transmission occurs via the faecal–oral route; oocysts are shed from infected animals and are taken up via contaminated water. Direct animal-to-animal transmission is unlikely because the oocysts shed in faeces must mature in the environment to become infective to the next host. Limited data indicate that the maturation process requires from days to weeks in favourable conditions.

Pathological findings

Altered mucosal architecture with shortening and widening of the intestinal villi due to diffuse oedema and infiltration by a mixed inflammatory cell infiltrate. Also observed is reactive hyperaemia with vascular dilatation and congestion of villous capillaries.

Clinical features

Infection can result in watery diarrhoea with anorexia and weight loss.

Diagnosis

Microscopic demonstration of oocysts in faeces is of high diagnostic value. However, wet preparation examination of fresh material either as the direct smear or as concentrated material is recommended rather than the permanent stained smear. PCR-assays have been developed for clinical diagnosis.

Treatment

There is no recommended treatment; however the drug of choice in humans is trimethoprim-sulfamethoxazole.

Control

Clean water supplies together with improved hygiene by ensuring correct disposal of animal faeces should limit this infection. Introducing measures to ensure passive transfer of colostral antibodies should minimize infection pressure.

Public health implications

Humans become infected via consumption of contaminated water and show clinical signs including watery diarrhoea with a median of six stools per day; anorexia, weight loss, fatigue, abdominal cramping, belching, abdominal bloating, vomiting, low-grade fever. Also, the disease has been associated with ownership of domestic animals and pets. The drug of choice is trimethoprim-sulfamethoxazole.

Cytauxzoonosis

Aetiology

Feline cytauxzoonosis is a tick-borne, fatal blood protozoal disease, caused by *Cytauxzoon felis*.

Epidemiology and geographical distribution

The organism occurs most frequently in North American cats and in the African ungulate animals. There is no age or sex predisposition. Cytauxzoonosis is seen more often during the summer months (May through September) when ticks are more likely to be found. Cats with access to the outdoors (especially wooded areas) are at higher risk of coming into contact with infected ticks and acquiring this disease.

Life cycle and pathogenesis

Ixodid ticks (*Dermacentor variabilis*) inoculate sporozoites of parasite directly into the bite wound in cats, whereas *Cytauxzoon* spp. in African ungulates are thought to be transmitted by *Rhipicephalus appendiculatus*. Young, stressed, or immunocompromised animals are thought to be at greatest risk. Organisms first invade macrophages, where they undergo schizogony. Released merozoites then invade erythrocytes in circulation. The severe clinical disease seen in cats with cytauxzoonosis is thought to be primarily attributable to large schizonts within macrophages obstructing blood flow (particularly in the lungs) and leading to disseminated intravascular coagulation and shock. A mild haemolytic anaemia also may develop due to the erythrocytic stage.

Pathological findings

Gross lesions include dehydration, pallor, icterus, hypopericardium, enlarged lymph nodes, splenomegaly and haemorrhages. Microscopically, accumulation of parasitized mononuclear phagocytes containing schizonts within the lumen of veins and venous channels of the liver, lungs, lymph nodes, and spleen, which makes these vessels appear occluded.

Clinical features

Clinical signs typical of haemolytic crisis such as anorexia, anaemia, laboured breathing, lethargy, dehydration, depression, icterus, pale mucous membrane. Cats usually die 2–3 days after body temperature peaks. Infection has a very poor prognosis.

Diagnosis

Diagnosis of cytauxzoonosis is made by locating the intraerythrocytic phase (piroplasms) in Giemsa-stained blood films or the tissue phase (schizont) in impression smears of the spleen. When detection of parasitized erythrocytes is difficult in the stained blood smear, fine-needle aspirates of the spleen, lymph nodes, or bone marrow may provide a diagnosis. In these cases, the large, merozoite-laden macrophages may be readily observed. Other methods used to diagnose cytauxzoonosis in cats include a direct fluorescent antibody test for detection of the tissue phase of the parasite and indirect immunofluorescent assay to detect serum antibody to the organism. However, these tests are largely experimental and generally are not available commercially. This infection should be differentiated from other causes of acute anaemia and severe disease.

Treatment

At present, there is no available treatment. Infection appears to result in death of the affected cat. Supportive therapy with parenteral fluids and broad-spectrum antimicrobial agents such as diminazene aceturate or imidocarb dipropionate (along with aggressive supportive care) may have beneficial effects.

Control

Tick control and confinement of cats indoors.

Public health implications

There is no information on cytauxzoonosis as a zoonotic disease.

Equine protozoal myeloencephalitis

Aetiology

Equine protozoal myeloencephalitis is a multifocal, progressive disease of the CNS, caused by *Sarcocystis neurona*. Another protozoan parasite, *Neospora hughesi* has also been implicated as a causative agent in some cases.

Epidemiology and geographical distribution

The disease is endemic in the United States, Canada and some Latin American countries. Disease is infectious but not contagious. The risk appears to be higher in young horses, but older horses can develop the condition. Any horse of any breed and any gender can be affected. The definitive host is the North American opossum (*Didelphis* spp.).

Life cycle and pathogenesis

Infective oocysts passed in the faeces of opossums contaminate the feed and water of horses and other intermediate hosts. Once ingested, the sporocysts excyst and release sporozoites, which penetrate the gut and enter arterial endothelial cells of various organs. Meronts mature and rupture the host cell, releasing merozoites into the bloodstream. This process ends with the formation of sarcocysts in the muscles in most sarcocystis infections. But in *S. neurona*, this sarcocyst formation is not common, only reported once in a foal, but the normal pathway of the parasite is to migrate to the neural tissues and replicate continuously via schizogony leading to inflammation and necrosis of the brain, brainstem, and spinal cord. Subsequent ingestion of infected muscle tissue by the predator definitive host completes the life cycle (Fig. 7.9).

Pathological findings

Grossly, the CNS lesions include multifocal areas of haemorrhage to light discolouration of the brain and spinal cord. Microscopically, non-suppurative myeloencephalitis characterized by marked mononuclear perivascular cuffing with necrosis and loss of neurons, with infiltration of monocyte, basophils, lymphocytes, and some eosinophils, with schizonts and merozoites in neurons, glial cells and leucocytes is observed.

Clinical features

Because the parasites affect any part of the CNS tissue, the clinical features can be variable. But commonly asymmetric spinal ataxia, focal, neurogenic muscle atrophy, intermittent lameness, gait abnormalities, and/or cranial nerve dysfunction is observed. Regional sweating may be observed if the sympathetic tracts of

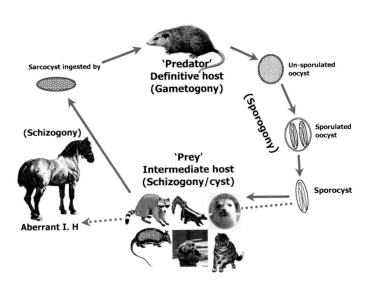

Figure 7.9 Life cycle of *Sarcocystis neurona*, the agent of EPM.

the spinal cord are affected. Head shaking, urinary incontinence and incoordination can occur. Horses may have a sudden onset of clinical signs, or disease may progress slowly over several months. There are no characteristic changes in blood or CSF.

Diagnosis

Diagnosis is based on clinical signs, exclusion of other neurological diseases, and the use of serological assays for detection of the parasite in serum or cerebrospinal fluid. Western blot analysis has high sensitivity but low specificity. Other serological tests such as ELISA, immunofluorescent assays, and direct agglutination test are also available. All these antibody tests are only measures of exposure to the parasite. PCR-based assays for rapid diagnosis are available. Intact merozoites rarely enter CSF; thus PCR testing of neural tissue can be used as a post-mortem test. Infected horses can have elevated CSF protein concentrations, increases in numbers of mononuclear cells, and high levels in CSF enzymatic activity.

Treatment

Antiprotozoal agents, including diclazuril, toltrazuril, ponazurial, nitazoxanide or a combination of a sulfonamide and pyrimethamine have shown promise. Potential side-effects of treatment with antifolate drugs include bone marrow suppression, anaemia, colitis and teratogenesis. Corticosteroids and other anti-inflammatory have been used with caution to avoid the development of immunosuppression.

Control

Prevent exposure to S. neurona by minimizing faecal contamination of feed by opossums. Prophylactic measures include killed S. neurona vaccine but it has limited success.

Public health implications

There is no information on equine protozoal myeloencephalitis as a zoonotic disease.

Giardiasis

Aetiology

Giardiasis is a diarrhoeal infection of the small intestine by protozoan parasite, Giardia spp.

Epidemiology and geographical distribution

Giardiasis is caused by the ingestion of infective cysts in contaminated water. Infection is transmitted by faecal–oral route; cysts shed from infected animals. It has been reported from cattle, sheep, goats, dogs, pigs, primates with a worldwide distribution.

Life cycle and pathogenesis

The life cycle of Giardia alternates between the cyst and the trophozoite forms, and both forms are found in faeces (Fig. 7.10). Cysts are more often found in non-diarrhoeal faeces, and they are the infectious stage of the parasite. The cysts are hardy and resistant to standard concentrations of chlorine used in water treatment and they can persist for several months in cold, moist environment. Infection begins when a new host ingests cysts in contaminated food, water, fomites or by the faecal–oral route. Mature cysts are able to survive the acidic environment of the stomach and migrate to the small intestine of the host. Exposure to stomach acid triggers a process called excystation, during which trophozoites are released from cysts. The trophozoites multiply asexually by binary fission in the small intestine and colonize the small intestine by attaching to the intestinal mucosa, which interfere with the absorption of food and result in clinical symptoms. As trophozoites migrate towards the large intestine, they retreat into the cyst form in a process called encystation. Cysts are released in faeces to continue the cycle.

Pathological findings

Abnormality of the small intestinal mucosa with crypt hyperplasia, resulting in flattening of the mucosa and the appearance of atrophy of villi (villous atrophy).

Clinical features

Most infections are asymptomatic but clinical signs may include faeces from affected animals as light coloured, greasy and soft with intestinal irritation, such as straining and mucus in the faeces, even though Giardia do not colonize the large intestine.

Diagnosis

Giardia can be diagnosed in faeces by the direct smear technique (phase microscopy or fluorescent antibody detection). The cyst form is best demonstrated by the zinc sulfate centrifugal technique. The cysts may be stained with Lugol's iodine solution to make the internal structures easily identifiable. During the reproductive stage, cells are about 12–15 µm long, 5–9 µm wide and contain two nuclei. Cysts are ovoid and contain four nuclei. Reproduce asexually by binary fission and form cysts for transmission. PCR-based assays as well as serology-based assays have been developed for rapid diagnosis.

Treatment

Several azole compounds (metronidazole, tinidazole, fenbendazole, albendazole, benzimidazoles) have been shown to be effective.

Control

Clean water supplies together with improved hygiene by ensuring correct disposal of animal faeces should limit this infection. Introducing measures to ensure passive transfer of colostral antibodies should minimize infection pressure.

Public health implications

This is a highly zoonotic pathogen that can produce severe diarrhoea, abdominal cramps, vomiting, foul flatus, with serious consequences, especially in individuals with weaker immune system.

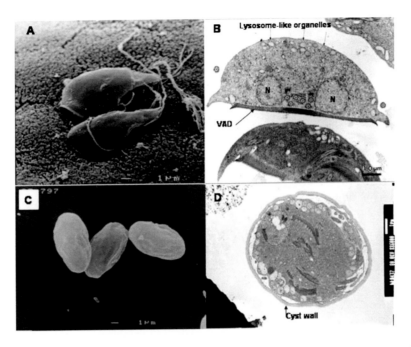

Figure 7.10 *Giardia* life cycle. (A) Scanning electron micrograph of trophozoites attached to intestinal epithelial microvilli courtesy B. Koudela (University of Brno Veterinary School), (B) Transmission electron micrograph of transversely sectioned trophozoites showing two nuclei and lysosome-like organelles courtesy D. Feely (University of Nebraska College of Dentistry), (C) Scanning electron micrograph of cysts courtesy B. Koudela (University of Brno Veterinary School), (D) Transmission electron micrograph of cyst showing the cyst wall filaments courtesy of B. Koudela (University of Brno Veterinary School). (Credit: Edward L. Jarroll, City University New York.)

Leishmaniasis (also known as Leishmaniosis)

Aetiology

Leishmaniasis is a disease caused by protozoan parasites that belong to the genus *Leishmania* and is transmitted by the bite of certain species of sand fly (subfamily Phlebotominae).

Epidemiology and geographical distribution

Leishmaniasis can occur in cutaneous, or visceral form. Disease can occur in various mammalian hosts but it is more common in humans and dogs. It is endemic in the Mediterranean countries and Latin America. Sandflies serve as the vector for infection of animals. Dogs, cats and rodents serve as reservoirs for human beings.

Life cycle and pathogenesis

The sandflies inject the infective stage, metacyclic promastigotes, during blood meals. These organisms are phagocytosed by macrophages and transform into amastigotes. Amastigotes multiply in infected cells and affect different tissues, depending in part on which *Leishmania* spp. is involved. These differing tissue specificities cause differing clinical manifestations of the various forms of leishmaniasis. Sandflies become infected during blood meals on an infected host when they ingest macrophages infected with amastigotes. In the sandfly's midgut, the parasites differentiate into promastigotes, which multiply, differentiate into metacyclic promastigotes, thus completing the cycle.

Pathological findings

Lesions occur mainly in anatomic sites where sandflies feed; around the muzzle, ears, and eyes. Microscopically, lesions include hyperkeratosis, parakeratosis, crusts, and granulomatous nodules in the periadnexal dermis.

Clinical features

Cutaneous forms involve skin ulcers on exposed areas of body with generalized alopecia with silvery white scales, or more severe lesions of nodules and ulcers. Diffuse cutaneous leishmaniasis produces disseminated and chronic skin lesions and is difficult to treat. In mucocutaneous forms, the lesions can partially or totally destroy the mucous membranes of the nose, mouth and throat cavities and surrounding tissues. Visceral leishmaniasis, also known as kala-azar, is characterized by high fever, weight loss, swelling of the spleen and liver and anaemia.

Diagnosis

For cutaneous leishmaniasis, margin of lesion reveal parasites, microscopically. In addition, PCR-based assays have been developed. For visceral leishmaniasis, parasites may be found in a splenic aspirate, liver biopsy or bone marrow biopsy, while demonstration of high levels of *Leishmania*-specific antibodies in serum using indirect immunofluorescence assays may provide a useful and straightforward method to diagnose this infection.

Treatment

For cutaneous leishmaniasis, pentavalent antimonials (sodium stibogluconate) and meglumine antimonite; while for visceral leishmaniasis, polyene macrolide antibiotics (amphotericin B), alkyl phospholipid (miltefosine) and aromatic diamidines (pentamidine isethionate) have shown improved prognosis.

Treatment and control

Reduction of biting insects should reduce transmission. Affected animals should be isolated and treated symptomatically.

Public health implications

Visceral leishmaniosis is a serious human disease that may be fatal if untreated. Children, infants, HIV-infected patients and those receiving immunosuppressive drugs are more susceptible. Transmission of *L. infantum* from dogs or wild canids to people via sandflies is the primary route of infection in zoonotic visceral leishmaniasis.

Neosporosis

Aetiology

Neosporosis is caused by an obligate intracellular protozoan parasite, *Neospora caninum*.

Epidemiology and geographical distribution

Neosporosis has been recognized in dogs, cattle, sheep, goats, deer, horses and experimentally rodents, pigs, monkeys and cats with a worldwide distribution. The dog and other canids (such as foxes) are the definitive host. Cattle are an intermediate host. It is a major cause of abortion in dairy cattle. The condition is predominantly a disease of dairy cattle, but sporadic abortions can occur in beef cows. The role of birds and wild rodents as intermediate hosts is suspected but has not yet been definitively demonstrated.

Life cycle and pathogenesis

Canids shed oocysts in their faeces after ingestion of infected tissues from intermediate hosts. Cattle become infected by eating oocysts that contaminate feed or pastures and then become infected (Fig. 7.11). Infection can then pass to her foetus. Cows that abort once are not protected from future abortion.

Pathological findings

Fetal lesions of multifocal non-suppurative encephalitis, myocarditis and periportal hepatitis are observed. Scattered foci of mixed inflammation with associated segmental myofibre necrosis in skeletal muscle, along with intracytoplasmic protozoal cysts.

Clinical features

Affected calves are often unable to stand and suckle and have abnormal reflexes. Abortion in cattle caused by *Neospora* is relatively common and of economic importance especially in dairy cattle. Midterm to late-term abortion (particularly between 3 and 8 months of gestation), but it may occur anytime from 3 months to term. Stillbirth or premature birth also occurs. Aborted calves might be found mummified. Occasionally, calves will have brain disease (encephalomyelitis) at birth. Repeat abortions possible in

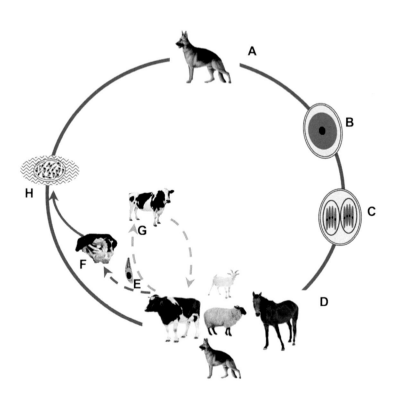

Figure 7.11 Transmission routes for *Neospora caninum* in nature. (A) definitive host; (B) non-sporulated oocyst passed in faeces; (C) sporulated oocyst in food, water or soil; (D) intermediate hosts (IH); (E) tachyzoite transmitted via placenta; (F) aborted infected foetus; (G) persistently infected calf; (H) bradyzoites-containing tissue cyst in IH. Continuous line indicates horizontal transmission and dashed line indicates vertical transmission.

the same cow. Infection in dogs can cause muscle wasting, progressive weakness and paralysis of one or both hind limbs, usually in pups under 6 months of age.

Diagnosis

This can be achieved based on clinical signs (progressive ascending neuromuscular dysfunction in young growing puppies), characteristic heart and brain lesions in aborted calf, and identification of parasite in the calf tissue by serology-based assays. Foetal brain and heart are the best specimens for diagnosis. The finding of a mixed inflammatory-neurogenic atrophy lesion within affected skeletal muscles should prompt a search for protozoa. An indirect fluorescent antibody test and ELISA of maternal serum and fetal fluids is of diagnostic value to detect antibodies. An immunoperoxidase test using specific antibodies can identify *N. caninum* in tissue sections or biopsy specimens.

Treatment

There is no treatment of any proven benefit in cattle. Trimethoprim–sulfadiazine may kill the parasite, but neuromuscular dysfunction in dogs will persist. Drugs used to treat toxoplasmosis (sulfadiazine, daraprim, clindamycin) showed some success in treating neosporosis.

Control

A vaccine based on whole killed tachyzoites is available for *Neospora* however its success is limited. Feed hygiene and calving hygiene should limit infection (e.g. dogs should not be allowed to defecate in cattle feed and by keeping cattle food and water away from dogs and foxes). Cull congenitally infected cattle or bitches. Prevention of farm dogs from scavenging aborted foetuses and afterbirth by not letting them wander freely, especially during the calving season should limit infection. Aborted foetuses, dead calves and afterbirth should be disposed of hygienically.

Public health implications

There is no information on neosporosis as a zoonotic disease.

Primary amoebic meningoencephalitis

Aetiology

Primary amoebic meningoencephalitis is a rare disease caused by opportunistic free-living amoeba, *Naegleria fowleri*.

Epidemiology and geographical distribution

Naegleria fowleri can cause primary amoebic meningoencephalitis a rapidly fatal disease of the CNS that occurs with a history of exposure to contaminated recreational, domestic, or environmental water sources. *N. fowleri* has been shown to produce infection in the majority of vertebrates, worldwide.

Life cycle and pathogenesis

N. fowleri exhibits three morphological forms including a feeding trophozoite, a dormant cyst, and a transient swimming flagellate (Fig. 7.12). The flagellate stage provides a useful diagnostic marker as it is not present in *Balamuthia* or *Acanthamoeba*. In the environment, *Naegleria* feed on bacteria and yeast and under nutrient deprivation, the trophozoite undergoes a transitory transformation to a flagellate stage, 'swims' to the water surface to seek a food source, and then reverts to the amoeboid form whereupon it feeds on bacteria. When rounded, they measure about 10–15 μm in diameter. Under harsh conditions, *Naegleria* switches into the cyst form, 8–12 μm in diameter that consists of smooth single-layered wall with pores sealed with a mucoid plug. The portal of entry of *Naegleria* is through the nasal passages. The amoebae attach to the nasal mucosa, follow the olfactory nerves and migrate through the cribriform plate to the brain resulting in death within 7–10 days. The factors that are responsible for the development of primary amoebic meningoencephalitis are unknown but the role of phospholipases has been suggested that may account for invasiveness and tissue damage *in vivo* and cytopathogenicity *in vitro*. haemolytic activity associated with the amoeba surface membrane also has been reported; however, designation of these phospholipases and other enzymes as unique virulence factors *in vivo* has yet to

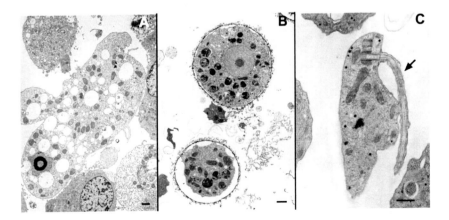

Figure 7.12 Transmission electron micrographs depicting *Naegleria fowleri* in its three states of transformation. (A) Trophozoite. (B) Cyst. (C) Flagellate. The arrow designates the flagellum. The bars represent 1 μm. (Credit: Francine Marciano-Cabral, Virginia Commonwealth University.)

be established. The pathogenic *Naegleria* escapes complement lysis and demonstrates the ability to respond chemotactically to nerve cells and nerve cell factors.

Pathological findings

Post-mortem examination often shows focal areas of granulomas proximal to the olfactory bulb and frontal portion of the brain.

Clinical features

Primary amoebic meningoencephalitis is an acute, fulminant and rapidly fatal infection of the brain. In the early stages patients may present with headache, fever and vomiting. The disease resembles purulent bacterial meningitis leading often to a misdiagnosis. Clinical manifestations of primary amoebic meningoencephalitis include sudden onset of severe bilateral headache, followed by nausea, vomiting, fever, stiff neck, diplopia, seizures and coma.

Diagnosis

The majority of cases of primary amoebic meningoencephalitis have been diagnosed post mortem by haematoxylin and eosin staining of brain tissue. Since disease progression is rapid, serological assays are not helpful since there is little possibility of measuring a rise in antibody titre. Direct microscopic examination of CSF as a wet-mount preparation may reveal motile trophozoites in CSF. PCR assays have been developed that allow for a more rapid, sensitive, and specific laboratory diagnosis. Laboratory findings indicate elevated leucocytes and analysis of CSF reveals pleocytosis with elevated polymorphonuclear leucocytes and elevated protein. A triplex real-time PCR assay based on the use of probes targeting regions of the nuclear small subunit ribosomal gene (18Sr RNA gene) has been developed for detection of *Naegleria*, *Balamuthia* and *Acanthamoeba* in the same sample with results obtained within 5 hours.

Treatment

Primary amoebic meningoencephalitis is almost always fatal; however, combined administration of amphotericin B intravenously, amphotericin B intrathecally and rifampin orally may improve survival rate.

Control

The majority of primary amoebic meningoencephalitis cases have resulted from exposure to water that is 26°C or warmer thus avoiding exposure to warm water, especially if it is shallow and/or stagnant (not moving) is helpful.

Public health Implications

There is no information on primary amoebic meningoencephalitis as a zoonotic disease. The exposure of hosts to contaminated water may attribute to this fatal infection in humans and animals. Avoid taking in water through the nose while swimming, diving, water skiing, or jumping into water. A nose clip can be used to prevent water being forced up the nose.

Rhinosporidiosis

Aetiology

Rhinosporidiosis is a chronic granulomatous infection of the mucous membranes caused by *Rhinosporidium* spp. Molecular techniques have recently demonstrated that this organism is an aquatic protistan parasite. It is currently included in a new class, the Mesomycetozoea.

Epidemiology and geographical distribution

Infection is generally associated with exposure to stagnant water, ponds, lakes, or rivers, but is also suspected to occur from dust or air. Generally limited to mucosal epithelium, it usually manifests as vascular friable polyps that arise from the nasal mucosa or external structures of the eye. It is endemic in India and Sri Lanka although cases have been reported in South America, Africa and the USA. It is reported in many animals including dogs, cats, bullocks, cows, heifers, bulls and buffalo.

Life cycle and pathogenesis

The life cycle begins with a trophocyte which will grow until it reaches about 50 μm in diameter. From that moment on, the nucleus undergoes a series of mitotic divisions. From about the seventh division, when the developing trophocyte is 100 μm in diameter and contains 128 nuclei, the envelope of the trophocyte is thickened by a deposit of cellulose which increases its total thickness to 8–9 μm over most of its surface and 15 μm at the site of the future spore. By the 14th division the sporangium is about 140 μm in diameter and contains 16,000 round endospores, each approximately 3 μm in diameter. Infection is initiated with the release of endospores into a host's tissues from its spherical sporangia. However, little is known about the mechanisms of sporangium formation and endospore release since this pathogen is intractable to culture. Infection usually results from a local traumatic inoculation with the organism. The disease progresses with the local replication of parasite and associated hyperplastic growth of host tissue and a localized immune response. The infection affects nasal mucous membranes and ocular conjunctivae of humans and animals, producing slowly growing masses that degenerate into polyps. The symptoms vary depending upon the stage of tumour development and site infected. The polyps are usually pink to purple and friable.

Pathological findings

Pathology is typically limited to the mucosal epithelium. Infection usually results from a local traumatic inoculation with the organism. Infection of the nose and nasopharynx, conjunctivae or associated structures is observed with structures of the mouth and upper airway may be sites of disease. Disease of the skin, ear, genitals, and rectum has also been described. Dissemination of infection can occur.

Clinical features

Nasal disease may present with unilateral nasal obstruction or epistaxis. Other symptoms may include local pruritus, coryza, rhinorrhea, and postnasal discharge. Eye involvement is initially asymptomatic. Increased tearing may be reported as the disease progresses. Photophobia, redness, and secondary infection may occur. Skin lesions begin as papillomas that gradually become verrucous. Soft polyps may develop on the nose or eye. These polyps are pink to deep red, are sessile or pedunculated, and are often described as strawberry-like in appearance. Because the polyps of rhinosporidiosis are vascular and friable, they bleed easily upon manipulation. This appearance results from sporangia, which is visible as grey or yellow spots in the vascular polypoid masses.

Diagnosis

Diagnosis is made by demonstrating organism on microscopic examination of smears of macerated tissue using Gomori methenamine silver, periodic acid–Schiff, as well as with standard haematoxylin and eosin staining.

Treatment

There is no recommended treatment. Local surgical excision is often successful in treating the disease.

Control

Avoid exposure to stagnant water.

Public health implications

Humans can be affected with this disease, but there is no evidence that supports the possibility of transmission of *Rhinosporidium* from animals to people. Humans and dogs become infected from common environmental sources.

Sarcosporidiosis

Aetiology

Sarcosporidiosis is caused by species of intracellular protozoan parasite, *Sarcocystis*.

Epidemiology and geographical distribution

Source of infection is faeces of carnivore, primarily farm dogs and cats fed raw meat or other carnivores if they have access to ruminant carcasses. It has been reported in the majority of vertebrates, birds and reptiles, worldwide.

Life cycle and pathogenesis

Sarcocystis spp. have an obligatory two-host life cycle with carnivores as definitive hosts and mostly omnivores or herbivores as intermediate hosts (Fig. 7.13). Intermediate hosts are infected following ingestion of water or food contaminated with sporocysts from the faeces of a carnivore. After ingestion, sporocysts penetrate the host's intestinal wall and proliferate in vascular endothelium before disseminating haematogenously. Dissemination leads to invasion of skeletal and cardiac muscle. Because humans are not typically preyed on, these cysts are not given the opportunity to progress through their typical life cycle and eventually disintegrate within the muscle. Definitive hosts are infected following ingestion of meat contaminated by infective oocysts. After ingestion, the oocysts sexually reproduce and mature in the intestinal tract. Infective oocysts are then shed via the stool (enteritis). The protozoa are in cysts within the myofibre and thus are protected from the body's surveillance. Hence, there is slight or no inflammatory response.

Pathological findings

Infected animals show non-suppurative encephalitis with neurological signs. Non-suppurative encephalitis, myocarditis, and hepatitis are observed in aborted foetus. In chronic cases, cysts are observed in carcass, while anaemia and elevated blood concentrations of enzymes associated with tissue damage is observed in acute disease.

Clinical features

Severity of disease is dose dependent. The vast majority of infections are subclinical, but the disease may become clinically

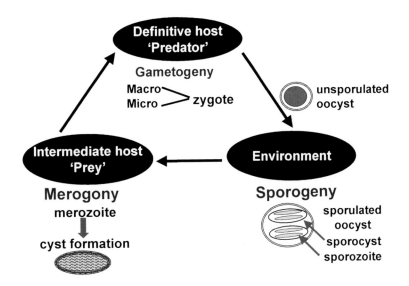

Figure 7.13 General life cycle of *Sarcocystis* sp.

apparent with sudden, overwhelming exposure to the parasite in a naïve animal. Reduced food intake, vomiting, diarrhoea, and depressed growth rate may be observed. Neurological disease and ataxia is common in sheep. Severe infection with some species results in carcass condemnation.

Diagnosis

The diagnosis requires demonstration of parasites microscopically in biopsy or post-mortem material. Sporocysts of different *Sarcocystis* spp. have an almost identical morphology, making it virtually impossible to distinguish between species. Molecular methods using PCR and serology-based assays are necessary to further identify the *Sarcocystis* oocysts at the species level.

Treatment

There is no specific treatment; however, the use of amprolium, monensin, or salinomycin may limit the infection.

Control

The farm dogs and cats should not be fed raw meat, together with proper disposal of carcasses and protecting the food supply of ruminants should help control this infection.

Public health implications

Humans can be infected with some *Sarcocystis* spp. following ingestion of the cysts in raw or undercooked infected meat. Individuals who practice poor hand hygiene, thus exposing themselves to faecal–oral transmission, are also at an increased risk of acquiring this infection. Metronidazole and cotrimoxazole have been used in eosinophilic myositis, although no specific outcomes have been studied. In one reported case, infection was treated with cotrimoxazole. Corticosteroids can be used to reduce inflammation associated with muscular involvement.

Theileriosis – Mediterranean coast fever

Aetiology

Theileriosis is a tick-borne disease caused by protozoan pathogen, *Theileria* spp.

Epidemiology and geographical distribution

It is an endemic disease of cattle, water buffalo, sheep, goats, wild animals and ruminants with a worldwide distribution. Disease is transmitted from infected animals to susceptible hosts via bite of the ticks (*Hyalomma* spp., *Rhipicephalus* spp., *Amblyomma* spp.).

Life cycle and pathogenesis

Theileria sporozoites are transmitted to animals in the saliva of the feeding tick. Inside the mammalian host, *Theileria* sporozoites undergo a complex life cycle involving the replication of schizonts in leucocytes and piroplasms in erythrocytes. Cattle that recover from *Theileria* infections usually become carriers for months or years. Iatrogenic transmission can also occur via blood (e.g. on re-used needles). Similar to East Coast fever, the damage is caused by both schizonts and piroplasms.

Pathological findings

Infected animals show anaemia and jaundice. Post-mortem examination show petechial and ecchymotic haemorrhages on the serosal surfaces of internal organs, and the body cavities may contain serous fluid. In acutely infected animals, the lymph nodes are usually enlarged and may be oedematous and haemorrhagic. The gastrointestinal tract can have signs of haemorrhagic enteritis, particularly in the small intestine. For East Coast Fever, pathological findings include pulmonary oedema, hydrothorax, hydropericardium, emaciation, haemorrhages, lymphadenopathy.

Clinical features

Clinical symptoms include fever, lymphadenopathy, wasting, anaemia and jaundice. Petechiae and ecchymoses may be found on the conjunctiva and oral mucous membranes. For east coast fever, clinical symptoms include fever, enlarged superficial lymph nodes, dyspnoea, wasting and diarrhoea.

Diagnosis

The diagnosis requires demonstration of schizonts in macrophages and lymphocytes especially in liver smears; piroplasms in erythrocytes. For east coast fever, demonstration of schizonts in lymphoblasts, and piroplasms in erythrocytes is needed. It should be differentiated from babesiosis, anaplasmosis, trypanosomiasis. ELISA and PCR-based assays have been developed for rapid diagnosis. It should be differentiated from babesiosis, anaplasmosis, trypanosomiasis, and malignant catarrhal fever.

Treatment

Early diagnosis with appropriate antimicrobial (buparvaquone) is effective. For East Coast fever, limited success has been observed with halofuginone, parvoquone and tetracyclines.

Control

In endemic areas, the tick burden should be decreased with acaricides and other methods of tick control such as rotational grazing. The transfer of blood between animals must also be avoided. Attenuated vaccine is available for this infection.

Public health implications

There is no information on theileriosis as a zoonotic disease.

Trichomoniasis

Aetiology

Trichomoniasis is a venereal disease of cattle, characterized primarily by early pregnancy loss and, occasionally, by abortion and pyometra. The causative agent is *Tritrichomonas foetus*.

Epidemiology and geographical distribution

The organism causes abortion in cattle. The bull acts as a carrier, with the parasite living on the surface of the penis or in the prepuce. When transmitted by coitus to the cow, the organism develops in the vagina and uterus, causing abortion or fetal resorption. Trichomoniasis has a worldwide distribution and is a major cause of infertility in naturally bred cattle in many countries.

Life cycle and pathogenesis

Parasite multiples by binary fission; consequently, large populations can be generated in a short period (Fig. 7.14). There are no cysts or any sexual stages known. Parasite is confined to all regions of the reproductive tract. In cows, the trophozoites attach to the surfaces of epithelial cells lining the reproductive tract and can be found in secretions from these sites, including the mild mucopurulent discharge associated with vaginitis and endometritis. Bulls carry the protozoa only on the penis and preputial membranes. Parasite does not affect either semen quality or sexual behaviour. A scant purulent preputial discharge may be noted within the first 2 weeks of infection, but generally, the infected bull serves as an asymptomatic carrier of the parasite. Older bulls tend to become permanent carriers of *T. foetus*, perhaps as a result of the development of epithelial crypts in the preputial cavity of older bulls. The pathogenesis of pregnancy loss is not yet well understood. A likely cause of abortion is the direct cytotoxic insult of maternal endometrium and/or fibroblasts and the fetal chorionic trophectoderm. Another potential virulence factor is the battery of extracellular cysteine proteinases that are elaborated by *T. foetus*. At physiological pH, these enzymes are very active against a wide variety of proteins including immunoglobulin, fibronectin and lactoferrin.

Pathological findings

The degree of autolysis in foetuses and placentas can vary from mild to marked. Placentas are oedematous, but otherwise unremarkable. Fetuses may have no discernible lesions; however, enlarged livers and non-inflated, enlarged, firm lungs may be present on some foetuses. Emphysematous bullae involving the splenic and hepatic capsules and the parietal peritoneum have been reported.

Clinical features

Overt clinical signs are rare as the apparent infertility due to embryonic death is the most common result. Pyometra and abortion often are the first signs of trichomoniasis noticed in a herd, but they occur in relatively few animals. When abortion occurs, it is usually within the first third to one-half of gestation.

Diagnosis

Because infection is inapparent in bulls and mild vaginitis is found only occasionally in cows, a definitive diagnosis requires the identification of parasites in infected animals. *T. foetus* is best located in preputial or vaginal secretions and, to a lesser extent, amniotic, allantoic, or abomasal fluids from the infrequently aborted fetuses. Microscopically, *T. foetus* is a slender, pear-shaped organism. A positive diagnosis requires demonstration of the organism in one or more infected animals. Diagnosis of bull consists of checking the breeding records and determining which bulls are infected.

Treatment

There is no recommended treatment; however, dimetridazole has been shown to be effective.

Control

Control necessitates resting the cows and allowing immunity to develop, treatment or elimination of infected bulls, and purchase of virgin bulls for breeding.

Artificial insemination can significantly reduce the infection, if appropriate procedures for bull testing and hygiene are practiced. The available vaccine (Trich Guard-Fort Dodge) is partially efficacious in the cow, but has no known efficacy in the bull.

Public health implications

Tritrichomonas foetus may also be an important cause of diarrhoea in cats. It can infect and colonizes the large intestine, and can cause prolonged and intractable diarrhoea. As a precaution, people in contact with infected cats are advised to take basic hygiene precautions to avoid ingesting the parasite. These precautions will also help to prevent the spread of the infection to other cats. *T. foetus* can produce disseminated infection in immunosuppressed individuals. The infected individual exhibited epididymitis and meningoencephalitis.

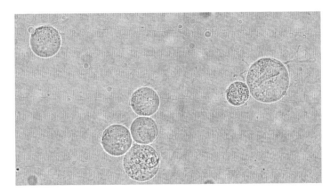

Figure 7.14 Microscopic observation of *T. vaginalis*. A small drop of fresh culture placed on a glass slide with 50% ethanol and visualized under the microscope (100×). (Credit: Bibhuti N. Singh and John. J. Lucas of SUNY Upstate Medical University, and Raina E. Fichorova of Harvard Medical School.)

Toxoplasmosis

Aetiology
Toxoplasmosis is a parasitic disease caused by *Toxoplasma gondii*.

Epidemiology and geographical distribution
The parasite infects most genera of warm-blooded animals, including humans, but the primary host is the felid (cat) family. Animals are infected by eating infected meat, or by ingestion of faeces of a cat with a worldwide distribution. Direct infection from handling cats is generally believed to be very rare.

Life cycle and pathogenesis
It is an important cause of abortion in ewes. Cats and other felidae are the definitive host where the mature parasite divides sexually in the intestinal mucosa (Fig. 7.15). Humans, dogs, cats, and many mammals become intermediate hosts following accidental ingestion of fertile oocysts shed in cat faeces. Fetuses can be infected transplacentally. Swine and rodents can acquire infection from ingestion of tissue stages of the parasite in carrion. Toxoplasmosis is often triggered by immunosuppression. Cats excrete the pathogen in their faeces for a number of weeks after contracting the disease, generally by eating an infected rodent.

Pathological findings
Granulomatous lesions in organs of all species, with abortions, placentitis, and focal necrotic lesions in brain, liver, and kidney of aborted foetus. Microscopically, variable degree of necrosis, haemorrhage, and leucocytic response, with a significant infiltrate of eosinophils.

Clinical features
Abortion and stillbirths in ewes is the major clinical manifestation. Other signs include encephalitis, pneumonia, and neonatal mortality. Ocular manifestation of toxoplasmosis has been described in many animal species, but especially in the cat. The role of *T. gondii* in causing anterior uveitis is controversial, since the parasites have not been identified in the globes.

Diagnosis
The diagnosis requires demonstration of parasite in tissues using immunohistochemistry, serology and/or PCR.

Treatment
Sulfamethazine and pyrimethamine can be used in abortion outbreaks.

Control
Control measures should include reduced exposure to oocysts (e.g. cats should not be allowed to defecate feed and by keeping

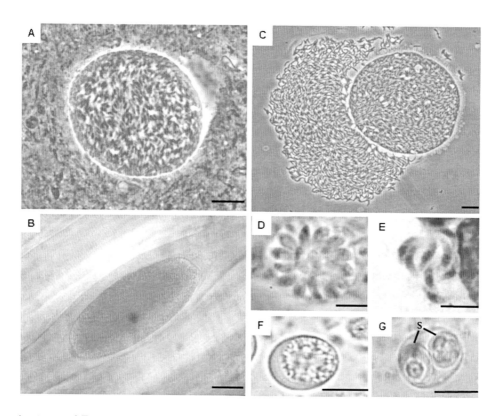

Figure 7.15. Life cycle stages of *T. gondii*. Scale bar 10 µm. (A) Tissue cyst in the brain of an infected mouse containing hundreds of bradyzoites. (B) Tissue cyst in a muscular cell of an infected mouse. Note the elongated aspect of the cyst. (C) Tissue cyst liberating hundreds of bradyzoites after pepsin digestion. Phase contrast. (D) Colonies of tachyzoites inside a fibroblast. Phase contrast. (E) Extracellular tachyzoites. Giemsa stain. (F) Unsporulated oocyst in cat faeces. (G) Sporulated oocyst with two sporocysts (S), each containing four sporozoites and a residual body. (Credit: Dardé Marie-Laure, Aubert Dominique, Derouin Francis, Dumètre Aurélien, Pelloux Hervé, Villena Isabelle, Trends Parasitol *18*, 355–359.)

food and water away from cats). In pregnant sheep, prophylactic feeding of monensin, decoquinate, and vaccination may have beneficial effects.

Public health implications

Highly zoonotic mainly via ingestion of infected meat and if the immune system is weak, it can result in congenital toxoplasmosis and can result in disseminated infection affecting the heart, liver, and the brain.

Trypanosomiasis – Nagana or African trypanosomiasis

Aetiology

Nagana or African trypanosomiasis is a disease of vertebrate animals, caused by several species of protozoan pathogen *Trypanosoma* (Table 7.1).

Epidemiology and geographical distribution

It is an endemic disease of all mammals in tropical Africa, as well as Central and South America but of greatest economic importance in cattle. The reservoir of parasites in wild populations of mammals is large, and the disease remains difficult to control. Some breeds of cattle, notably the N'Dama, a West African *Bos taurus* breed, has shown resistance to nagana. This contrasts with the susceptibility shown by East African *Bos indicus* cattle such as the zebu.

Life cycle and pathogenesis

During a blood meal on the mammalian host, an infected tsetse fly (genus *Glossina*) injects metacyclic trypomastigotes into skin tissue. The parasites enter the lymphatic system and pass into the bloodstream. Inside the host, they transform into bloodstream trypomastigotes, and are carried to other sites throughout the body, reach other blood fluids (e.g. lymph, spinal fluid), and continue the replication by binary fission that lead to anaemia with or without tissue invasion. The tsetse fly becomes infected with bloodstream trypomastigotes when taking a blood meal on an infected mammalian host. In the fly's midgut, the parasites transform into procyclic trypomastigotes, multiply by binary fission, leave the midgut, and transform into epimastigotes. The epimastigotes reach the fly's salivary glands and continue multiplication by binary fission. These parasites undergo cyclical development in tsetse flies but they can also be transmitted mechanically by other biting flies.

Pathological findings

Not definitive but include pallor, emaciation and enlargement of liver, spleen and lymph nodes.

Clinical features

Clinical features include fever, apathy, pale mucous membranes, swollen lymph nodes, emaciation, weight loss, cachexia and death.

Table 7.1 Major species of the genus *Trypanosoma* and associated infections

Trypanosoma spp.	Host	Disease
T. brucei *T. congolense* *T. simiae*	Majority of vertebrates	Nagana (fever, weakness, lethargy, swollen lymph nodes, weight loss, anaemia and can be fatal)
		Transmitted by tsetse flies
		Diagnosis can be made by demonstrating parasites in blood
		Antimicrobials: samorin, berenil, ethidium
		Integrated methods involving tsetse fly control, prophylaxis, good husbandry and use of trypano-tolerant breeds. There is no vaccine available
T. evansi	Majority of vertebrates	Surra (fever, weakness, lethargy, enlargement of liver, spleen and lymph nodes, weight loss and anaemia
		Transmitted by horse-flies, and also by the vampire bat, *Desmodus rotundus*, in South America
		Diagnosis can be made by demonstrating parasites in blood
		Antimicrobials: samorin, berenil, ethidium
T. suis	Pigs, sheep, goats	Chronic form of Surra
		Transmitted by tsetse flies
T. equiperdum	Horses and other Equidae	Dourine or covering sickness (mainly genital signs including a mucopurulent urethral discharge, penile paralysis, but cutaneous and nervous signs can be found with 50–70% mortality
		Sexually transmitted (does not require a vector). The organism can be found in genital organs and secretions
		Diagnosis can be made by isolation of the organism
		Antimicrobials as for nagana but chronic cases unresponsive to trypanocides
		Control measures include elimination of reactors, control of breeding and movement of animals in affected areas or endemic countries

Diagnosis

The diagnosis can be made by demonstrating parasite in blood and progressive anaemia.

Treatment

Trypanocides such as isometamidium chloride (samorin), suramin, diminazene aceturate (berenil), homidium bromide (ethidium), and antrycide can have protective effects.

Control

Integrated methods involving tsetse fly control, prophylaxis, good husbandry and use of trypano-tolerant breeds will help limit this infection. There is no vaccine available.

Public health implications

Trypanosoma brucei is the causative agent of sleeping sickness in humans with fatal consequences.

Further reading

Aucott, J.N. and Ravdin, J.I. (1993). Amebiasis and 'nonpathogenic' intestinal protozoa. Infect. Dis. Clin. North Am. 7, 467–485.

Barr, S.C. (2009). Canine Chagas' Disease (American Trypanosomiasis) in North America. Vet. Clin. North Am. Small Anim. Pract. 39, 1055–1064.

Bondurant, R.H. (2005). Venereal diseases of cattle: natural history, diagnosis, and the role of vaccines in their control. Vet. Clin. North Am. Food Anim. Pract. 21, 383–408.

Corbeil, L.B. (1999). Immunization and diagnosis in bovine reproductive tract infections. Adv. Vet. Med. 41, 217–239.

Dubey, J.P. (2005). Neosporosis in cattle. Vet Clin North Am Food Anim Pract. 21, 473–483.

Dubey, J.P. and Lindsay, D.S. (2006). Neosporosis, Toxoplasmosis, and sarcocystosis in ruminants. Vet. Clin. North Am. Food Anim. Pract. 22, 645–671.

Dubey, J.P., Lindsay, D.S. and Lappin, M.R. (2009). Toxoplasmosis and other intestinal coccidial infections in cats and dogs. Vet. Clin. North Am. Small Anim. Pract. 39, 1009–1034.

Dubey, J.P., Lindsay, D.S., Saville, W.J., Reed, S.M., Granstrom, D.E. and Speer, C.A. (2001). A review of Sarcocystis neurona and equine protozoal myeloencephalitis (EPM). Vet. Parasitol. 95, 89–131.

Dubey, J. P., Speer, C. A., Fayer, R. (1989). Sarcocystosis of Animals and Man. CRC Press, Boca Raton, FL, USA.

Dubey, J.P., Schares, G., Ortega-Mora, L.M. (2007). Epidemiology and control of neosporosis and Neospora caninum. Clin. Microbiol. Rev. 20, 323–367.

Elsheikha, H.M. (2008). Congenital toxoplasmosis: priorities for further health promotion action. Publ. Health. 122, 335–353.

Elsheikha, H.M. (2009). Has Sarcocystis neurona Dubey et al., 1991 (Sporozoa: Apicomplexa: Sarcocystidae) cospeciated with its intermediate hosts? Vet Parasitol. 163, 307–314.

Elsheikha, H. and Khan, N. A. (2010). Protozoa traversal of the blood–brain barrier to invade the central nervous system. FEMS Microbiol. Rev. 34, 532–553.

Felleisen, R.S. (1999). Host–parasite interaction in bovine infection with Tritrichomonas fetus. Microbes Infect. 10, 807–816.

Holman, P.J. and Snowden, K.F. (2009). Canine Hepatozoonosis and Babesiosis, and Feline Cytauxzoonosis. Vet. Clin. North Am. Small Anim. Pract. 39, 1035–1053.

Hunfeld, K.P., Hildebrandt, A. and Gray, J.S. (2008). Babesiosis: recent insights into an ancient disease. Int. J. Parasitol. 38, 1219–1237.

Jolley, W.R. and Bardsley, K.D. (2006). Ruminant Coccidiosis. Vet. Clin. North Am. Food Anim. Pract. 22, 613–621.

Khan, N. A. (2006). Acanthamoeba: biology and increasing importance in human health. FEMS Microbiol. Rev.30, 564–595.

Khan, N. A. (2008). Acanthamoeba and blood–brain barrier: the breakthrough. J. Med. Microbiol. 57, 1051–1057.

Khan, N. A. (2008). Emerging Protozoan Pathogens, Taylor & Francis.

Khan, N. A. (2008). Microbial Pathogens and Human Diseases, Science Publishers.

Khan, N. A. (2009). Acanthamoeba: Biology and Pathogenesis, Caister Academic Press.

Matin, A., Siddiqui, R., Jayasekera, S. and Khan, N. A. (2008). Increasing importance of Balamuthia mandrillaris. Clinic. Microbiol. Rev. 21, 435–448.

O'Handley, R. M., Olson, M.E. (2006). Giardiasis and cryptosporidiosis in ruminants. Vet. Clin. North Am. Food Anim. Pract. 22, 623–643.

Payne, P.A. and Artzer, M. (2009). The biology and control of Giardia spp. and Tritrichomonas fetus. Vet. Clin. North Am. Small Anim. Pract. 39, 993–1007.

Rae, D.O. and Crews, J.E. (2006). Tritrichomonas fetus. Vet. Clin. North Am. Food Anim. Pract. 22, 595–611.

Rosenblatt, J.E. (2009). Laboratory diagnosis of infections due to blood and tissue parasites. Clin. Infect. Dis. 49, 1103–1108.

Schuster, F.L. and Ramirez-Avila, L. (2008). Current world status of Balantidium coli. Clin. Microbiol. Rev. 21, 626–638.

Schwebke, J.R. and Burgess, D. (2004). Trichomoniasis. Clin. Microbiol. Rev. 17, 794–803.

Scorza, A.V., Lappin, M.R. (2004). Metronidazole for the treatment of feline giardiasis. J. Feline Med. Sun. 6, 157–160.

Siddiqui, R. and Khan, N. A. (2008). Balamuthia amoebic encephalitis: an emerging disease with fatal consequences. Microb. Pathog. 44, 89–97.

Smith, H., Nichols, R.A. (2006). Zoonotic protozoa—food for thought. Parasitologia. 48, 101–104.

Stramer, S.L., Hollinger, F.B., Katz, L.M., Kleinman, S., Metzel, P.S., Gregory, K.R. and Dodd, R.Y. (2009). Emerging infectious disease agents and their potential threat to transfusion safety. Transfusion 49, 1S–29S.

Tan, K.S. (2008). New insights on classification, identification, and clinical relevance of Blastocystis spp. Clin. Microbiol. Rev. 21, 639–665.

Uilenberg, G. (2006). Babesia—a historical overview. Vet. Parasitol. 138, 3–10.

Vial, H.J. and Gorenflot, A. (2006). Chemotherapy against babesiosis. Vet. Parasitol. 138, 147–160.

Section IV

Diseases Associated with Arthropods

8

Diseases Caused by Insects

Heinz Sager and Hany M. Elsheikha

Gasterophilus infestation

Aetiology

- *Gasterophilus intestinalis*: common horse bot
- *Gasterophilus nasalis*: throat botfly
- *Gasterophilus haemorrhoidalis*: nose botfly.

Adults are brown, hairy and bee-like, about 18 mm long, with one pair of wings. The reddish mature larva (bot) is 2 cm long. The narrow hooked anterior end tapers from a broad, rounded body. There is a single row of spines per segment on *Gastrophilus nasalis* larvae, and two rows per segment on *G. intestinalis* and *G. haemorrhoidalis*.

Epidemiology and geographical distribution

G. intestinalis and *G. nasalis* are common in most parts of the world where horses are raised. *G. haemorrhoidalis* is less common. *G. intestinalis* and *G. nasalis* are the main species present in Western Europe.

Life cycle and pathogenesis

Larvae over winter attached to the mucosa of the stomach of the host and can be so numerous that the stomach tissue cannot be seen. In late winter or early spring they release their hold and are passed in the faeces. The larvae burrow into the ground and pupate. The adults emerge in 3–10 weeks, depending on temperature. Egg laying begins in early summer. The female flies dart onto the horse and cement eggs singly onto individual hairs. Eggs of the three major species differ in colour and placement. *G. intestinalis* lays pale yellow eggs on the forelegs and shoulders, up to 1000 per female fly. Moisture and friction from the horse licking itself cause the eggs to hatch in about 7 days. *G. nasalis* lays about 500 yellow eggs around the chin and throat, which hatch in a week without stimulation. The female *G. haemorrhoidalis* lays 150 black eggs around the lips of the horse, which hatch in 2–3 days. After hatching, *G. intestinalis* larvae are licked into the host's mouth, but *G. nasalis* and *G. haemorrhoidalis* larvae burrow under the skin to the mouth. After a month wandering in the mucosa of the tongue

and cheeks, the larvae of all three species migrate to the stomach, where they moult into third instars, which can remain attached to the stomach and intestine for 8–10 months.

Pathological findings

The burrowing first- and second-stage *Gatsrophilus* larvae in the tissues of the tongue and mouth may result in tunnelling production associated with various pathological lesions, which are dependent on the degree of larval burrowing behaviour and the healing process. The attachment of third-stage larvae causes ulceration at the site of attachment with fibrosis. The cephalic portion of embedded larvae may found surrounded by a cellular exudate infiltrated with red blood cells and inflammatory cells.

Clinical features

Gasterophilus infestation is associated with impaired swallowing, gastrointestinal ulcerations, haemorrhage, gut obstructions or volvulus, rectal prolapse, anaemia, diarrhoea, and digestive disorders. High-intensity larval infestations have been implicated in gastric ulceration and rupture, intramural gastric suppuration, peritonitis following gastroduodenal perforation, and gastro-oesophageal reflux. Immature *G. nasalis* may burrow into the spaces around the teeth and can cause necrosis of the gums. The annoyance from adult flies may be of more significance than the presence of bot larvae in the stomach. Deposition of eggs by adult flies causes nervousness. Horses may stand with their chins and lips against the flanks of other animals for protection from the flies.

Diagnosis

Myiasis in horses is commonly detected by the visual inspection of larvae at slaughter, observation of eggs on the hair of the horses or third instars in the rectum of the horses or in their faeces. Eggs may be identified by colour and site, and larvae by the arrangement of the spines.

Treatment

Trichlorphon and dichlorvos have been commonly used to treat this parasite. The broad-spectrum macrocytic lactones, e.g. ivermectin and moxidectin, are also effective.

Control

Removal of eggs by frequent grooming and providing shelter from *Gastrophilus* flies will help control these parasites. Regular treatment with ivermectin is necessary to provide good control of the bot fly.

Public health implications

There are a few reports of human myiasis associated with *Gasterophilus* larvae causing subcutaneous crawling or ophthalmo-myiasis.

Flea infestation

Aetiology

Fleas are small (about 6 mm long), bilaterally compressed, wingless, blood-sucking insects. Males are generally smaller than females. They are the most common cause of skin disease in dogs and cats worldwide. The flea species commonly found on companion animals are *Ctenocephalides felis* (the cat flea), *Ctenocephalides canis* (the dog flea), and *Spilopsyllus cuniculi* (the rabbit flea). The cat flea, *C. felis*, is found worldwide on many wild and domesticated animal species, and is the most common flea of dogs and cats in Europe and the USA. *C. canis* also may parasitise both dogs and cats, but it is less prevalent than *C. felis*. The rabbit flea, *S. cuniculi* is found naturally on rabbits and hares, but rarely on dogs or cats. It has a worldwide distribution and acts as a carrier of myxomatosis virus and other pathogens.

Epidemiology and geographical distribution

Fleas are widely distributed but are much more common in warm, humid environments. In Temperate climates, fleas are only a problem during the warmer summer months. In warmer climates, fleas can cause disease all year round. Fleas are vector of other organism like tapeworms. The presence of segments of *Dipylidium caninum* in the perianal area of the animal or in faeces indicates the presence of fleas.

Life cycle and pathogenesis

The metamorphosis of the flea includes the egg, larva, pupa and adult stages (Fig. 8.1). Three of the four stages of the flea's life cycle are spent off the host. Development of the immature flea stages take place in the pet's environment, particularly in areas where the animal lies. When environmental conditions are favourable, fleas have a great reproductive potential. The life cycle can be completed, from hatching of an egg to the laying of the next generation of eggs, in up to 28 days under optimal conditions. Fleas are not host specific and can attack other animals and humans.

Pathological findings

Non-specific pattern of superficial to deep eosinophil-rich perivascular to interstitial dermatitis.

Clinical features

Non-flea allergic animals may have fleas but show no dermatological signs. Flea allergic animals show itching, irritation, acute pruritus, erythema, and dermatitis. Anaemia occurs particularly in puppies and kittens. Dermatitis may results in crusty lesions.

Diagnosis

History of exposure, clinical signs, and finding of adult fleas or their droppings (Fig. 8.2). A wet paper test allows visualization

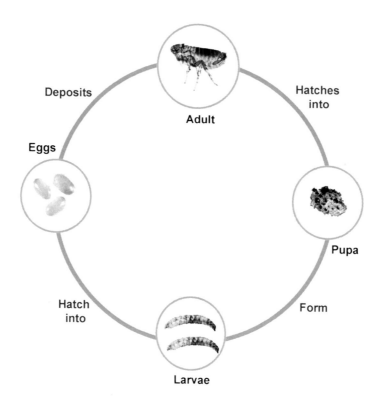

Figure 8.1 Stages of the life cycle of fleas.

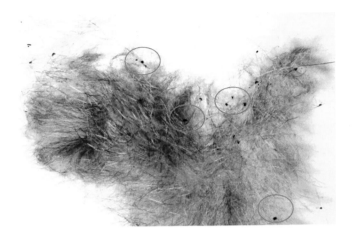

Figure 8.2 Flea dirt (circled) in the fur of a cat.

of pet's partly digested blood in flea faeces, which produces red streaks from haemoglobin present in the flea dirt when the coat is brushed onto wet paper. However, identification of fleas or flea 'dirt' may be difficult especially in a cat that is over grooming or a dog that is being regularly shampooed. Intradermal allergy or *in vitro* allergy testing with flea antigens. Flea infestation should be differentiated from food allergy, atopy, pediculosis, cheyletiellosis, demodicosis, dermatophytosis, superficial pyoderma, and alopecia.

Treatment
Fleas are amenable to treatment with several compounds. All topical insecticides should be used according to label directions. In general, the use of organophosphate preparations on puppies younger than 16 weeks or on kittens younger than 6 months should be avoided. Any product containing lufenuron, fipronil or imidicloprid as its active ingredient should not be administered to or used on nursing animals. Pyrethrin-based products are generally safe for frequent application.

Control
Successful flea control can be challenging. Topical treatments should be coordinated with in-home environmental flea control. Because most of the flea's life cycle is spent off the host, it is important to treat both the environment and the animal. The use of insecticides (compounds that contain chlorpyrifos, malathion, or diazinon as their active ingredient) labelled for outdoor flea control is still the best and most economical approach. Such approaches must incorporate repeated applications at 2-week intervals throughout the flea season where temperature and humidity are favourable for flea reproduction.

Public health implications
Humans can be infested with *C. felis*, causing itching, especially in sensitive people.

Flies

Aetiology
Gadflies (Tabanidae) belong to the order of Brachycera, while all flies of relevance for cattle are part of the order of Cyclorrhapha. These include flies of the family of Muscidae, as well as blowflies (Calliphoridae, Sarcophagidae and Oestridae), and bot flies (*Hypoderma*). Biting midges (Ceratopogonidae), blackflies (Simulidae) and mosquitoes (Culicidae) belong to the order Nematocera. These will be discussed separately in a later section.

Epidemiology and geographical distribution
Flies are mainly active during mild or warm climatic conditions, i.e. during summer. Larvae or pupae are able to hibernate. Under ideal conditions the development from egg to the adult stage may require 1–2 weeks, while the adult females may survive for 2–4 weeks. Flies are able to travel distances of several kilometres. Flies feed either on blood (b) or secretions (s). Most of them act as mechanical vectors of pathogens. Flies can be divided into species that are active in stables [like *Musca domestica* (s) (Fig. 8.3), *M. autumnalis* (s), *Stomoxys calcitrans* (b) (Fig. 8.4), *Fannia canicularis* (s)] and on pastures [like the Tabanidae (b), *Hydrotaea irritans* (s), *Haematobia irritans* (b) (Fig. 8.5) and *H. stimulans* (b)].

Life cycle and pathogenesis
The adult females lay eggs in organic material, like dung. Of special interest are blowflies, which deposit their eggs or larvae in carcasses and meat, but also in exposed or soiled wounds. The larvae may moult several times before they pupate. Several fly generations can be expected during a season, while Tabanidae and the head fly (*Hydrotea irritans*) in general only produce one generation per year. Myiasis is caused by blowfly larvae. The mechanical disruption of the tissue by mouth hooks and the production of proteolytic enzymes and toxins are responsible for signs like fever and increased respiratory frequency and heart rate. The migration under the skin accompanied by massive inflammatory reactions may lead to toxaemia and general exhaustion. In severe cases,

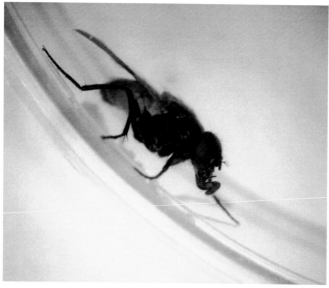

Figure 8.3 The house fly *Musca domestica* is a nuisance fly (5–8 mm). Its mouthparts allow licking-sucking food uptake.

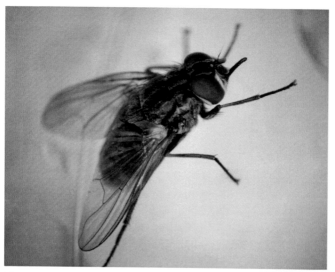

Figure 8.4 The stable fly *Stomoxys calcitrans* has piercing mouthparts. The stable fly has a size of 7–8 mm.

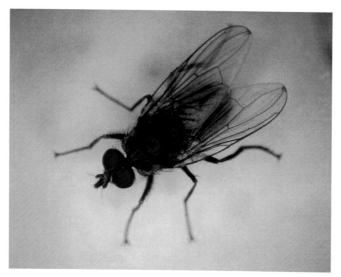

Figure 8.5 The horn fly *Haematobia irritans* has a size of 3–4 mm. The mouthparts consist of the proboscis and pedipalps and allow the uptake of blood.

when not treated on time, the animals may die. However, this is more often observed in sheep than in cattle.

Pathological findings

The lesions caused by gadflies and blood feeding flies are painful as they stab relatively deep into the skin ('pool feeder'). The saliva contains anticoagulant components which may cause local swelling. Mass attacks of gadflies may also cause considerable blood losses. Of major impact is the permanent disturbance of the animals, resulting in reduced food uptake, weight and production losses. The mechanical transmission of pathogens is important, especially in milk-producing animals, where mastitis may be due to the presence of flies.

Clinical features

Gadflies and blood feeding flies cause painful skin lesions and the salivary excretions may cause local swelling. High numbers of flies may cause blood loss and weight and production losses. Blowflies cause myiasis, i.e. the deposition of eggs or larvae in wounds, fleece or heavily soiled and folded skin sites. The larvae feed on necrotic tissue, lymph and plasma proteins. Infection is accompanied by fever, increased respiratory frequency and heart rate, absence of appetite and apathy. Flies may act as vectors of pathogens like viruses, bacteria (e.g. *Hydrotaea irritans* is responsible for the transmission of *Corynebacterium pyogenes* and *Streptococcus dysgalactiae*, the causative agents of 'summer mastitis'), protozoan and filarial parasites. Either on pasture or in stables, cattle may show nervousness; or in the case of blood feeding flies bleeding stab wounds. In the case of myiasis, the animals show fever, tachypnoea and tachycardia, anorexia and apathy.

Diagnosis

Flies may be found easily on the animals. Myiasis is more difficult to diagnose. An accurate examination of the animal for presence of lesions is indispensable. Larvae can be collected and sent to specialized laboratories for species differentiation (based on key morphological criteria, such as the morphological appearance of the stigmatic plates of the third-stage larvae). *Cochliomyia hominivorax* (New World screw-worm fly) is diagnosed based on the presence of pigmentation of the tracheal trunks. If no flies are found on the animals, other blood feeding parasites, namely mosquitoes may be considered. In the case of myiasis with lacking history of fly infestation, viral or bacterial infections causing fever and bad general condition need to be excluded.

Treatment

Treatment is usually applied topically. Treatment of cutaneous myiasis requires the mechanical removal of all larvae – if possible – from the wound followed by local treatment with an insecticide (e.g. an organophosphate or synthetic pyrethroid). Additional symptomatic treatment against the effects of toxins and potential bacterial secondary infections are required in most cases. Although growth regulators like cyromazine or dicyclanil for the control of blowflies are registered only for sheep, their use might be envisaged for cattle in high-risk situations (off-label use, please refer to the local authorities).

Control

Effective fly control on pasture is difficult. Repellents can be used and may result in reduced fly numbers. In most cases pyrethroids are used as pour on, spray on or ear tags. Anthelmintic treatment with macrocyclic lactones seems to result in a partial reduction of the fly burden, at least of blood feeding flies. In case of severe problems, the animals should be placed on pasture during the night and put into stable for the day. The control of flies in stables should be based on good hygiene (elimination of breeding sites) and on the use of growth inhibitors, e.g. spinosad or lambda-cyhalothrin. The fight against adult flies is relatively inefficient, but traps (adhesive strips) and fly screens still may help to reduce the burden. Procedures such as docking and castration should be performed before the fly season; dead carcasses should be disposed of hygienically.

Public health implications

Gadflies and flies are pests for humans. In rare cases problems may occur due to deposition of eggs on the conjunctivae (ophthalmomyiasis). The larvae normally die within one week, but need to be removed surgically.

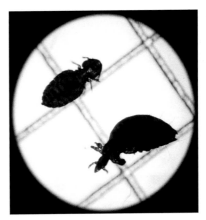

Figure 8.6 Adult biting lice of *Bovicola bovis* spp.

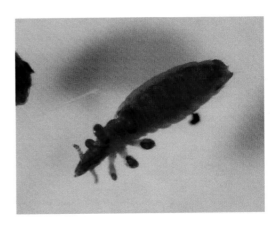

Figure 8.7 *Linognathus vituli* is a blood-sucking louse; the head has a smaller diameter than the thorax.

Table 8.1 Louse species on domestic animals

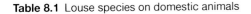

Cattle

Bovicola bovis, chewing
Haematopinus eurysternus, sucking
Haematopinus quadripertusus, sucking
Linognathus vituli, sucking
Solenopotes capillatus, sucking

Buffalo

Haematopinus tuberculatus, sucking

Sheep

Bovicola ovis, chewing
Linognathus africanus, sucking
Linognathus ovillus, sucking
Linognathus pedalis, sucking

Horses

Bovicola equi, chewing
Haematopinus asini, sucking

Dogs

Linognathus setosus, sucking
Linognathus piliferus, sucking
Trichodectes canis, chewing

Cats

Felicola subrostratus, chewing

Louse infestation (pediculosis)

Aetiology

Domesticated animals are commonly infested with lice of the orders Anoplura (sucking lice) and Mallophaga (chewing lice) (Table 8.1). Lice are insects spending the whole life cycle in the fur/hair/wool of different animal species. Whereas chewing lice *Bovicola bovis* (Fig. 8.6) feed on debris of hair and epidermis, sucking lice feed on blood. Three major species of the latter are of relevance for cattle: *Haematopinus eurysternus*, *Linognathus vituli* (Fig. 8.7) and *Solenoptes capillatus*.

Epidemiology and geographical distribution

The lice are highly host specific and are fully adapted to live continuously in/on the fur/hair of the host. Lice may be a problem year-round on dogs and cats but are more commonly a problem in the winter months on cattle, sheep, and horses. They can only survive a few days in the environment. Transmission occurs by direct contact between animals or via grooming equipment, harness or bedding. Infection peaks are found in late winter and early spring when animals are in the stable, while the infestation is drastically reduced during pasture season. Animals in poor condition that are kept together in large numbers and are not groomed regularly often have heavy burdens.

Life cycle and pathogenesis

Adult lice lay their operculated eggs, referred to as 'nits', cemented to the hair or wool of the host. The eggs hatch, and the small larvae are similar to the adults (incomplete metamorphosis). They develop into nymphs and then into adults; the entire life cycle requires 3–5 weeks, depending on the species.

Pathological findings

Gross lesions consist of papules, crusts, and secondary excoriations with lice and eggs visible on the lesions. Due to pruritus, affected animals start to scratch leading to abrasions and lesions in the skin that open the door for secondary bacterial infections. In severe cases the skin lesions may become purulent.

Clinical features

Light infection with lice may remain asymptomatic. Animals may show itching and uneasiness. Superficial abrasions may be caused by rubbing. A high louse burden is often linked with a pre-existing health problem. Therefore massive louse proliferation is normally observed solely on weakened and sick animals. Signs are pruritus, scaling and hair loss. Affected animals often loose weight. Anaemia occurs in extremely high infestations by sucking lice. Typically calves in a bad health status and with scrubby coat are presented (young animals are mainly infected with *Linognathus*, while older animals more often suffer from *Bovicola* and *Haematopinus*). The louse infestation is often a secondary problem due to a primary disease. In many cases only a few individuals show such drastic signs while lice might be detected on healthy animals only in low numbers and accidentally.

Diagnosis

This can be made by a through clinical examination. Lice and eggs can be detected by examination of the body surface eventually by use of a loupe (Fig. 8.8). The eggs have a shiny appearance and are attached to the hairs. Chewing species are fawn in colour and sucking lice become blue-black when they are filled with blood.

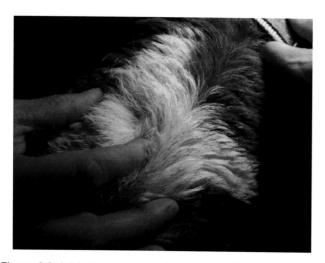

Figure 8.8 Adult lice as well as the eggs sticking to the hair of cattle's neck can be easily detected on the animals without special equipment. A good light and eventually a loupe may help to identify the parasites.

Dark coat may hamper the identification of lice. A differentiation between chewing and sucking lice can be easily made by comparing the head diameter to the thorax. Lice of the order Mallophaga have broad heads, and those of Anoplura have pointed heads. As mentioned above, severely affected animals often suffer from a primary disease which needs to be diagnosed and treated. Louse infestation has to be differentiated from mange, fungal and bacterial skin diseases.

Treatment

Treatment consists of dust, plunge-dips, pour-ons (backline treatments), spot-ons, sprays, sponge-on dips, or shampoos, depending on the host and environmental conditions. Successful treatment can be achieved with pyrethroids (pour on, spray on, washing) or with macrocyclic lactones (applied topically for both chewing and sucking lice and systemically for sucking lice). As eggs are not killed, pyrethroid-treatment needs to be repeated after 7–10 days. Macrocyclic lactone treatment may fail against infestation caused by the chewing lice because they are less exposed to the active ingredient compared with sucking lice. Residues in milk and meat have to be considered when treating. Existing underpinning conditions have to be treated accordingly.

Control

Compliant use of host-targeted louse control products, together with knowledge of louse life cycles, is necessary to control lice on the animal, in the home, and in outdoor environments. Bedding and grooming equipment from infested animals should be cleaned and disinfected.

Public health implications

None, the lice are very host specific.

Midges, mosquitoes

Aetiology

Mosquitoes belong to the order of Nematocera, which include three families of relevance for cattle: Culicidae (mosquitoes/gnats), Simulidae (blackflies) and Ceratopogonidae (biting midges).

Epidemiology and geographical distribution

Midges and mosquitoes have a worldwide distribution. All of them are blood-suckers and can act as vectors of diseases. The development of mosquitoes includes eggs, larvae and pupae before adults emerge. Environmental requirements are strongly dependent on the genera. Female mosquitoes, biting flies and blackflies require blood for their egg production. While mosquitoes (Culicidae) and biting midges (*Culicoides*) are mainly active at dusk and during night, blackflies (*Simulium*) can have its blood meals during the day.

Life cycle and pathogenesis

Mosquitoes (Culicidae), represented by the three genera *Aedes*, *Culex* and *Anopheles*, need still water for their life cycle. Females place their eggs on the water, while larvae and pupae are located under the water surface. Several generations of Culicidae may develop between spring and autumn. *Simulidae* attach their eggs to stones or plants in flowing oxygen-rich water. The eggs and life stages of *Culicoides* are adapted to water with rich plant life or a moist dung environment. Of major importance are mass attacks of Simulidae in spring on pastures near to streams or rivers, when the warm temperatures allow a fast development of the hibernating eggs or larvae.

Pathological findings
Especially after *Simulium* mass attacks generalized petechial bleeding and oedema may be observed on the chest, belly, udder, scrotum and perineum.

Clinical features
Mosquitoes are pests. The stab is painful and causes itching. Animals become anxious and may show local skin swelling, especially when exposed to mass attacks. Special attention has to be paid to large clusters of blackflies. Allergic reactions to toxins of the salivary gland may cause generalized petechial bleeding and oedema formation. In some cases death may occur due to a cardiovascular collapse. Diseases which might occur in Europe and which are transmitted by mosquitoes include bluetongue (Orbivirus, transmitted by the biting midges *Culicoides* sp.) and onchocercosis (*Onchocerca gutturosa*, transmitted by *Simulium* sp.). Many other viruses can be transmitted, especially arboviruses, of which the importance in many cases is not yet known. Cattle on pasture are mainly affected. Animals may show pruritus, petechiae and/or local inflammatory skin reactions. Due to anxiety, the animals may show loss in weight and milk production.

Diagnosis
Mosquitoes (Fig. 8.9) may be found on the animals (depending on the activity peak of the dominating genera). Mosquitoes may act as transmitter of various viral, bacterial or parasitic diseases which also need to be diagnosed. Lesions should be differentiated from those caused by infection with haematophageous flies, or caused by allergic reactions (atopy, food and flea).

Treatment
Chemotherapy with repellent active ingredients like pyrethroids may considerably reduce the parasite burden. These products are applied topically as pour on or spray on or as ear tags. The duration of protection is influenced by the weather as, for example, rainfall may shorten the length of protection, especially for pour on-treated animals.

Control
The ideal would be avoidance to exposure. This can be partially achieved by pasturing during day (to overcome infections predominated by Culicidae and Culicoides) or during the night (*Simulium*). However, in many cases this is not feasible or a mixed fly population is causing problems.

Public health implications
The public health significance of mosquitoes is great because mosquitoes are important vectors for severe diseases like malaria, yellow and Dengue fever and river blindness (onchocercosis). However, due to control and surveillance programmes and to climatic conditions in Europe, the major impact for humans is the local inflammatory reactions against mosquito bites.

Oestrus ovis infestation (sheep nasal flies)

Aetiology
Oestrus ovis (nasal bot) infestation is common in sheep, and occurs when the adult greyish *O. ovis* fly, about the size of a honeybee, emerges from spring through fall and deposits first-stage larvae around the nostrils of the sheep.

Epidemiology and geographical distribution
Oestrus ovis has worldwide distribution and is associated with a severe parasitosis of small ruminants, with emphasis especially in the Mediterranean areas of Europe and Africa. Although *O. ovis* is primarily a myiasis of sheep, it sporadically affects goats, dogs, and sometimes, humans especially shepherds. Goats are relatively resistant to *O. ovis* infection. The adult fly is active during warm months, and the parasite may overwinter for a period of time either as a first instar larva in the upper airways in the host or as a pupa in the ground to avoid climate extremes.

Life cycle and pathogenesis
The larva is the pathogenic stage of this parasite. The first instar larvae deposited on the nostrils of the sheep by adult flies migrate up the nasal passages into the sinuses, where they develop to become third instar larvae for weeks to months before being sneezed out onto the pasture to pupate. This type of parasitism in which living tissues are invaded by larvae of flies is known as myiasis. The adult fly has rudimentary mouthparts and is not able to feed; thus the larvae must ingest enough nutrients while in the host to support the life of the adult fly.

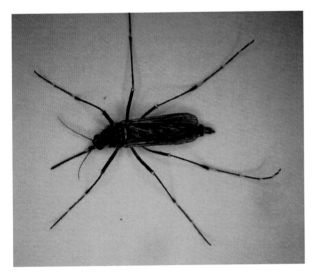

Figure 8.9 Female *Aedes* sp. with typically long antennae and piercing mouthparts.

Pathological findings

The larvae cause direct irritation to the nasal passages and sinuses, and this irritation may predispose animals to the development of secondary bacterial rhinitis, sinusitis, and/or pneumonia. Inhalation of parasite antigens can produce interstitial pneumonia.

Clinical features

Both larvae and adult stages can lead to decreased productivity by decreasing the time spent grazing by affected animals. Infestation of the nasal cavity with the larvae (bots) irritates the tissues, causing rhinitis, sneezing, mucopurulent nasal discharges, and obstruction of the airflow. Adult flies cause annoyance by flying around the heads of animals. Secondary bacterial infection and pneumonia may develop. Rarely, larvae of *O. ovis* penetrate the cranial vault through the ethmoidal plate, causing direct or secondary bacterial meningitis.

Diagnosis

Diagnosis is usually tentative, based on clinical signs. Diagnosis is based on the presence of these larvae in the nose or sinuses. Endoscopy is helpful in making a diagnosis. Bots of *O. ovis* can be found easily if the head is cut to expose the nasal passages. Third instar larvae are yellow-white in colour and have a dark dorsal-transverse stripe with rows of spines on the ventrum of each segment. Laterally, there are well-developed inter-segmental fleshy humps. Differential diagnosis to consider include nasal foreign bodies, fungal rhinitis, sinusitis, trauma, actinomycosis, actinobacillosis, allergic rhinitis, nasal adenocarcinoma, bluetongue disease or scrapie.

Treatment

Ivermectin is used in the late summer to prevent the build-up of heavy infestations and again in the winter to kill overwintering larvae.

Control

Control is aimed at regular strategic treatment with effective anthelmintics to prevent long-term infection with the larvae.

Public health implications

Humans can be incidentally infected, with conjunctival infection the most common form of disease in humans.

Warble flies (heel fly, hypodermosis)

Aetiology

Bovine hypodermosis is a myiasis caused by larvae of the bot flies *Hypoderma bovis* and *Hypoderma lineatum* (Diptera, Oestridae), and is characterized by cutaneous nodules (commonly called 'warbles' or 'grubs') under the skin in the dorsal and lumbar regions, mainly during spring and summer. Warble flies rarely lay their eggs on the horse, but larvae may migrate and reach the dorsum, and sometimes migrate to unusual locations.

Epidemiology and geographical distribution

This myiasis is widespread in the northern hemisphere: North America, i.e. Canada and USA, several European countries, such as Germany, Greece, Italy and Romania. Warble flies can be found in Central Europe from the beginning of January until the end of June, the third-stage larvae stay in the skin for 8–14 weeks. Due

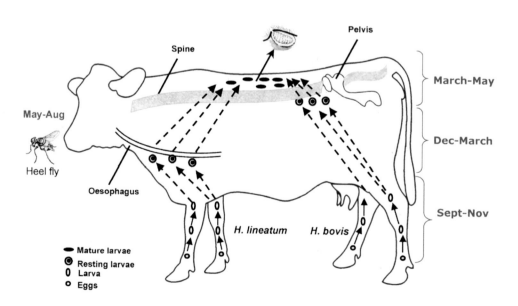

Figure 8.10 Life cycle of the warble fly (*Hypoderma* spp.).

to control measures, hypodermosis has been drastically reduced in many countries, while others like the UK are completely free of this disease. However, in Mediterranean countries, bot flies, dominated by *H. lineatum* are still common.

Life cycle and pathogenesis

The life cycle (Fig. 8.10) begins when the female bot flies deposit eggs on the hairs of cattle at pasture between May and September. While females of *H. bovis* may cause panic in cattle herds by the buzzing sound of their approach, this phenomenon is not known for *H. lineatum*. The further development of the hatched larvae differs between the two species: larvae of *H. bovis* penetrate the skin and migrate towards the vertebral column. They are normally found in the epidural fat tissue between early December to March. Then they continue their migration towards the skin of the back. They form the typical warble-like tumour – with a respiratory hole – inside which they mature to the third larval stage (L3), which leave the skin, fall on the ground and pupate. Within 2 weeks or up to 2 months they develop to the adult fly. The biology of *H. lineatum* is similar; however, the migration through the body does not include a stay in the epidural fat tissue. Larvae of *H. lineatum* are mainly found in the oesophagus (where they stay up to 7 months) before they reach the skin. Warble fly infestation is the cause of severe economic losses to the livestock industry as it can impair milk production, weight gain and hide quality.

Pathological findings

Migrating larvae of *H. bovis* do not cause any tissue damage, unless they get killed. This is of major importance when they are located in the epidural fat where an inflammatory reaction could cause severe neurological signs. In contrast, larvae of *H. lineatum* induce inflammatory processes, bleeding and oedema when migrating into the submucosa of the oesophagus. The further development of the larvae of both species in the subcutis of the back leads to fibrinous exudation, encapsulation and fistula formation (warble tumour). Microscopically, the larvae are located in a cavity filled with fibrin and a few eosinophils and bordered by granulation tissue containing clusters of eosinophils.

Clinical features

Warble tumours are the dominating finding of infection with bot flies. The painful swelling of the skin is filled with a larval stage. Immunosuppression (increasing the risk of mastitis, pneumonia and other infectious diseases) and production losses caused by hypodermosis are of economic relevance but are not specific for this disease. The warble tumours which are present between January and June are the most important finding. The tumours are painful and have a respiratory hole. Larvae can be pressed out of the pocket.

Diagnosis

Diagnosis can easily be done by the presence of warble tumours (subcutaneous nodule, often with a breathing pore) on the back of the animal. The lesions can be poulticed or surgically lanced to express the fly. Larvae can be identified and differentiated morphologically by their respiratory openings. A serological test (ELISA) can be used to identify infected animals during the body migration phase of the larvae. The early diagnosis allows a prophylactic treatment and prevents skin damage. Warble tumours need to be differentiated from any kind of skin lesions. However, the seasonality and the detection of fly larvae are pathognomonic.

Treatment

Organophosphates are about 89% effective if applied during the autumn, but less efficient for spring treatments. Treatment can be done with macrocyclic lactones, either as subcutaneous injection (0.2 mg/kg) or as pour-on (0.5 mg/kg). Larvae need to be mechanically removed from the warble tumours. Treatment with macrocyclic lactones needs to be done before December. Later treatment may cause severe problems due to the potential localization of the *H. bovis*-larvae in the epidural fat. If they are killed when at this site, they can stimulate a hypersensitivity reaction by the animal. This causes inflammation, swelling and pressure on the spine and may lead to paralysis of the hind legs.

Control

The economic importance due to damage of the skin and production losses has led to rigorous measures to control this parasite including restriction of animal movement on infected farms, prophylactic treatment in endemic areas, and treatment of imported cattle on arrival. In UK and Ireland both *Hypoderma* spp. have been eliminated and prophylactic treatment of imported cattle with avermectins prevents the re-introduction of this parasite.

Public health implications

None.

Acknowledgements

We would like to thank Dr Peter Bates, the director of Veterinary Medical Entomology Consultancy (VMEC), Surrey, England, for critical reading.

Further reading

Arther, R.G. (2009). Mites and lice: biology and control. Vet. Clin. North Am. Small Anim. Pract. 39, 1159–1171.

Blagburn, B L. and Dryden, M.W. (2009). Biology, Treatment, and Control of Flea and Tick Infestations. Vet. Clin. North Am. Small Anim. Pract. 39, 1173–1200.

Cortinas, R. and Jones, C.J. (2006). Ectoparasites of cattle and small ruminants. Vet. Clin. North Am. Food Anim. Pract. 22, 673–693.

Kwochka, K.W. (1987). Fleas and related disease. Vet. Clin. North Am. Small Anim. Pract. 17, 1235–1262.

Maroli, M. and Khoury, C. (2004). Prevention and control of leishmaniasis vectors: current approaches. Parassitologia. 46, 211–215.

Marsella, R. (1999). Advances in flea control. Vet. Clin. North Am. Small Anim. Pract. 29, 1407–1424.

Moriello, K.A. (2003). Zoonotic skin diseases of dogs and cats. Anim. Health Res. Rev. 4, 157–168.

Rust, M.K. (2005). Advances in the control of *Ctenocephalides felis* (cat flea) on cats and dogs. Trends Parasitol. 21, 232–236.

Rust, M.K. and Dryden, M.W. (1997). The biology, ecology, and management of the cat flea. Annu. Rev. Entomol. 42, 451–473.

Scheidt, V.J. (1988). Flea allergy dermatitis. Vet. Clin. North Am. Small Anim. Pract. 18, 1023–1042.

Stromberg, B.E. and Moon, R.D. (2008). Parasite control in calves and growing heifers. Vet. Clin. North Am. Food Anim. Pract. 24, 105–116.

Taylor, M.A. (2001). Recent developments in ectoparasiticides. Vet. J. 161, 253–268.

Diseases Caused by Acarines

Heinz Sager and Hany M. Elsheikha

Mite infestation

Overview

Mites are ectoparasites of a wide range of birds, domesticated and wild animal species. Some have a zoonotic significance. Mites are members of the phylum Arthropoda. The mites commonly found on domesticated animals are listed in Table 9.1. *Demodex* spp. and *Psorobia* spp. are host specific, and these species will not cross-infest other hosts. However mange mites (*Chorioptes* spp., *Psoroptes* spp. and *Sarcoptes* spp.) are no host specific and can cross-infest a large number of hosts. Mites live on the host continuously and infest other animals by contact. The life cycles of mites are all slightly different because some burrow, whereas others live on the surface of the skin. *Sarcoptes* spp. and *Notoedres cati* females burrow in the skin and deposit eggs. The eggs hatch into six-legged larvae, which develop and moult to eight-legged protonymphs and tritonymphs, which develop and moult into adults. The entire cycle requires 9–17 days.

Species of the genera *Chorioptes, Psoroptes, Psorergates, Otodectes* and *Cheyletiella* have similar life cycles except that they do not burrow to deposit eggs. *Demodex* spp. generally live in the hair follicles. Identification of mites is based on the morphological appearance of adults and generally requires a thorough skin scraping. Treatment consists of dusts, plunge-dips, pour-ons (backline treatments), sprays, sponge-on dips, shampoos or injections of macrocyclic lactones.

Demodectic mange (follicular mange)

Aetiology

Mites of *Demodex* spp. infest hair follicles of all species of domestic animals. The disease causes little concern but in cattle and goats there may be significant damage to the hide and, rarely, death may result from gross secondary bacterial invasion. Mites infesting the different host species are considered to be specific and are designated as *Demodex bovis* for cattle, *D. ovis* for sheep, *D. caprae* for goats, *D. equi* for horses, *D. phylloides* for pigs, and *D. canis* in dogs.

Epidemiology and geographical distribution

Demodicosis may occur worldwide in farm animals of any age, especially those in poor condition but most cases in cattle occur in adult dairy cattle in late winter and early spring. The entire life cycle is spent on the host. Adult mites invade the hair follicles and sebaceous glands, which become distended with mites and inflammatory exudates.

Life cycle and pathogenesis

The life cycle consists of the egg, larval and two nymphal stages. The disease spreads slowly and transfer of mites is thought to take place by contact, probably early in life. Calves can acquire mites from an infected dam in half a day. However in horses grooming instruments and rugs may transmit infection. Invasion of hair follicles and sebaceous glands leads to chronic inflammation; loss of the hair fibre and in many instances the development of secondary staphylococcal pustules or small abscesses. It is these

Table 9.1 Mite species of domestic animals

Psoroptes spp.	Found on the bodies of cattle, sheep and horses and the ears of sheep, horses, goats, and rabbits
Sarcoptes scabiei	Varieties are found on the bodies of cattle, sheep, horses, goats, swine, and dogs
Chorioptes spp.	Species occur on the bodies of cattle, sheep, goats, and rabbits
Psorobia spp.	Species occur on the bodies of cattle and sheep
Otodectes cynotis	Occurs in the ears of dogs, cats, and other related animals
Notoedres cati	Occurs on the heads of cats
Cheyletiella spp.	Occur on the bodies of dogs, cats, and rabbits
Demodex spp.	Occur in hair follicles of dogs, cats, cattle, sheep, humans, and horses

foci of infection that cause the small pinholes in the hide which interfere with its industrial processing as well as reducing its value dramatically.

Pathological findings

Grossly, localized demodecosis consists of one to several small scaly, erythematous, alopecic areas on the face or forelegs. Generalized demodecosis involves large areas of the body; lesions consist of larger coalescing patches of erythema, alopecia, scales, and crusts. Microscopically, lesions show epidermal hyperkeratosis, lymphoplasmacytic perifolliculitis, and intraluminal mites. The characteristically elongated mites are usually easy to find in large numbers in the waxy material that can be expressed from the pustular lesions. Mites are much more difficult to isolate from squamous lesions. Lesions in hides can be detected as dark spots when a fresh hide is viewed against a strong light source. However, lesions may not be readily seen until the hair has been removed and the skin has been soaking for some time.

Clinical features

The important sign is the appearance of small (3 mm diameter) nodules and pustules that may develop into larger abscesses, especially in pigs and goats. The small lesions can be seen quite readily in short-coated animals and on palpation feel like particles of 'bird-shot' in the hide. In severe cases there may be a general hair loss and thickening of the skin in the area, but usually there is no pruritus and hair loss is insufficient to attract attention. The contents of the pustules are usually white in colour and cheesy in consistency. In large abscesses the pus is more fluid. In cattle and goats the lesions occur most commonly on the brisket, lower neck, forearm, and shoulder, but also occur on the dorsal half of the body, particularly behind the withers. Larger lesions are easily visible but very small lesions may only be detected by rolling a fold of skin through the fingers. In horses the face and around the eyes are predilection areas. Demodicosis in pigs usually commences on the face and spreads down the ventral surface of the neck and chest to the belly. There is little irritation and the disease is observed mainly when the skin is scraped at slaughter. The disease may be especially severe in goats, spreading extensively before it is suspected and in some instances causing deaths. Severe cases in goats commonly involve several skin diseases such as mycotic dermatitis, ringworm, besnoitiosis and myiasis. Demodicosis is rare in sheep. In this species pustules and scabs appear on the coronets, nose, tips of the ears, and around the eyes, but clinical signs are not usually seen and mites may be found in scrapings from areas of the body not showing lesions. Clinical signs associated with demodectic mite infestation in dogs include erythema and alopecia (Fig. 9.1), which is related to inflammation caused by the migratory and feeding behaviours of the developing mites

Diagnosis

Demonstration of the mite in the skin lesion is satisfactory. In most farm animals the lesions are difficult to see externally and only the advanced ones will be diagnosed. The commonest error is to diagnose the disease as a non-specific staphylococcal

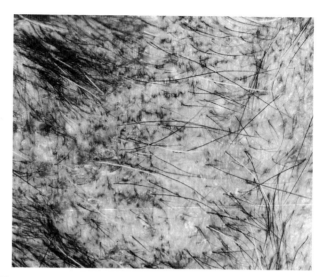

Figure 9.1 Close-up photograph depicting lesions in the abdominal skin of a dog infested with *Demodex canis*.

infection. In cattle and goats the disease often passes unnoticed unless the nodules are palpated. Deep-seated ringworm in horses has much in common with demodicosis.

Treatment

Repeated dipping or spraying with the acaricides recommended for other manges is usually carried out but is more to prevent spread than cure existing lesions. Ivermectin does not eradicate the infection in dogs, possibly because of the difficulty in getting the acaricide to the mite, has been reported to cure 98% of beef bulls when used at 0.3 mg/kg. Ivermectin in a premix, fed for 7 consecutive days, has been reported to clear the infestation in pigs.

Control

Control measures are rarely applied. Spaying of females with generalized demodicosis or with a history of infection has been suggested because of the inheritable predisposition of the disease.

Public health implications

It is extremely rare for *D. canis* to infect humans. Most of the public health issues surrounding canine demodicosis involve the use of Amitraz during treatment as poisoning can occur if it is accidentally ingested.

Itch mites

Aetiology

Two species of the genus *Psorobia*, formerly *Psorergates*, namely *Psorobia ovis* (sheep) and *Psorobia bos* (cattle).

Epidemiology and geographical distribution

Itch mite has been recorded as a parasite of cattle in the UK and sheep in Australia, New Zealand, South Africa, the United States, Argentina and Chile. Amongst sheep, merinos are most commonly affected. The highest incidence is observed in this breed, particularly in areas where the winter is cold and wet. There is a marked seasonal fluctuation in the numbers of mites; the numbers are very low in summer, commence to rise in the autumn, and peak numbers are found in the spring. Spring or summer shearing exacerbates the decline in numbers.

Life cycle and pathogenesis

The entire life cycle of this mite, eggs, larvae, three nymphal stages, and adults, takes place entirely on the host. In sheep the cycle takes 2–3 weeks. All stages occur in the superficial layers of the skin. Clinically, the disease resembles louse infestation, but may be distinguished on the smaller proportion of the flock affected (10–15%), the less severe irritation and tendency of the sheep to bite those areas it can reach. Hence lesions are confined to parts of the flank and the hindquarters and the wool tufts have a chewed appearance. Only the adults are mobile on the skin surface and they affect spread of the disease by direct contact. Sheep on poor nutrition have significantly higher mite populations, more scurf and greater fleece derangement.

Pathological findings

Hyperkeratosis, desquamation, and increased numbers of mast cells. The irritation appears to be a hypersensitivity reaction and results in biting and chewing of the fleece on the flanks and rump behind a line approximately from the elbow to the hips.

Clinical features

Mite feeding activity, in addition to excreta causes skin irritation leading to rubbing and biting of the affected parts principally the sides, flanks, and thighs and, sometimes shedding, of the fleece. Wool over these areas becomes thready and tufted and contains dry scales. The skin shows no gross abnormality other than an increase in scurf.

Diagnosis

Diagnosis depends on finding the mites in a skin scraping. The mites have a seasonal incidence and may be very difficult to find in summer and autumn. For best results the scraping should be made on the ribs or shoulder in winter or spring. Scrapings are usually teased out in oil and examined microscopically without digestion. A number of scrapings may be needed from each sheep before mites can be demonstrated.

Treatment

There is no compound available that will eradicate itch mite after a single treatment. Arsenic, lime sulfur, or finely divided sulfur have been used and markedly reduce the number of mites. However, arsenic is no longer used in most countries. Phoxim, an organophosphorus compound, has good activity but two dippings 1 month apart are necessary to eradicate infestations. Amitraz causes a marked reduction in mites that can be maintained for some months. A single subcutaneous injection of 0.2 mg/kg ivermectin freed sheep of mites up to 56 days post-treatment. Other macrocyclic lactone products, in various formulations, have also been shown to have good efficacy.

Control

Dipping sheep after shearing will suppress the mite population, keep the infestation rate low.

Public health implications

Transient infestation of humans may occur. The mites do not reproduce on humans, but reinfestation may continue as long as contact with infested animals continues.

Mange mites (scabies)

Aetiology

Mange mites include parasitic mites of the families Sarcoptidae and Psoroptidae. Mange in cattle is caused by the genera *Psoroptes* (Fig. 9.2), *Sarcoptes* (Fig. 9.3) and *Chorioptes* (Fig. 9.4). *Chorioptes* and *Psoroptes* are surface feeders (i.e. live on the surface of the skin). *Sarcoptes* are superficial burrowers. All three have distinct morphological and biological characteristics. The adults are extremely small and can be seen only with the aid of a microscope.

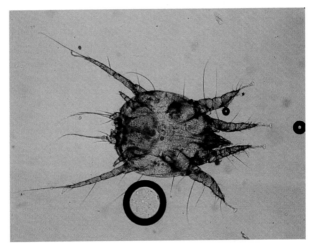

Figure 9.2 *Psoroptes* sp. The male has a size of 500–650 μm (female measures 600–800 μm). The leg suckers have a long segmented pedicel.

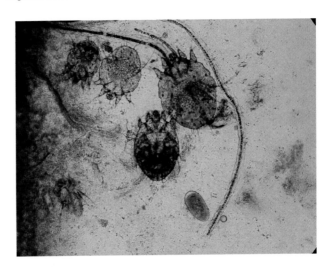

Figure 9.3 Skin scraping with different stages of *Sarcoptes* sp. Adult male measures 200–280 μm, female 300–500 μm. The leg suckers have a long pedicel without segments.

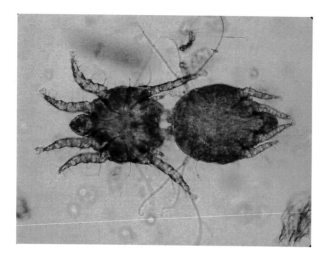

Figure 9.4 *Chorioptes* sp. The male is slightly smaller (300–450 µm) than the female (400–600 µm). Typically, the leg suckers have a short pedicel without segments.

Epidemiology and geographical distribution

Mites-causing scabies have a worldwide distribution. The mites are fully adapted to a life in and on the skin of their host. Their survival in the environment is rather short: *Sarcoptes*, maximum 18 days; *Psoroptes*, maximum 17 days; *Chorioptes*, maximum 28 days. *Chorioptes* and *Psoroptes* occur commonly in cattle and sheep but less so in goats.

Life cycle and pathogenesis

In general the mites develop in and on the skin. The entire life cycle takes place on the host and includes eggs, larvae, two nymph-stages (protonymph and tritonymph) and the adult females and males. The full development requires on average about 2–3 weeks. Mites are transmitted by direct contact between animals, in some cases, especially for *Psoroptes*, various objects (like brushes, barriers etc.) may harbour the parasites and are of relevance for the spread within a herd. The skin lesions are caused by immune reactions (allergic reactions) against mite antigens.

Pathological findings

Due to pruritus, affected animals start to scratch and opening lesions to secondary bacterial infections. In severe cases the skin lesions may become purulent. Gross lesions include erythematous macules, papules, crusts, and excoriations. Chronic lesions are scaly, lichenified, and hairless. Microscopically, dermatitis with eosinophils, mast cells, and lymphocytes; epidermal acanthosis, hyperkeratosis, parakeratosis, and crusting.

Clinical features

The clinical picture is linked to the genera, their biology and their predilection sites. Mange caused by *Sarcoptes bovis* starts at head, neck and spreads all over the body. It is characterized by scaly, crusts, hair loss and thickening of the skin. *Psoroptes ovis* causes hyperkeratosis on the back line and inner side of the legs, lateral of chest and neck and on the head. *Chorioptes bovis* is mainly focusing on the caudal part of the body where it causes hair loss and crusty skin areas (Fig. 9.5). In all cases the signs are dependent on

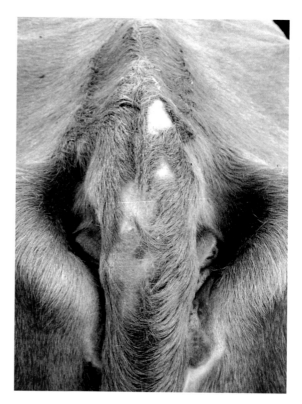

Figure 9.5 Skin lesion in a cattle caused by infestation with *Chorioptes* mite.

the infestation burden, the severity of the immune reaction and secondary bacterial infections (often due to lesions after extensive scraping). The infestation starts with pruritus and is accompanied with weight and production losses. Infestation may occur all over the year, but mite infestation is mostly of clinical relevance during winter and when the animals are in stable (close contact between animals, humid environment). Animals show pruritus and more or less pronounced skin lesions like scaly, crusts and hair loss.

Diagnosis

Confirmation is obtained by microscopic examination of skin scrapings (that need to be collected at the border between lesion and healthy skin, as deep as possible with a scalpel blade or sharp spoon). They can be identified and morphologically distinguished under the microscope. Serological tests (ELISA) exist and have proven to have a high sensitivity and specificity (so far only for *Sarcoptes* and *Psoroptes*). Mange has to be differentiated from louse infestation, fungal and bacterial skin diseases. Mites in skin scrapings have to be differentiated from food mites.

Treatment

Most effective treatment can be achieved with macrocyclic lactones (note: residues in milk in lactating cows). This can be avoided with eprinomectin formulation. Alternatively, pour on, spray on or washing with organophosphates, carbamates, amitraz or pyrethroids is possible, but has to be repeated in intervals of 7–14 days (to kill newly hatched larvae).

Control

As mites may survive in the environment for a limited time, the treatment of the animals has to be accompanied with cleaning and disinfection of the stable and objects in contact with cattle.

Public health implications

Symptoms in humans may occur: in exceptional cases the mites may cause inflammatory reactions on the skin which will disappear, as soon as the contact with infested animals stops.

Tick infestation

Overview

The ticks found on domesticated animals are not host specific, although they do have host preferences, and their distribution is subject to environmental conditions. The species, and their host ranges, are listed in Table 9.2. Ticks are identified as being soft or hard ticks. The hard ticks are generally classified as one-, two-, or three-host ticks. Some ticks may complete the cycle in a relatively short period (*Rhipicephalus* spp.), whereas other ticks (*Dermacentor* spp.) require 2 years, with 1 year between each stage before they reattach to a host.

Ixodidiosis

Aetiology

Ticks may act as causative agent of disease or may be carriers and vectors of pathogens like viruses, bacteria, protozoa and even helminths. In Europe, cattle are mostly affected by ticks of the widespread genera *Ixodes* (Fig. 9.6), *Haemaphysalis*, *Dermacentor* and *Rhipicephalus* (Fig. 9.7). Many tick species can affect livestock. *Ixodes ricinus* is the most frequent representative and will be discussed in more detail.

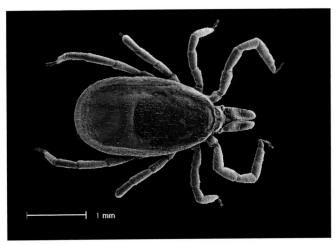

Figure 9.6 Dorsal view of a female *Ixodes ricinus* tick.

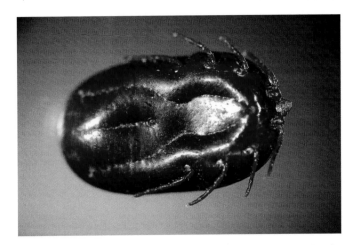

Figure 9.7 Ventral view of an engorged *Rhipicephalus* sp. female tick.

Table 9.2 Common tick species of livestock

Cattle	Sheep	Pigs
Ornithodoros spp.[1]	*Ornithodoros* spp.[1]	*Ornithodoros* spp.[1]
Otobius spp.[1]	*Otobius* spp.[1]	
Rhipicephalus spp.[2]	*Rhipicephalus* spp.[2]	*Rhipicephalus* spp.[2]
Ixodes spp.[2]	*Ixodes* spp.[2]	*Ixodes* spp.[2]
Hyalomma spp.[2]	*Hyalomma* spp.[2]	*Hyalomma* spp.[2]
Amblyomma spp.[2]	*Amblyomma* spp.[2]	*Dermacentor* spp.[2]
Dermacentor spp.[2]	*Dermacentor* spp.[2]	
Haemaphysalis spp.[2]	*Haemaphysalis* spp.[2]	
Boophilus spp.[3]	*Boophilus* spp.[3]	

[1]Soft tick belong to the family Argasidae, the rest are hard ticks belonging to the family Ixodidae.

[2]Three-host life cycle.

[3]One-host life cycle. In recent literature *Boophilus* has been re-named to *Rhipicephalus*.

Epidemiology and geographical distribution

Ixodes ricinus can be found in shady habitats with sufficient humidity. They prefer coppice, bush and underbrush. Larvae normally climb up to 30 cm off the ground while nymphs and adults may reach up to 1 m. *I. ricinus* ideally develops at temperatures between 17–20°C and a relative humidity of 80–95%. It is therefore mostly active in the mild climate of spring and autumn. Most relevant pathological findings in Europe are caused by tick-transmitted agents: babesiosis, caused by *B. divergens*, and anaplasmosis (tick-borne fever), caused by *Anaplasma phagocytophilum*. Other diseases can occur (see Chapter 10 for more details).

Life cycle and pathogenesis

The adult female drops to the ground after the blood meal, produces one to several thousand eggs and dies. The tick development includes one larval (three pairs of legs) and one nymph stage (four pairs of legs) before the adult stage is reached. Most European ticks change the host for each stage, which extends the life cycle to several years, due to host finding and climatic conditions. While larvae mainly infest small mammals, birds and reptiles, the later stages (nymphs and adults) prefer larger mammals, including humans. The full life cycle in middle Europe takes 2 years but may be considerably extended under unfavourable climatic conditions.

Pathological findings

Local cutaneous reactions vary in severity with the tick and its secretions, and host resistance. Gross lesions consist of focal erosions, erythema, and crusted ulcers with alopecia and nodules. Microscopic lesions include epidermal and dermal necrosis, and perivascular to diffuse inflammation at the margins of the necrotic area. The exudate is composed of eosinophils, macrophages and lymphocytes. Cutaneous basophil hypersensitivity likely contributes to the reactions induced by tick bites.

Clinical features

Ticks localize mainly on head and ears as well as on the perineum and the inner part of fore and hind legs. Attachment may result in thickening of skin (hyperkeratosis) and local skin inflammation with ulcers. In case of high infestation anaemia, weight loss and reduced milk production may be observed. *Ixodes ricinus* is transmitter of infective agents such as *Trypanosoma*, *Theileria*, *Babesia*, *Dipetalonema* larvae, the tick-borne encephalitis virus (TBE) and *Borrelia burgdorferi*, which causes borreliosis (Lyme disease) in humans. In most cases tick infestation in Europe does hardly cause clinical signs and is often not noted. Problems may occur in the case of local inflammation and by secondary bacterial infection of the penetration site. Severe diseases may be due to tick-transmitted pathogens.

Diagnosis

Ticks (Fig. 9.8) can be easily identified on animals, mainly on the favoured spots like udder, inguinal region, head, ears and cervix. For species differentiation the ticks can be sent to specialized labs. Ticks can be easily identified on the animals, especially engorged

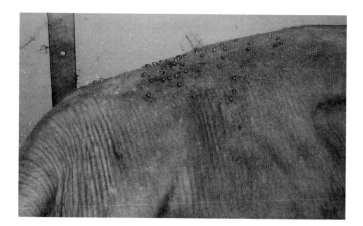

Figure 9.8 Ticks can be easily identified on cattle. High infection loads may cause skin irritation, pruritus and inflammation.

adult females. Mating often occurs on the host while the female is sucking blood. The male has a scutum that covers his whole back. *Ixodes ricinus* can be easily identified by the inverted U-shaped perianal groove.

Treatment

Systematic treatment of cattle against ticks is rare in Europe. A decision on required treatments has to be based on the severity of clinical signs and production losses and on the expenses and risks (costs, residues etc.) of treatment. Acaricides can be applied by pour on, spray on, washing or injection. Registered active classes are pyrethroids and macrocyclic lactones. The latter are also used for anthelmintic treatment. It is described that cattle dewormed with macrocyclic lactones have less tick infestation when put on pasture.

Control

Control of ticks should target the infested animals and the animal's surrounding environment. The former is more challenging because most ticks of veterinary significance use more than one host other than the infested animal to complete their life cycle. Reducing exposure to ticks by being informed about endemic species in the local area and avoiding periods when most ticks are active may reduce the animal and the animal owner's risk of exposure.

Public health implications

Ticks can infect humans and transmit pathogens. Of most relevance are *Borrelia burgdorferi* (Lyme disease), Flaviviridae (Tick Borne Encephalitis) and *Ehrlichia*. *Babesia divergens* is worth mentioning as it may cause clinical signs in splenectomized and immunosuppressed patients, which may be misdiagnosed as malaria. Infestation of domestic animals with ticks should alert their human owners that they too are at risk of tick exposure and thus potential exposure to tick-borne diseases (see Chapter 10). Humans in contact with tick-infested animals should inspect themselves for similar infestation and remove ticks as soon as possible before engorgement occurs and before the transmission of infectious agents to humans occur.

Acknowledgements
We would like to thank Dr Peter Bates, the director of Veterinary Medical Entomology Consultancy (VMEC), Surrey, England, for critical reading.

Further reading
Arther, R.G. (2009). Mites and lice: biology and control. Vet. Clin. North Am. Small Anim. Pract. *39*, 1159–1171.

Bates, P.G. (1993). Alternative methods for the control of sheep scab. Vet Rec. *133*, 467–469.

Blagburn, B. L. and Dryden, M.W. (2009). Biology, Treatment, and Control of Flea and Tick Infestations. Vet. Clin. North Am. Small Anim. Pract. *39*, 1173–1200.

Cortinas, R. and Jones, C.J. (2006). Ectoparasites of cattle and small ruminants. Vet. Clin. North Am. Food Anim. Pract. *22*, 673–693.

Drummond, R.O. (1985). New methods of applying drugs for the control of ectoparasites. Vet. Parasitol. *18*, 111–119.

Fadok, V.A. (1984). Parasitic skin diseases of large animals. Vet. Clin. North Am. Large Anim. Pract. *6*, 3–26.

Ghubash R. (2006). Parasitic miticidal therapy. Clin. Tech. Small Anim. Pract. *21*, 135–144.

Hicks, M.I. and Elston, D.M. (2009) Scabies. Dermatol. Ther. *22*, 279–292.

Hiepe, T. (1988). Advances in control of ectoparasites in large animals. Angew Parasitol. *29*, 201–210.

Mumcuoglu, K.Y. and Gilead, L. (2008). Treatment of scabies infestations. Parasite *15*, 248–251.

Tick-borne Diseases

10

Hany M. Elsheikha

Background

Ticks are giant acarids (phylum Arthropoda), which have a major veterinary and public health impact. They represent an obstacle in economic growth especially in developing countries. Due to their feeding behaviour ticks inflict considerable physical damage and irritation which disrupt the foraging of livestock, thereby reducing productivity and fitness, and lowering defences against other diseases (e.g. tick-borne fever predisposes lambs to tick pyaemia). Wounds induced by tick bites are open to invasion by secondary bacterial and fungal, and other opportunistic infections. Tick infestation may also cause tick paralysis, thought to be due to a neurotoxin elaborated by the tick's ovaries, and introduced into the host with saliva while the tick is feeding. This condition is generally characterized by progressive, ascending, flaccid motor paralysis with muscle in-coordination and ataxia.

Ticks are among the most important vectors of pathogens affecting livestock, companion animals and humans. Ticks have been implicated as a vector of Texas cattle fever (*Babesia bigemina*) for more than a century. Since then, the number of newly recognized pathogens and health hazards associated with ticks increased dramatically. Of an estimated 899 tick species that exist worldwide, about 10% are implicated in the transmission of pathogens. Ticks and tick-borne diseases (TBDs) in Europe have recently shown expansion in their distribution, which indicates that the interaction between ticks and hosts is more common than it is actually recognized. This is largely due to changes in tick habitats caused by shifts in landscape, via reforestations, climatic changes and changes in habitat structure of wildlife. TBDs may also spread through increased travel of animals. There is a recent evidence of new diseases arriving into UK due to pets travelling with their owners such as canine babesiosis. Additionally, current emphasis in some countries on sustainable agriculture and extensification is likely to lead to an increase in tick populations with increased risk of TBDs.

Ticks are divided into two major families: the Ixodidae (hard ticks) and the Argasidae (soft ticks). Hard ticks (ixodids) are so named because of the hardened shield-like structure or scutum found on their backs (Fig. 10.1). In female hard ticks, the scutum covers approximately the anterior third of the body, with the remainder consisting of leathery cuticle to allow for expansion during blood-feeding. In male hard ticks the scutum extends the length of the body. In contrast, soft ticks have no scutum; their whole body is leathery. Soft ticks are transient feeders, rarely achieve great population densities and do not inflict a burden on

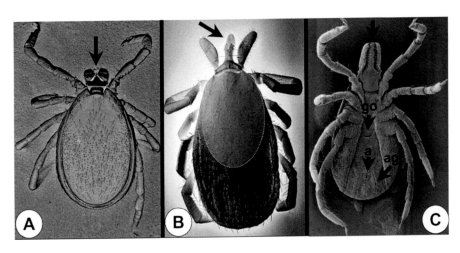

Figure 10.1 *Ixodes ricinus*: Dorsal view of adult male (A) and female (B) showing the morphological features of this species. Note, the gnathosoma (arrow), scutum (shaded) covers the dorsum entirely in the male and partially in the female. (C) Ventral view of an adult tick showing the genital opening (go), the anal groove (ag) arching behind the anus (a).

mammalian animals. The family Ixodidae includes a number of species of interest, most of which belonging to the genera *Ixodes*, *Amblyomma*, *Dermacentor*, *Haemaphysalis* and *Rhipicephalus*. This family is the most important from a medical and veterinary point of view. This chapter focuses on *Ixodes ricinus*, the most prevalent tick species in the UK and Europe, with especial emphasis on diseases transmitted by this tick species to animals and humans.

Biology of *Ixodes ricinus*

Ixodes ricinus (also known as European sheep tick, pasture tick, or deer tick) are ectoparasites of a wide range of medium- to large-sized mammals, e.g. sheep, cattle, deer, dogs and humans. Its life cycle comprises four stages (egg, larva, nymph and adult) and development from egg to adult can take up to six years, depending on the weather and hosts' availability. *I. ricinus* is a three-host-tick (Fig. 10.2). Each tick stage (i.e. larva, nymph and adult female) feeds on a different host. Both larva and nymph infect smaller animals (e.g. rabbits), birds (e.g. chickens) and even reptiles. Adults prefer ungulates (ruminants). All life stages quest by climbing to the tips of the vegetation and waiting for a suitable host to brush against them. Larvae and nymphs must each take a blood meal to develop to the next stage. Tick feeding behaviour at each life stage plays a significant role in the risk for TBDs. When feeding on an infected host, tick larvae, nymphs, and adults can take up one or more pathogens, which might be transmissible to susceptible hosts during subsequent blood meals. The seed ticks (larvae) attach to a passing small animal (usually rodents) to feed for a few days, and then drop back into the ground vegetation where they digest their blood meal, moult into nymphs and seek a new host. Nymphs will bite any mammal they encounter. Adults attach to a final host, usually larger mammals or humans. Males rarely feed, and only occur on the host when searching for females. After mating and feeding, adult females drop from the host, lay their eggs (1000–2000), and die. The nymphs' small size (approximately 1 mm) allows them to feed undetected on the hosts long enough to transmit various pathogens. Adult ticks are larger and more likely to be detected and removed before disease transmission.

Ecology of *Ixodes ricinus*

The geographic distribution of *I. ricinus* ranges from 60° to 40° northern latitude, i.e. from southern Scandinavia to the Mediterranean Sea. Also, it occurs in some regions of Asia and North Africa. In Germany, Ireland and the British Isles *I. ricinus* is the most common species of the tick population. British hotspots include Thetford Forest in Norfolk, the New Forest in Hampshire, the Lake District, the Yorkshire Moors, the Scottish Highlands and the uplands of Wales. *I. ricinus* can also present in open habitats such as pasture. The distribution and abundance of *I. ricinus* are not static in time and space, but are related to various factors such as the presence of wooded, forested or brushy habitat and the abundance of suitable hosts for all life stages of the ticks. Tick habitat varies according to climate, temperature, moisture and biotope. *I. ricinus* is hydrophilic (favour moisture) and free-living stages are susceptible to heat and desiccation and cannot survive relative humidity of less than 80% for any length of time. *I. ricinus* is usually found in vegetations that maintain high humidity. Larvae normally stay closer to the ground as they are more sensitive to humidity than mature stages, whereas adults may be found on vegetation even as high as 1.5 m. This is one reason why larvae are more often found to infest smaller animals than nymphs and adults. *I. ricinus* can acquire water from humid air by ingestion of hygroscopic material secreted by the salivary glands. This mechanism enables unfed ticks to climb up to the tips of vegetation – where they can ambush passing hosts – for several days before having to descend to the vegetation base in order to rehydrate. Although *I. ricinus* ticks can be found throughout the year, they are particularly active during spring and early summer, and again from late summer into autumn.

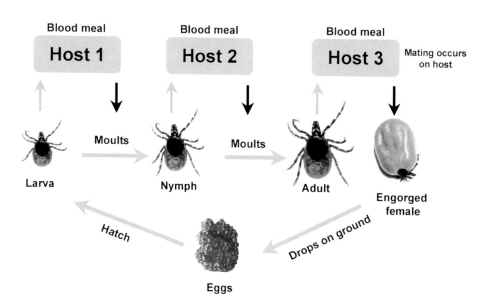

Figure 10.2 The life cycle of *Ixodes ricinus*, showing the three-host cycles.

Hard ticks are efficient disease carrying vectors

Humans and animals may become ill because of infection by numerous species of arboviruses (arthropod-borne viruses), bacteria, and protozoa transmitted by ticks. Hard ticks are very successful ectoparasites and have a remarkable ability to transmit a wide variety of pathogens than any other arthropods. Their important role in disease transmission is reinforced by the fact that ticks have a worldwide distribution, can adapt to diverse environments, and feed for extended periods of time and on a variety of vertebrate hosts as they develop from juveniles to adults. Ticks have a slow life cycle that takes several years. Because of this remarkable longevity, ticks can carry TBDs over prolonged period of time, thereby not only serving as vectors but also act as reservoir hosts for the pathogens they carry. Ticks have salivary glands that play a major role in tick biology because of their extraordinary physiology, and their role in enhancing pathogen transmission and establishment, and secretion of bioactive products of various critical functions. The haematophagous capacity of ticks along with the lack of digestive enzymes in their gut favours the survival of ingested pathogens.

Different species of hard ticks transmit different infectious agents. But, only diseases transmitted by *I. ricinus* will be considered. There are two mechanisms by which *I. ricinus* can facilitate transmission of pathogens to susceptible hosts: (1) transovarian/vertical (adult female egg/larva) transmission, in which the infective organism is transmitted from the female to her offspring, e.g. *Babesia divergens.*; and (2) transsstadial (stage-stage) transmission, which occurs between stages of the tick's life cycle.

Ixodes ricinus-borne diseases in humans

Ixodes ricinus ticks have non-specific feeding habits; they not only feed on species that are reservoirs for multiple tick-borne pathogens (e.g. small mammals) but also can bite humans. This indiscriminate feeding habit of *I. ricinus* increases the opportunities of pathogens' transmission to humans.

- *Anaplasma phagocytophilum* – the agent of human granulocytotropic anaplasmosis, previously known as human granulocytotropic ehrlichiosis.
- *Coxiella burnetii* (Q-fever) – there is little evidence that a human subject has been infected with *Coxiella* following a bite by an infected *I. ricinus* despite reports of the bacterium in ticks in some countries.
- *Francisella tularensis* – the agent of a rare zoonotic infection called tularaemia. The disease is endemic in North America, and parts of Europe and Asia. Small animals such as rabbits and hares serve as reservoir hosts.
- *Borrelia burgdorferi sensu lato* – the agent of Lyme borreliosis (LB). LB is a multisystem disorder that is treatable with antibiotics, but may lead to severe complications of the neurological system, the heart, and the joints.
- Tick-borne encephalitis (TBE*)* – viral TBE is endemic in most European countries, and > 3000 cases are reported annually for Europe, including the Baltic states.

- *Babesia* spp. – human babesiosis is a significant emerging tick-borne zoonotic disease. There are several species of *Babesia* that can infect humans, but *B. microti* (a rodent species) and *B. divergens* (a bovine species) are the most prevalent aetiological agents of human babesiosis in the USA and Europe, respectively.

Ixodes ricinus-borne diseases in animals

Herein, I provide a brief overview of the most common *I. ricinus*-borne diseases that have relevance to the animal health and welfare.

Babesiosis (red-water fever)

In the UK and northern Europe, bovine babesiosis is caused by the intraerythrocytic protozoan parasite *Babesia divergens* (Fig. 10.3). This disease is usually first reported in May/June when the tick host first becomes active. *B. divergens* produces a disease syndrome similar to *B. bigemina* and *B. bovis*; however, the cerebral form is rarely seen. Red-water fever is often only noticed at the onset of haemoglobinuria, when the disease is far advanced. Babesiosis is not only a cause of significant loss to the cattle industry; it can also infect immunocompromised humans. Diagnosis is based on clinical signs, history of recent exposure to ticks and microscopic examination of blood smears.

Treatment

Mild cases may recover without treatment. More severe cases need treatment. This is often best combined with a preventative treatment for the unaffected cattle. Therapy and transfusion generally save affected animals even at an advanced stage of the

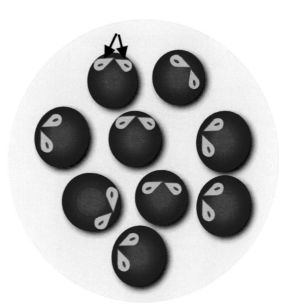

Figure 10.3 Illustration of the intraerythrocytic protozoan *Babesia divergens* in a blood smear. Merozoites are pear shaped (arrows) and often occurs in pairs, joined at the tip, a result of binary schizogony.

disease. Imidocarb dipropionate and diminazene aceturate are the most widely used drugs. But, imidocarb is most toxic when given intravenously. Hence, intramuscular or subcutaneous administration is generally recommended. Also, imidocarb is associated with residue problems especially if used for chemoprophylaxis, which has led to its withdrawal in several European countries. Blood transfusion is recommended for animals with acute anaemic anoxia, indicated by jaundice or pale mucous membranes, and a body temperature of less than 38°C. Long-acting oxytetracyline has no therapeutic effect if given when the parasitaemia has become patent. The continuous prophylactic treatment will allow sufficient numbers of parasites to multiply for antibodies to be produced, while clinical effects are absent. However, the continuous administration of oxytetracycline is too costly and risky because of the likelihood of the development of resistance in bacterial pathogens. Vaccine is not yet available in UK. Attempts to control *B. divergens* infections by stimulating non-specific immunity failed.

Lyme borreliosis (Lyme disease)

Lyme disease is caused by a Gram-negative spirochaete bacterium called *Borrelia* burgdorferi s.l. (Fig. 10.4). Reservoir animals are small rodents, hares and birds. Lyme disease has gained increasing attention as an emerging zoonotic disease problem. However, there is very little evidence that it poses a significant veterinary problem in Europe despite the sales of the dog vaccine. This multisystemic disease causes fever, lameness, stiff joints, arthritis, fatigue, renal failure, heart disorders, meningitis, and other neurological signs. Once the host contracts Lyme's disease, urgent treatment with antibiotics is required. Differential diagnosis can be difficult, and co-infection, particularly with *Babesia* spp. or *Ehrlichia* spp., can occur.

Treatment

Doxycycline or amoxicillin is the drug of choice. However, doxycycline should not be used in very young pups because it can cause teeth staining. Other drugs that are effective include azithromycin, cephalexin, amoxicillin, tetracycline, penicillin G, and chloramphenicol. Non-steroidal anti-inflammatory drugs may also be used for symptomatic treatment. The current vaccine consists of killed *B. burgdorferi* in adjuvant, and is used for dogs.

Tick-borne fever (anaplasmosis)

Tick-borne fever (TBF) is a febrile disease of cattle, sheep and horses in the UK and other countries. It is caused by a bacterium called *Anaplasma* (*Ehrlichia*) *phagocytophilum* (Fig. 10.5). Anaplasmosis leads to fever, anorexia, joint pain and swelling. The disease suppresses the immune system in young lambs, predisposing infected animals to other infections, such as louping-ill, tick pyaemia. There is no colostral protection, so in areas where disease is circulating; young lambs are at greatest risk of disease. Adults are more resistant as immunity builds up as animal age.

Treatment

The short-acting oxytetracyclines are regarded as the most effective option. If dairy cattle are treated with oxytetracyclines within a few days of infection, the pyrexia is reduced quickly and milk yield restored. Other antibiotics such as penicillin, streptomycin, and ampicillin do not prevent relapses. Sulfamethazine is also useful. Treatment with long-acting tetracyclines may be used as a prophylactic measure in enzootic areas.

Tick pyaemia of sheep

This disease affects lambs born on or introduced to a tick-infested area, usually at the time of the maximal tick activity (usually in the spring). The disease is caused by the bacterium *Staphylococcus*

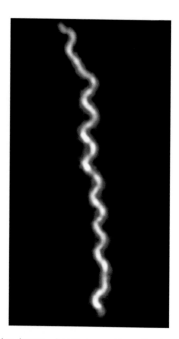

Figure 10.4 Spirochaete bacterium *Borrelia burgdorferi*, the causative agent of Lyme disease.

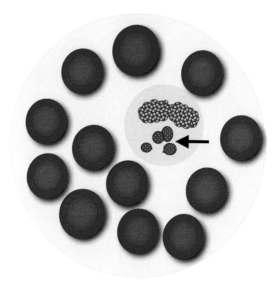

Figure 10.5 Illustration of a peripheral blood smear demonstrating variably sized basophilic inclusions representing a cluster of *Anaplasma* (*Ehrlichia*) *phagocytophilum* (arrow) contained within vacuoles within the cytoplasm of a leucocyte.

aureus, an inhabitant of the normal skin, which enters the blood stream by the biting action of the blood-sucking nymphal stage and adult females. This infection can result in skin abscesses, but in immunosuppressed animals (such as those with TBF) the bacteria can spread into the joints and spinal column causing arthritis or even paralysis. Lambs may be affected by both tick pyaemia and joint-ill on the same premises, especially if the ewes are in poor condition and have insufficient colostrum. Diagnosis is based on the history, necropsy findings, and bacterial culture of infected joint.

Treatment

Parenteral administration of penicillin or tetracycline can be effective especially if the lesions are not too advanced. Local treatment of affected joints is often unsatisfactory, because by the time lesions are noticed abscess formation may be advanced and irreversible damage to the joint may have occurred. Prophylactic administration of long-acting antibiotics, to which particular strains of *S. aureus* agents are sensitive, can be used, though care should be taken not to under-dose, which could promote bacterial resistance. Long-acting tetracyclines are effective against both *S. aureus* and the rickettsial agent of TBF. Thus, treatment of tick pyaemia with oxytetracycline may delay the development of immunity to the TBF agent.

Louping-ill (ovine encephalomyelitis, infectious encephalomyelitis of sheep, trembling-ill)

Louping-ill (LI) is an acute viral disease primarily of sheep caused by a neurotropic single-strand RNA flavivirus. It is characterized by a biphasic fever, depression, ataxia, muscular incoordination, tremors, posterior paralysis, coma and death. LI is a tick-transmitted disease whose occurrence is closely related to the distribution of *I. ricinus*. LI is a disease of all ages of sheep and can infect other hosts such as grouse. Louping-ill virus is transmissible to humans. LI is endemic in rough upland areas in Scotland, northern England, Wales and Ireland. Although cases of LI can occur at any time of the year, the disease is most prevalent during the periods of maximal tick activity between April and June and again in September. Colostrum protects lambs in areas where ewes have been exposed to the virus and therefore clinical signs will generally be seen in weaned lambs. Young lambs, which have not received sufficient colostrum, are also susceptible to disease, as are naïve sheep of any age brought into an area where disease is circulating. All stages of ticks, larva, nymph and adult, acquire the virus by feeding on a viraemic host. Diagnosis is based on clinical grounds, history of a recent exposure to tick in an endemic area, serological assays and RT-PCR.

Treatment

If there is evidence that susceptible animals have been exposed to the disease, the administration of the louping-ill antiserum within 48 hours of exposure to the infection is useful. Vaccination is probably the single most important means of controlling LI in areas endemic for the disease. Vaccination should take place at least 1 month before exposure to infection. A formalin-inactivated commercial vaccine is available that has been used successfully for many years in endemic areas. Two doses of vaccine with an interval of 2–8 weeks between injections are recommended to achieve optimal protection to natural infection. Vaccination of pregnant ewes during the last trimester is advocated to ensure that lambs receive maximal levels of passively acquired antibodies and are protected during the initial critical months of life. Unlike sheep, cattle affected with LI may respond favourably to good nursing and symptomatic treatment.

Management and control

One of the most common approaches to the control of TBDs is the control of tick vectors. Effective control of tick populations should include the strategic use of acaricides, exploitation of natural exposure augmented with vaccination and the use of tick-resistant breeds of animals. Tick control also involves targeting animals and addressing the animal's environment.

Chemical treatment of infested animals

Widespread destruction of tick habitats is ecologically unacceptable, environmentally non-sustainable and may be counterproductive because pockets of ticks usually survive to parasitize fully susceptible hosts. The most practicable approach is the application of synthetic acaricides to animals with slow-release devices or as pour-ons with high residual activity during the periods of greatest exposure. Many acaricidal/insecticidal products are useful against ticks, including but not limited to:

- *phenylpyrazole*: high safety margin in dogs as well as cats due to a selective action on invertebrate GABA receptors (gamma amino-butyric acid receptors);
- *formamidine*: selective action on octopamine receptors;
- *pyrethroids*: their long-term effect varies (from some days to several weeks) according to pharmaceutical forms;
- *organophosphates* (licensed products not available in the UK): these molecules have no long-term effect and are usually used more in treatment rather than prevention.

Environmental control

The indiscriminate and improper use of acaricides has resulted in selection of resistant ticks, environmental pollution, and toxicity to humans and other non-target organisms. Thus, control of ticks should consider alternative non-chemical approaches.

- *Agronomic measures* to destroy tick areas via:
  - restricting animals to low-ground, tick-free pastures especially for the first few weeks of life;
  - keeping grass and weeds cut short in tick infested areas.
- *Zoological measures/biological control* with the use of tick predators such as the oxpecker birds of genus *Buphagus* in Africa. Also, the use of entomopathogenic fungi *Metarhizium anisopliae* and *Beauveria bassiana* has been reported.
- *Pheromone-based* anti-tick products can be exploited to aid tick control.
- *Tick-resistant animals* (genetically resistant animals) that show a heritable ability to become resistant to tick infestation can be

an important element of many tick control strategies, e.g. *the one-host cattle tick Rhipicephalus (Boophilus) microplus.*

• *Vaccinations*, of which only one, to the author's knowledge, is a commercially available tick vaccine [against cattle ticks (*Rhipicephalus microplus*)], and even then only in Australia and Cuba. Continued improvements in genetic analysis, identification, isolation, and the delivery of putative immunogens, may eventually lead to the development of more vaccines against other tick species. Development of effective vaccines against multiple tick species may be possible by using highly conserved tick-protective antigens, antigens showing immune cross-reaction to different tick species, or a combination of key protective antigens. Tick antigens exposed naturally to the host during tick feeding and those concealed have both shown promise as candidate vaccine antigens.

Important things to consider when designing a tick control programme

Even though acaricide-based infection control remains important, the development of resistance could limit this approach. Indeed, widespread and increasing resistance to most available acaricides threatens global livestock industries and public health. Any control programme that features the use of acaricides should consider the following measures in order to delay the rate of selection for resistant ticks.

• Reduce dependence on pesticides and use only when necessary.
• Consider some protective measures to reduce or eliminate exposure of animals to tick infestations.
• Spraying of acaricides should be considered for ticks with limited ranges (gardens, kennels etc.).
• Use a narrow-spectrum acaricides where possible.
• Rotate acaricides where appropriate.
• A single treatment will kill adult ticks, but eggs and larvae may still around.
• Monitor the level of tick infestation to optimize the timing of acaricide use and to determine the need for additional treatments.
• Delay the move of animals for 1–2 days after treatment.
• Administer the acaricides effectively (use at the rate recommended, do not mix, check method of application).
• Avoid introducing resistant acarines – maintain biosecurity of premises and herds.

Perspectives

The importance of ticks has long been recognized due to their ability to transmit diseases to animals and humans. Ticks are vectors of a variety of pathogenic agents, including species of bacteria (*B. burgdorferi*, *Rickettsia* spp., *Ehrlichia* spp.), viruses (TBE virus – family Flaviviridae), and parasites (*Babesia* spp.). Infections with tick-borne pathogens can cause severe to life-threatening illnesses, however, prompt diagnosis and early treatment of these diseases is often associated with a reduced risk of severe complications or fatalities. The public health importance of these illnesses will become more significant as human behaviours continue to alter the habitats of tick and reservoir species, resulting in increased transmission of known TBDs and the emergence of previously unrecognized zoonotic infections. Despite the veterinary and zoonotic importance of TBDs, relatively little research has been carried out on the ticks and diseases associated with them, and many questions regarding the epidemiology and the host's response remain unanswered. A better understanding of the tick species' biology and host–parasite interactions is fundamental to improved control mechanisms and new trends in management of TBDs. A major challenge for the control of several TBDs is the development of acaricide resistance, although the real extent of the problem is unknown. Vaccination is a feasible tick control approach that offers a cost-effective, environmentally friendly alternative to chemical control. However, identification of tick-protective antigens remains the limiting step in vaccine development. Characterization of the tick genomes will have a great impact on the discovery of new protective antigens.

Acknowledgements

I wish to thank Professor Gray Jeremy from University College of Dublin for thoughtful comments and critical reading.

Further reading

Bowman, A.S. and Nuttall, P. (2008). Ticks: biology, disease and control. Cambridge University Press. 506 pp.

Fritz, C.L. (2009). Emerging tick-borne diseases. Vet. Clin. North Am. Small Anim. Pract. *39*, 265–278.

Gray, J.S. (2002). Biology of *Ixodes* species ticks in relation to tick-borne zoonoses. Wien. Klin. Wochenschr. *114*, 473–478.

Gray, J.S., Dautel, H., Estrada-Peña, A., Kahl, O. and Lindgren, E. (2009). Effects of climate change on ticks and tick-borne diseases in europe. Interdiscip. Perspect. Infect. Dis. *2009*, 593232.

Jongejan, F. and Uilenberg, G. (2004). The global importance of ticks. Parasitology *129*, S3–S14.

Otranto, D., Dantas-Torres, F., and Breitschwerdt, E.B. (2009). Managing canine vector-borne diseases of zoonotic concern: part one. Trends Parasitol. *25*, 157–163.

Parola, P., Paddock, C.D. and Raoult, D. (2005). Tick-borne rickettsioses around the world: emerging diseases challenging old concepts. Clin. Microbiol. Rev. *18*, 719–756.

Scharlemann, J.P., Johnson, P.J., Smith, A.A., Macdonald, D.W. and Randolph, S.E. (2008). Trends in ixodid tick abundance and distribution in Great Britain. Med. Vet. Entomol. *22*, 238–247.

Shaw, S.E., Day, M.J., Birtles, R.J., and Breitschwerdt, E.B. (2001). Tick-borne infectious diseases of dogs. Trends Parasitol. *17*, 74–80.

Smith, T. (1893). Investigations into the nature, causation, and prevention of Texas or Southern cattle tick fever, pp. 177–304. Bureau of Animal Industries, bulletin no. 1. U.S. Department of Agriculture, Washington, D.C.

Yaramis, A., Soker, M. and Bilici, M. (2000). Amitraz poisoning in children. Hum. Exp. Toxicol. *19*, 431–433.

Diagnostic Parasitology

Laboratory Diagnosis of Parasitic Infections 11

David J. Bartley and Hany M. Elsheikha

Introduction

Accurate diagnosis of parasitic infections is a prerequisite for successful treatment and control of these pathogens. Errors in the diagnosis can lead to the initiation of unnecessary therapies, or delays in initiating the correct therapy. Thus, the clinicians must maintain a sharp index of suspicion and must rely on detailed history and clinical manifestations, to raise the possibility of a parasitic disease. Even though the diagnosis can be difficult, and definitive identification of the parasites can be challenging particularly in the non-endemic settings. Therefore, laboratory testing for detection and identification of the parasitic agents is required to complement clinical judgement, enhance the clinician's ability to select specific anti-parasitic drugs, and ultimately improve patient care. A wide range of laboratory procedures are available for the diagnosis of parasitic infections. These procedures vary in methodology, expense, availability, sensitivity, and specificity. In this chapter, the standard techniques used in the laboratory diagnosis of parasitic infections are discussed.

Faecal examination

This section will outline some of the methodologies used in the collection, processing and analysis of faecal material for identification of, predominantly, helminths commonly involved in PGE in ruminants (Fig. 11.1). Techniques commonly used in the detection of anthelmintic resistance will also be covered.

Collection, storage and preservation of faecal samples

Faecal collection

It is essential that good practice is followed in all stages of the collection, processing and analysis of faecal material in order to ensure that viable and representative samples are examined safely and effectively. When collecting and examining faecal material it is important to adopt good hygiene and it is essential to take precautions to reduce the likelihood of transmitting zoonotic infections to the sample handler and others. Basic precautions include the use of gloves, face and eye protection, as well as other appropriate protective clothing.

When collection is not solely for disease diagnosis, but, for example, for monitoring purposes, it is important to decide on the most suitable time to collect samples, and, for livestock owners with large flocks/herds, the most appropriate cohort. The best results for lambs/calves are often obtained from animals that have grazed for at least 6 weeks on contaminated pasture: these will normally provide more eggs in the samples than is usually present in material collected from adult animals. If samples from lactating ewes are required, samples taken when the lambs are about 4–6 weeks old will usually provide the most eggs. Samples should be taken at least 4 weeks after the animals' last non-persistent oral drench (such as a benzimidazole or ivermectin) or 8 weeks after treatment with a persistent anthelmintic such as moxidectin or doramectin.

Composite (mob) samples

With production animals, it may be practicable and economical to gather samples from a group (mob) of animals. Fresh mob samples can be collected by concentrating animals in a corner of the field and allowing them to stand for a few minutes. Very fresh samples (steamers) can then be collected from the ground into individually numbered polythene bags. Depending on the size of the flock/herd, between 10 and 15 samples (2 g minimum size or similar quantities of diarrhoea) should be collected from each class of animal to be examined. Mix the faeces in each bag by kneading together. Take a 2-g subsample from each of the samples and this will form the pooled material. Homogenize the pooled sample thoroughly and remove a 10-g subsample of the pooled material. Add the faeces to the sample containers and fill the container with water, leaving only a small air space. Published work showed that treatment efficacies based on composite samples collected in this manner could be as accurate as those generated by individual sampling and separate analysis of each sample.

Faecal storage

Fresh samples (preferably obtained directly from the rectum) are optimal, and material can be stored as anaerobically as possible for transportation.

Consumables

Sample bag, plastic gloves, air-tight container.

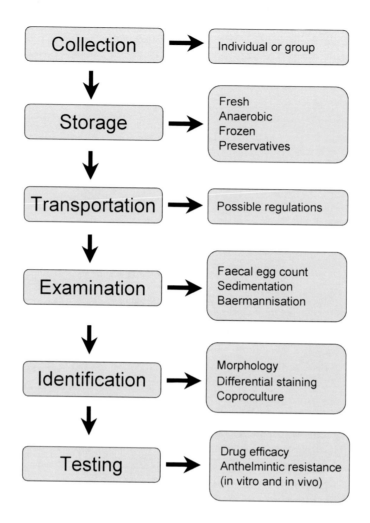

Figure 11.1 Flow diagram of the main steps used in faecal examination.

Protocol

Collect fresh faecal samples from a representative proportion (10%) of the animals of interest (not just from either the sick or healthy-looking animals). For the storage system to work properly, dung samples must have been observed to be freshly passed or collected directly from the rectum. Place the sample into an air-tight container, preferably with a screw-on lid, and add water to leave only a small air space. Screw the lid on tightly and shake the container vigorously for 1 min. If sending the sample via a courier or postal service, see section on biological sample transportation.

Occasionally, excess gases can be produced by microbial fermentation/activity within stored faecal material containers. These gases may be inflammable and cause pressurization of the containers. Exploding containers may result in the dissemination of pathogenic aerosols and infectious shards of plastic/glass. Hence the use of glass containers should be avoided.

Faecal preservation

Preservation of faeces can be done with 10% formalin. Also, faeces can be preserved using refrigeration or freezing. Freezing is inadvisable with samples collected from grazing ruminants. The process leads to a low recovery (mean approximately 22%) of eggs when processed using salt floatation media. Recovery of *Haemonchus contortus*, *Teladorsagia circumcincta* and *Trichostrongylus colubriformis* eggs was consistently low at a range of different concentrations and with a number of different parasite species in all frozen samples compared with samples examined fresh (Table 11.1).

Transportation regulations within the UK

Transportation of biological samples is regulated (International Air Transport Association) and requires the sender to consider whether the material is likely to contain pathogens (bacteria, viruses, rickettsiae, parasites or fungi) and other agents such as prions which can cause disease in humans or animals. Transported

Table 11.1 Faecal egg count analysis of subsamples of ovine faecal material when examined fresh and following freezing at –20°C (unpublished data)

Species	Sample type examined		Yield (%)
	Fresh (EPG*)	Frozen (EPG*)	
Teladorsagia circumcincta	69	15	21
Trichostrongylus colubriformis	432	85	20
Haemonchus contortus	6390	1392	22

*Eggs per gram of faeces.

material must be packaged and transported according to the appropriate guidelines (further information can be found at various sites, e.g. http://www.who.int.

Faecal examination

Faecal specimens should be first inspected visually for consistency, colour, evidence of blood, mucus, undigested food particles, and worm segments. Blood indicates intestinal or gastric bleeding. Some species of parasite are readily identifiable from gross morphology of the whole parasite, or segments thereof, found in the faecal matter. For example nematodes such as ascarids, and large bowel worms can be expelled from the host intact. Proglottids of cestodes such *Monezia expansa* may also be recognized in the faeces (Fig. 11.2).

For those parasites where only the egg, oocyst or larval stages are mostly observed in the faeces, there are a number of detection methods. But, for the microscopic examination of faeces for parasitic infection, there is no all-purpose technique. For reliable diagnosis of enteric parasites, a combination of several techniques is required. A simple wet mount or stained smear is often inadequate. Repeated specimen collections and testing are often necessary to optimize the detection of parasites that are shed intermittently or in fluctuating numbers. Concentration of specimens by sedimentation or flotation techniques may be required to detect low numbers of egg (worms) or cysts (protozoa) in faecal specimens. The most commonly used techniques rely on flotation media such as saturated sodium chloride (NaCl) solution to isolate and/or cleanse the parasitic life stages prior to counting; some of these methods are outlined below.

Flotation media

Sodium chloride solution with a specific gravity (SG) of around 1.2 (± 400 g sodium chloride per 1000 ml water) is commonly used for the detection of nematode and cestode eggs and protozoal oocysts in faeces. Although, when examining faeces for trematode eggs, zinc sulfate (SG 1.18–1.4; ± 420–500 g zinc sulfate chloride per 1000 ml water) or magnesium sulfate (SG 1.28; ± 500 g $MgSO_4$ per 1000 ml water) may be preferable due to the denser nature of these eggs. When making up the solution for the flotation step, if a hydrometer is unavailable, continue to add the appropriate salt crystals until they no longer dissolve.

Micrometry

When measuring helminth eggs, it is useful to use an ocular micrometer attached to a stereo microscope fitted with ×4, ×10 and ×40 objectives. A ×100 objective is useful if examining for protozoan parasites. Lengths and breadths can be accurately measured at a magnification of ×100, though higher magnifications can be used.

Faecal egg counts (FEC)

A number of variations of the FEC technique exist, and all provide an indication of the number of eggs being shed by a particular animal; however, these differ in sensitivity, speed of generation of results and the level of expertise required (Table 11.2).

Direct smear method

Consumables
Physiological saline (0.85% NaCl w/v), microscope slide, coverslip.

Equipment
Compound microscope.

> **Protocol**
> Add a few drops of water or physiological saline (0.85% NaCl w/v in distilled water) to a small quantity of faeces and draw along the slide with a coverslip until a thin covering of faeces is evident (Fig. 11.3). The technique allows for the qualitative, though not quantitative, assessment of eggs and larvae and is best used in cases when large numbers of parasites are expected.

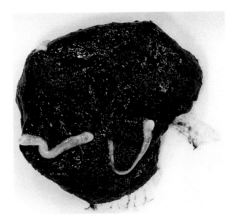

Figure 11.2 Faecal pat with *Monezia expansa* segments.

Table 11.2 Comparative properties of several faecal egg count techniques (✓poor – ✓✓moderate – ✓✓✓good)

Method	Smear	Coverslip	McMaster	Moredun
Speed	✓✓✓	✓✓	✓✓✓	✓✓
Versatile	✓	✓✓	✓✓	✓✓
Reliable	✓	✓✓	✓✓✓	✓✓✓
Sensitive	✓	✓✓	✓✓	✓✓✓
Expertise	✓✓	✓✓	✓✓	✓✓
Material	✓✓	✓✓	✓✓	✓✓
Low cost	✓✓✓	✓✓	✓✓	✓✓
Total	**13**	**14**	**16**	**16**

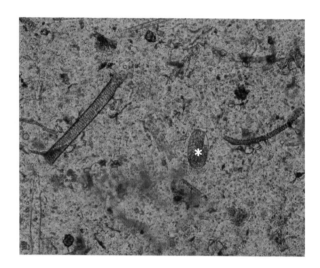

Figure 11.3 Example of faecal smear, strongyle egg (*).

Coverslip method

Consumables

Saturated sodium chloride solution, measuring cylinder, beaker, tea strainer/1 mm mesh, coverslip, microscope slide.

Equipment

Balance, compound microscope.

Protocol

Take a volume of faeces (±3 g) and dilute in a flotation medium such as saturated NaCl or ZnSO4 (±42 ml). Thoroughly mix the suspension and pass through a 1-mm sieve (tea strainer) or suitable mesh and collect the filtrate whilst discarding the debris. Resuspend the mixture and pour into a test tube producing a positive meniscus. Place a coverslip over the top of the test-tube, ensuring that no air bubbles are present. The tube can either be centrifuged at 1000 rpm (203 g) for 2 min or left on the bench for 15–20 min. The eggs will stick to the coverslip. Lift the coverslip off vertically and place on a microscope slide.

Original McMaster method

The most commonly used method is the McMaster technique which relies on flotation media such as saturated sodium chloride solution (NaCl) to isolate and/or cleanse the eggs or larvae prior to counting. A diagrammatic representation of the McMaster slide can be seen in Fig. 11.4. The sensitivity of the McMaster technique is generally 50 eggs per gram (EPG).

Consumables

Shaker jar containing approximately 45 glass balls, saturated sodium chloride solution, measuring cylinder, beaker, tea strainer/1 mm mesh, Pasteur pipette and bulb, McMaster counting slide.

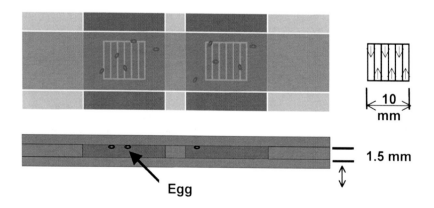

Figure 11.4 Diagrammatic representation of McMaster slide and recommended counting pattern.

Equipment
Balance, compound microscope.

> **Protocol**
> Place the glass balls in a shaker jar and add 42 ml of saturated NaCl. Add 3 g of faeces to the jar, lid and shake until all the faecal matter is broken down. Pour the mixture over a 1 mm sieve into a beaker and discard the retentate/debris. Thoroughly stir the filtrate and draw around 0.15 ml into a Pasteur pipette. Carefully run into one side of the counting chamber of a McMaster counting chamber. Repeat this step and fill the second chamber. Count all the eggs under the two grids (see Fig. 11.4), under a compound microscope at ×100 magnification. Multiply the total number of eggs under the two grids by 50 to calculate the number of eggs per gram.

Modified McMaster method

Consumables
As per McMaster method plus polythene bag, vacuum line, centrifuge tubes.

Equipment
Bench-top centrifuge.

> **Protocol**
> Take a 4.5 g subsample of the faecal sample into a polythene bag. Add 40.5 ml of tap water and rub bag thoroughly between fingers and thumb to macerate the material. Pour the mixture through a 1 mm sieve into a beaker, stir the filtrate and dispense a 10-ml sample into a centrifuge tube. Centrifuge the tube for 2 min at 1000 rpm (203 g). Remove the supernatant using a vacuum line and add 10 ml of saturated NaCl solution to the tube. Gently invert the tube ensuring even distribution, draw 0.15 ml of the sample into a Pasteur pipette and carefully run into one side of the counting chamber of a McMaster counting chamber. Repeat these steps and fill the second chamber. Count all the eggs under the two chambers. Multiply the total number of eggs under the two grids by 10 to calculate the number of eggs per gram.

Moredun flotation method

Consumables
10 ml pipette, saturated NaCl solution, beaker, tea strainer/1 mm mesh, polyallomer centrifuge tubes, artery forceps, 4 ml disposable microcuvette, cuvette lids, Miller square eye piece graticule (Electron Microscopy Sciences).

Equipment
Balance, centrifuge, compound microscope.

> **Protocol**
> Add 10 ml water per gram of faeces to the sample bag and emulsify. Thoroughly resuspend faecal sample prior to taking a 10-ml subsample using a 10-ml pipette with approximately 1 cm removed from tip. Dispense subsample through a 1-mm sieve into a beaker. Wash the retentate with approximately 5 ml of water into beaker. Squeeze retentate on strainer to remove excess liquid and discard retentate. Pour filtrate into a centrifuge tube and spin for approximately 2 min at 1000 rpm (203 g). Remove the supernatant using a vacuum line and add approximately 10 ml of saturated NaCl solution, gently re-suspend the pellet (caution: vigorous mixing will lead to the inclusion of an excessive amount of faecal debris). Centrifuge at 1000 rpm for 2 min. Using artery forceps clamp the tube just below the meniscus and pour the contents of the upper chamber into a cuvette, rinse the upper chamber of tube using approximately 1 ml saturated sodium chloride solution and add to the cuvette. Gently invert the cuvette several times and fill with saturated sodium chloride until there is a small positive meniscus. Carefully slide a cuvette lid on from the side to prevent air bubbles. Count the eggs within the cuvette (see section below about counting).

Data collation and explanation of eggs per gram calculation for Moredun flotation method

Step 1
A quick examination of the sample will enable an estimation of the egg density and therefore which is the most appropriate square of the Miller square eye piece graticule (Fig. 11.5) to use in calculating the numbers of eggs per gram:

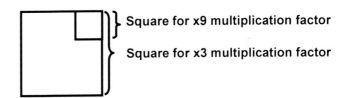

} Square for x9 multiplication factor

} Square for x3 multiplication factor

Figure 11.5 Diagrammatic representation of Miller square eye piece graticule, the small square is exactly 1/3 of the width of the larger square.

1 = All of the cuvette is examined and counted, used when very low numbers of egg are present in the sample.

3 = The sum of the two traverses (counted areas in Fig. 11.6A) is the equivalent of examining one-third of the cuvette, used when low to moderate numbers of eggs are present in the sample.

9 = The sum of the two traverses (counted areas in Fig. 11.6B) is the equivalent of examining one-ninth of the cuvette, used when moderate to high numbers of egg are present in the sample.

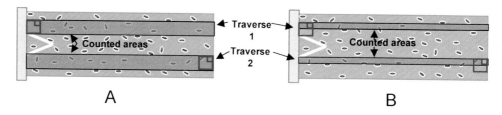

Figure 11.6 Diagrammatical representation of areas examined (traverse 1 and 2) in a faecal egg count using multiplication factors of 3 (A) and 9 (B).

Step 2
Individual counts of all of the eggs that fall within the designated squares in each of the traverses (Fig. 11.6).

Step 3
Sum of the individual traverse counts (step 3) multiplied by the multiplication factor (step 2, i.e. 1, 3 or 9).

Examples
A 3 g sample, examined with a multiplication factor of 9 with individual traverse counts of 12 and 8

$$= (12 + 8) \times 9 = 180 \text{ eggs per gram}$$

A half-gram sample, examined with a multiplication factor of 3 with individual traverse counts of 4 and 3

$$= [(4 + 3) \times 3] \times 2 = 42 \text{ eggs per gram}$$

Note: In samples of ≥ 1 gram only the eggs recovered from one gram of faeces gets examined. Counts for *Nematodirus* species are calculated independently of other strongyle counts using the same procedure.

Results can be expressed as eggs per gram of wet faeces (EPG_{ww} as demonstrated) or as a count per gram dry matter (EPG_{DM}). A subsample of faecal material should be thoroughly dried to determine percentage dry residue.

$$EPG_{DM} = EPG_{ww} \times (\text{faeces wet weight} \div \text{faeces dry weight})$$

Step 4
Subjective assessment of the numbers, but not identification, of coccidian oocysts is made for each sample:

1 = Small numbers of oocysts present.
2 = Moderate to high numbers of oocysts present.
3 = Very high numbers of oocysts present.

Step 5
The presence of eggs and larvae of other pulmonary and gastrointestinal parasites are recorded for each sample, in this case:

M – *Monezia* eggs
T – *Trichuris* eggs
S – *Strongyloides* eggs
L – lungworm larvae
F – fluke eggs (NB: usually needs a denser floatation medium than NaCl to determine the presence of fluke eggs).

It may be useful to determine whether eggs are viable or dead, particularly if using eggs in further tests. Indicators of viability are that eggs have intact shells with defined internal cellular integrity or motile larvae inside (Fig. 11.7A). Dead/non-viable eggs lack any definable internal structure and may have damaged shells (Fig. 11.7B).

Problems associated with FECs
Below are some problems associated with FECs.

- The consistency of faecal material can influence egg counts; watery diarrhoea can cause a dilution effect, whereas very dry faeces or constipation can cause a relative concentration of parasite numbers. Eggs can be expelled from hosts at different rates throughout the day, therefore if following a group of animals over time, it is best to obtain each sample at a similar time of day.

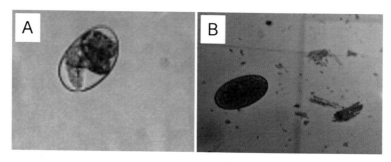

Figure 11.7 Viable (A) and dead (B) strongyle eggs.

- Eggs can be distributed unevenly throughout sample and this is thought to be of particular issue in horse and cattle samples. Therefore, ensure that samples are thoroughly homogenized/mixed before taking subsamples for enumeration of eggs.
- When assessing anthelmintic treatment efficacy, the time interval chosen for sample collection post treatment can influence the interpretation of results. With ruminants, faecal samples need to be collected between 7 and 17 days post treatment depending on the class of anthelmintic used. Ten days post treatment (PT) is most often used when looking at the action of the benzimidazoles, 17 days PT for avermectins although seven days PT is preferred if looking at the action of levamisoles (imidazothiazoles).
- Some parasites such as *F. hepatica* have a natural intermittent shedding pattern of eggs; therefore the absence of eggs is not necessarily an indication of lack of parasites. Also keep in mind that immature stages of parasites do not shed eggs, and in parasites where inhibition at an early stage of development is commonplace, such as with cyathostomins in horses or *Ostertagia osertagi* in cattle, accurate determination of worm burdens can be very difficult at certain times of the year.
- The immune responses of adult hosts may also lead to an inhibition of parasite development. A relaxation of immunity can occur around parturition in some hosts (notably sheep) with an associated increase in parasite development or acquisition of new infections, with a resultant increase in FEC.
- Worm size and fecundity can be affected by the total parasite burden (different and same species) within a host. This density dependent effect on the shedding of eggs may be a problem when examining FECs post treatment when surviving worms may shed more eggs per capita than was occurring before treatment.

Sedimentation methodologies

Trematodes – malachite green/methylene blue staining

Consumables
Beaker, tea strainer/1 mm mesh, centrifuge tube, Pasteur pipette and bulb, microscope slide.

Equipment
Compound microscope.

Protocol

Take a subsample of the faecal material and mix thoroughly with water. Pour suspension over a 1 mm sieve to remove large particulate matter, pass the filtrate through a finer sieve (nominal aperture 250 μm) into a conical flask. Let the filtrate stand for 3 min, remove the supernatant and transfer to a centrifuge tube. Add a few drops of malachite green (5%) or methylene blue (1%) aqueous solution and mix. Transfer the remaining sediment to a microscope slide and examine the entire sample under a dissection microscope, with both stains the fluke eggs 'glisten' and are easily recognizable against the dark background (Fig. 11.8).

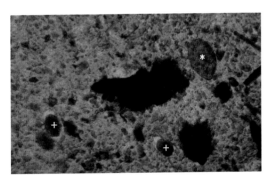

Figure 11.8 Strongyle (+) and *Fasciola* (*) eggs following sedimentation and treatment with malachite green.

Baermannization methodologies

Lung worm

Consumables
Gauze, funnel fitted with tap, retort stand, microscope slide, test tube, Pasteur pipette and bulb.

Protocol

Fill the supported funnel with tap water (approximately 22°C, max. 30°C). Enclose the faecal material within the gauze and submerge in the water until all of the faeces are covered. Leave the apparatus (Fig. 11.9) to sit for 12–18 hours to allow the larvae to migrate from the faeces. Open the tap at the bottom of the funnel and collect the first 10-15 ml of water into a test tube. Allow the larvae to resettle and remove the supernatant. Examine the sediment for larvae.

The examination of fresh material is advisable. If faecal material is allowed to sit in aerobic conditions at room temperature for more than 18–24 hours any trichostrongylid or *Strongyloides* eggs present in the sample may hatch and make diagnosis more difficult.

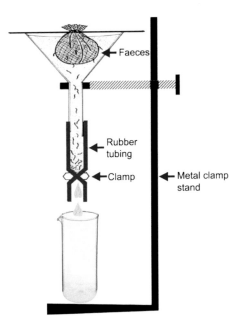

Figure 11.9 Baermann apparatus for separation and enrichment of nematode larvae from faeces, soil, or minced tissues of an animal.

Parasite species identification

Identification based on morphology and/or size

Some eggs are easily distinguishable via morphological means (Figs. 11.10 and 11.11), though many of the ruminant trichostrongylid parasites need to be differentiated by size or coprocultured to produce infective third-stage larvae which can be identified on the basis of a variety of aspects, for example length of the retained L2 cuticle sheath (Fig. 11.12).

Coproculture method

Consumables
Polythene bags, sieve 1 mm aperture, bucket, culture tray.

Equipment
Incubator, vacuum line.

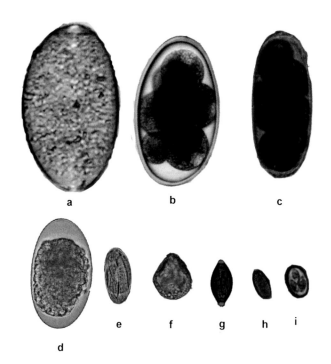

Figure 11.11 Key for commonly identified small ruminant nematode eggs/oocysts: (A) *Fasciola hepatica*, (B) *Nematodirus filicolis*, (C) *Nematodirus battus*, (D) Strongyle species, (E) *Strongyloides papillosus*, (F) *Monezia expansa*, (G) *Trichuris ovis*, (H) *Eimeria entricata*, (I) Coccidian oocyst.

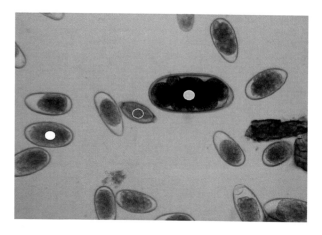

Figure 11.10 Commonly observed eggs from field-derived small ruminant faecal samples. Trichostrongylid egg (white closed circle), *Trichuris* (white open circle) and *Nematodirus* egg (grey closed circle).

> **Protocol**
> Place faeces in culture tray or suitable receptacle to a maximum depth of approximately 3 cm and loosely seal tray inside polythene bag. Puncture bag to allow airflow. Incubate the tray at 22°C for 10 days. Flood the tray with tepid tap water (22°C) and soak for between 2 and 4 hours. Sieve the fluid through a 1.0-mm sieve and collect filtrate. Sediment the filtrate for 2 hours at 4°C and then reduce the volume using a vacuum line and Baermannize (see Fig. 11.15).

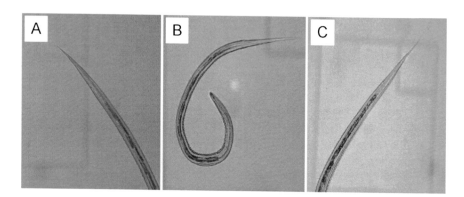

Figure 11.12 Short (A), medium (B) and long (C) 'tails'/sheaths used as one of the determining factors in speciating infective larvae.

Differential stains

Peanut agglutinin test

A lectin derived from peanuts (*Arachis hypogaea*) has been shown to preferentially bind to the surface of *H. contortus* eggs. When the lectin is conjugated with fluorescein isothiocyanate (FITC) it can be used as a diagnostic tool to identify these eggs. Unfortunately, at present this is the only lectin that is known to preferentially bind to eggs of a single species.

Consumables

Fluorescein isothiocyanate (FITC)-labelled peanut agglutinin (PNA; Vector Laboratories), phosphate-buffered saline (PBS), 1.5 ml Eppendorf tubes, microscope slide, pipette.

Equipment

Microcentrifuge, whirly mixer, microscope fitted with UV blue filter (wavelength 495 nm).

Protocol

Add 10 µl of FITC-labelled PNA to 990 µl of PBS and thoroughly mix to produce a 'working' solution. Collect a 'clean' preparation of eggs for examination, either by recovering from the faecal egg count or by mass extraction (see following section). Thoroughly mix the egg suspension and pipette 10 µl onto a slide and count the number of eggs present, repeat three times. Determine egg number and adjust suspension by sedimentation or dilution to 500 eggs per ml. Thoroughly mix the egg suspension and pipette 200 µl into an Eppendorf tube.

Add 200 µl of PNA/PBS solution to the Eppendorf, vortex, and incubate for 1 hour at 20°C. Add 1 ml of PBS, vortex and then centrifuge at 6000 rpm for 2 min. Remove the supernatant with a pipette. Repeat these steps three times.

Place 10-µl aliquots onto a microscope slide and count eggs under normal /transmission and UV light. Calculate the percentage of eggs fluorescing, and hence the number of *H. contortus* present (Fig. 11.13).

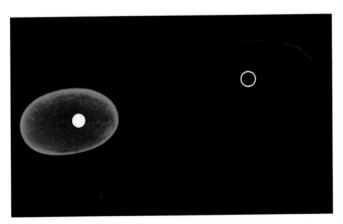

Figure 11.13 Strongylate eggs following peanut agglutinin staining. *Haemonchus contortus* egg showing fluorescence (solid circle) and other strongyle egg showing no fluorescence (open circle).

Mass egg extraction

Differential sieving

Consumables

Polythene bags, Beckmann polyallomer centrifuge tubes, saturated sodium chloride solution.

Equipment

1 mm, 500 µm, 212 µm, 75 µm and 38 µm aperture sieves, centrifuge, compound microscope.

Protocol

Add water to the faeces and emulsify until the faeces is a liquid suspension. Wash the suspension over a sequential tower of sieves; for example, for trichostrongylid eggs 1 mm, 500 µm, 212 µm, 75 µm and 38 µm aperture sieves will suffice. Collect the retentate from the 38 µm sieve into a centrifuge tube. Centrifuge at 1000 rpm (203 g) for approximately 2 min. Remove the supernatant and re-suspend the faecal pellet with 10 ml of saturated NaCl solution. Centrifuge at 1000 rpm (203 g) for approximately 2 min. Pour the supernatant over a 38 µm sieve and wash off the excess saturated NaCl solution with water.

Density gradient centrifugation

Consumables

38 mm sieve retentate containing nematode eggs to be cleaned, saturated sucrose solution (3:2 w/v), sucrose solutions (saturated sucrose diluted 1:4 with water; diluted 1:6 with water and diluted 1:8 with water, 10 ml syringe, beakers, 50 ml centrifuge tubes, Pasteur pipette and bulb.

Equipment

Centrifuge, 38 mm sieve.

Protocol

Carefully layer 9 ml of the sucrose solutions into the 50 ml centrifuge tube forming four distinct layers (Fig. 11.14). Gently layer 9 ml of the 38 mm sieve retentate containing nematode eggs to be cleaned on top of the sucrose gradient. Centrifuge the tube at 2000 rpm (814 g) for 15 min. The eggs form a discrete layer after centrifugation which can be removed using a Pasteur pipette. Wash the eggs over a 38 mm sieve with water to remove any sucrose.

Baermannization method

Consumables

Polythene bags, high wet strength paper, filter holder, elastic band, 250 ml beakers or jam jar, 250 ml culture flasks.

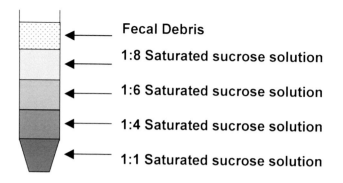

Figure 11.14 Saturated sucrose gradient for cleaning faecal samples.

Protocol

Place layers of high wet strength paper over filter holder and attach with elastic band (Fig. 11.15). Note: If cleaning larval suspension use single layer paper, if extracting from faecal filtrate use two layers. Fill the 250-ml beaker or jam jar with tepid water (approximately 22°C). Pour the chilled filtrate or larval suspension through the paper of the Baermann apparatus, ensuring that the sample is distributed evenly over the paper and removing any excess water. Immerse the Baermann apparatus in the warm tap-water in the beaker and leave standing at room temperature for two hours.

Methods of studying anthelmintic efficacy and resistance testing

Methodologies for the *in vivo* and *in vitro* examination of anthelmintic sensitivity from the field and in the laboratory are well detailed. Standardization of the techniques conducted to assess anthelmintic activity against endo- and ectoparasites of production and companion animals has been published by both the World Association for the Advancement of Veterinary Parasitology (http://www.waavp.org/node/25) and VICH (http://www.vichsec.org/en/guidelines.htm) (overview in Table 11.3).

The precise methodologies for the detection of anthelmintic resistance (AR) in small ruminants can be found in more details in published reviews, whilst work is being conducted to standardize methods in cattle (http://www.parasol-project.org, last accessed 10SEP08). General parasitological-based techniques such as controlled efficacy tests (CET, drench and slaughter), FEC reduction tests (FECRT), egg hatch test (EHT) and larval development test (LDT) have been used in the initial reporting and subsequent surveying of BZ and ML resistance in ruminants and are outlined below.

In vivo tests

In vivo tests are the cornerstone of AR detection in the field. Two tests are commonly cited in the literature; the FEC reduction test (FECRT) and the controlled efficacy test (CET). The first technique is most commonly utilized by scientists, veterinarians and producers alike.

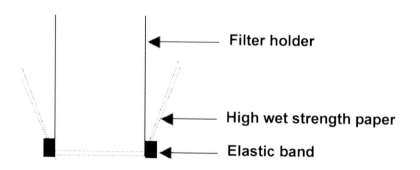

Figure 11.15 Baermann filtration apparatus.

Table 11.3 VICH and WAAVP guidelines for assessing the efficacy of anthelmintics in livestock

Host	VICH guideline	WAAVP reference
General requirements	VICH GL7	–
Bovines	VICH GL12	Vet. Parasitol. *58*,181–213
Ovines	VICH GL13	Vet. Parasitol. *58*,181–213
Caprines	VICH GL14	Vet. Parasitol. *58*,181–213
Equines	VICH GL15	Vet. Parasitol. *103*, 1–18
Porcines	VICH GL16	Vet. Parasitol. *141*, 138–49
Poultry	VICH GL21	Vet. Parasitol. *116*, 159–173

VICH, Veterinary International Co-operation on Harmonization; WAAVP, World Association for the Advancement of Veterinary Parasitology.

Full faecal egg count reduction test

The FECRT has been used world-wide to characterize and assess anthelmintic efficacy and/or survey for the presence/absence of AR in sheep, goats, cattle, horses, pigs and chickens. The World Association for the Advancement of Veterinary Parasitology (WAAVP) has described appropriate FECRT methodology for small ruminants to assess the efficacy of anthelmintic treatments. The 'full' test uses reductions in the FEC of treated animals compared with untreated control animals, with samples being collected after a specific period of time depending upon the drug class being investigated. Where having groups of animals left untreated is unacceptable it is possible to assess treatment efficacy by comparative analysis of pre- and post-treatment FECs. Resistance is inferred if the reduction in FEC is less than 95%, with lower confidence intervals of less than 90%.

In brief, the test involves taking rectal faecal samples from all animals to be examined and performing FECs on them. Animals are allocated into groups, of at least 15 animals, for each treatment and an untreated control, ensuring minimal difference in group mean FEC. Groups are randomly assigned an anthelmintic treatment or left untreated to act as controls. Each animal is dosed with its designated anthelmintic on the basis of body weight, ensuring that each animal receives its full dose. The group mean FECs are calculated for the pre-treatment samples. The optimal time for re-sampling of treated animals is 3–7 days, 8–10 days and 14–17 days post treatment for the LEV, BZ, and ML, respectively, to avoid possible false positive/negative results. Levamisole has no label claim against juvenile worms and therefore resampling needs to be conducted before maturation of surviving immature stages occurs, whereas suppression of egg production may occur for up to 10 and 14 days post treatment with BZ and ML, respectively. The mean FECs of the groups are calculated for the post-treatment samples. The efficacy is estimated using one of a range of standard formulae, where C_1 and C_2 are the FEC of untreated control animals pre- and post treatment, respectively, and T_1 and T_2 are the FEC of the treated animals pre- and post treatment respectively:

$$[1 - (T_2/C_2)] \times 100 \text{ using arithmetic means}$$

$$[1 - (T_2/T_1)(C_1/C_2)] \times 100 \text{ using geometric means}$$

$$[1 - (T_2/T_1)(C_1/C_2)] \times 100 \text{ using arithmetic means}$$

$$[1 - (T_2/T_1)] \times 100 \text{ using arithmetic means}$$

Consumables

5, 10, 20 and 50 ml syringes, anthelmintic and dosing sheets giving appropriate recommended dose rate for the animal, bags for collecting samples, marker spray to identify treated animals, recording sheets for body weight and observations (consumables and equipment to conduct faecal egg count).

Equipment

Weight crate/balance and compound microscope.

Protocol

For ruminants, ideally weigh and faecal sample a minimum of 15 animals for each treatment group and controls. Assign animals into anthelmintic treatment groups and control groups randomly or balanced for weight and FEC. Dose each animal in the treated groups with its designated anthelmintic on the basis of body weight, ensuring that each animal receives its full dose. Conduct FECs using salt flotation for each animal and record the egg per gram (EPG) count. Calculate the groups' mean FECs for the pre-treatment samples. Faecal sample all the animals between 7 and 17 days PT. Ten days PT is most often used when looking at the action of the benzimidazoles, 17 days PT for avermectins though 7 days PT is preferred if looking at the action of levamisoles. Repeat the egg count procedure and again record the EPG count for each animal. Calculate the groups' mean FECs for the post-treatment samples. Estimate efficacy using a standard formula outlined above.

Post-drench efficacy test

The post-drench efficacy test (PDET) is where some information on anthelmintic efficacy can be determined at a fraction of the cost of a FECRT. The PDET looks at the FECs of animals following treatment at the allotted times as identified above. If eggs are present it is assumed that the treatment is not working fully efficiently and requires further investigation. Unfortunately, due to the lack of FEC data pre-treatment, it is impossible to determine the true efficacy of treatment.

Controlled efficacy test

This test, also known as 'drench and slaughter', assesses treatment efficacy in infected animals compared with untreated control animals by estimation of total worm burdens post mortem and can be used with field infected or artificially challenged animals. The CET can be used to assess all stages of parasitic life cycle, from day one post-artificial infection to infections carried by naturally infected animals. To ensure that findings are both biologically and statistically relevant, groups should contain a minimum of five animals per drug compound, plus a control group. Rectal faecal samples and FECs need to be conducted on all animals prior to treatment to allow appropriate allocation of animals with minimal difference in group mean FEC if examining adult egg laying populations. Treatment groups should be allocated randomly and animals need to be weighed and treated according to body weight. Notes should be made of any treatment errors or immediate adverse reaction to the anthelmintic. After a specified time, the animals are euthanized and the gastrointestinal tract removed and processed according to the appropriate protocol. Total worm burden estimations allow calculation of the efficacy of the treatments using either arithmetic or geometric means in the formulae as detailed above. The test is generally only used in research laboratories to characterize new isolates of parasites or to assess novel treatments, due to the prohibitively expensive running costs or to assess the effect of new anthelmintics for licensing purposes.

Consumables

5, 10, 20 and 50 ml syringes, anthelmintic and dosing sheets giving appropriate recommended dose rate for the animal, bags for collecting samples, marker spray to identify treated animals, recording sheets for body weight and observations. Consumables and equipment to conduct faecal egg count may be required if treatments against egg laying stages are being examined.

Equipment

Weight crate/balance and compound microscope.

Protocol

Animal requirements

Group of at least five animals per drug compound plus one control group of minimum six animals. To be housed indoors at day −1.

Procedure for day −1

Take rectal faecal sample from all animals when brought into housing. Perform FEC on all samples. Allocate animals into groups with minimal difference in group mean FEC. Allocate groups to treatment randomly.

Procedure for day 0

Weigh and treat animals according to body weight. Note any treatment errors or immediate adverse reaction to drug.

Procedure for day +14

Perform necropsy to remove gastrointestinal tract. Perform worm burden estimation.

Abomasal processing

Take the abomasum and remove mesenteric fat before processing. Open lengthways along the greater curvature, working over the bucket to collect the contents. Rinse any surface adherent material into the bucket with warm physiological saline (0.85% NaCl) and top up to approximately 5 litres with warm 0.85% physiological saline. Incubate for 4–6 hours at 37°C.

Intestinal processing

Take the intestine and run through fingers to expel contents. As with the abomasum, remove as much excess mesenteric fat before processing. Open the intestine longitudinally and rinse any surface adherent material into the bucket with saline, toping up to approximately 5 litres with warm 0.85% physiological saline. Incubate for 4–6 hours at 37°C.

Following incubation thoroughly rinse the organ in the bucket and rub the entire surface to ensure the removal of any retained debris, mucus and worms. Remember to pay particular attention to the folds of the abomasum. Discard the tissue and top up the contents/saline digest suspension to 5 litres with 0.85% physiological saline.

Re-suspend thoroughly and remove two 250-ml aliquots. Pool the two aliquots into a pre-labelled 500-ml container to give a 10% abomasal wash and saline digest subsample, fix subsample with 20 ml of formalin and archive for worm burden analysis.

1% pepsin/HCl can be used in place of physiological saline where inhibited or juvenile nematode stages are being quantified. Caution must be observed when using this digestive medium.

Calculate efficacy using arithmetic or geometric means in the formula:

Efficacy = 100 × [(mean worm burden control group) − (mean worm burden treated group) ÷ (mean worm burden control group)]

Interpretation of results

There needs to be clear guidance with regards to the interpretation/significance of those findings. It is clear that slowing the selection, development and spread of AR within livestock is a complex and multifaceted problem and sadly, there are no simple blueprint solutions. However, it may be possible to simplify the FEC and PDET systems by introducing a three tier system such as the traffic light system. In the latter system, a green classification (low egg counts/high drench efficacy) requires no action, an amber classification (moderate egg counts/moderate drench efficacy) raises some concerns and a red classification (high egg counts/low drench efficacy) requires urgent action (Fig. 11.16). This type of system is not without its problems, primarily in being too broad in its recommendations, but has been shown to work well with systems such as the one use for the detection of anaemia, i.e. FAMACHA©.

In vitro bioassays

Most *in vitro* bioassays examine the response of a developmental stage(s) of the parasites to xenobiotic/anthelmintic treatment when administered in a dose-dependent fashion. From the dose response, it is possible to determine the concentration of anthelmintic required to inhibit a known percentage of the population from completing their normal development, e.g. ED_{50} is the concentration of compound required to inhibit 50% of eggs from developing and hatching within an egg hatch test.

Egg hatch test (EHT)

The *in vitro* EHT assesses the ability of eggs to hatch in different concentrations of thiabendazole (TBZ). Approximately 100 strongyle eggs are incubated in final concentrations of TBZ of 0.05, 0.1 and 0.3 μg/ml for 48 hours at 22°C in 24-well cluster plates. Helminthological iodine is used to stop the test and prevent further hatching of eggs. The numbers of eggs and larvae are counted and the data are used to determine the ED_{50} estimation. Estimates of greater than 0.1 μg/ml are indicative of resistance.

Consumables

24-well cluster plate; thiabendazole (TBZ), dimethylsulfoxide, distilled water, helminthological iodine (250 g of potassium

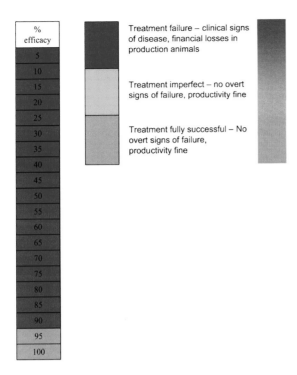

Figure 11.16 Graphical representation of system for presenting treatment efficacy results.

iodide, 50 g of iodine; add to 500 ml of tap water, dissolve; store at room temperature), fresh nematode egg suspension.

Equipment
Pipettes to dispense 10–1000 ml; inverted/stereo microscope.

Protocol
Prepare working concentrations of thiabendazole (TBZ) suspended in dimethylsulphoxide (DMSO). Possible suggested concentrations for investigating TBZ resistance in the majority of ruminant trichostrongylid eggs are shown below.

Working TBZ concentration (µg/ml)	Final TBZ concentration (µg/ml)
60	0.3
20	0.1
10	0.05
0	0

Extract eggs from fresh faecal material (less than 4 hours from rectal collection) or from anaerobically stored material (see above). Adjust concentration of egg suspension to 1000 eggs per ml. Add 10 µl of working stock solution to the wells of the cluster plate followed by 1890 µl of distilled water. Administer the water as two aliquots of 945 µl to ensure even distribution of the drug.

Thoroughly mix the egg suspension and add 100 µl to each well of the plate. Label the culture plate to show the concentration used in each well. Place the culture plate in a 100% relative humidity chamber (or lunch box with sealable lid) and incubate at approximately 25°C for 48 hours. Following incubation add 50 µl of helminthological/lugols iodine to each well.

Count the number of eggs and hatched larvae using an inverted or stereo microscope (it may be necessary to transfer the contents of each well into a small Petri dish since the edges of wells may be obscured from view depending on the quality of illumination of the microscope).

Calculate mean numbers of eggs (E) and first-stage larvae (L1) at each concentration and the percentage hatch using the standard formula:

$$\text{Percentage hatch} = [L1 \div (E + L1)] \times 100$$

The percentage of eggs which fail to hatch at each drug concentration are corrected for natural mortality using data from control wells and transformed using arcsin transformation and plotted against drug concentration. The resulting log dose response line enables the ED50 to be estimated (i.e. the concentration of TBZ required to prevent 50% of the eggs from hatching). In ovine and caprine derived samples, if the ED50 estimate is greater than 0.1 µg/ml, then the population is presumed to be resistant to benzimidazoles.

Larval development test (LDT)
The *in vitro* LDT assesses the ability of eggs to hatch, develop and moult through two larval stages to become third-stage larvae (L3) in the presence of increasing BZ and LEV concentrations. Work performed in Australia showed that the LDT was unreliable at detecting ML resistance with field-derived material, particularly with *T. circumcincta*. Details of how to conduct the technique can be found in published manuscripts.

Larval migration inhibition test
The larval migration test, like the larval motility test, assesses effects on somatic musculature but avoids the need for potentially subjective assessment of activity by examining the ability of anthelmintic-treated L_3 to migrate through mesh filters. The test has been trialled with a range of anthelmintics (macrocyclic lactones and/or levamisoles) on a number parasitic nematode species from a range of hosts, e.g. pigs, sheep and equids.

Consumables
Fresh infective larvae suspension, sodium hypochlorite (sterilizing solution, sodium hypochlorite NaOCl), microscope slide, phosphate buffered saline, 24-well cluster plate, pure anthelmintic powder (macrocyclic lactone or levamisole) is preferable if available although commercially available compounds can be used if necessary, DMSO, distilled water, tapering plastic tubing (Two sizes, one to fit tightly inside other to create fixed collar for mesh, approximate maximum diameter 15 mm), 25 µm nylon mesh (40 mm × 40 mm per well), helminthological iodine.

Equipment

Pipettes to dispense 10–1000 ml; inverted/stereo microscope.

Protocol

Ensure that the test L3 are fresh and healthy; if necessary re-Baermannize the larvae immediately prior to the test. Prepare stock drug solutions, suspend in DMSO if using pure compounds (suspend commercial products in distilled water), a recommended starting range of concentrations is 1000, 500, 250, 125, 62.5, 31.25 μg/ml. Prepare the filters (Fig. 11.17).

Exsheath the L3 by placing them in a conical bottomed centrifuge tube, add NaOCl (5% v/v) and invert the tube to mix the solution, take a subsample of suspension and place on microscope slide, observe L3 until approximately 95% have exsheathed (Fig. 11.18). Centrifuge remaining L3 for 2 min at 1000 rpm (203 g) and remove supernatant. Resuspend larvae in PBS to wash off the NaOCl and re-centrifuge as before. Repeat this process a further two times or until the chlorine smell is removed.

Count the exsheathed L3 and adjust the concentration such that 100 μl suspension contains approximately 100 L3. Dispense 100 μl containing the larvae into a series of labelled eppendorf tubes, 25 μl of the stock drug solutions and make up to 1 ml with distilled water and incubate for 2 h at 37°C.

Following 2 h incubation, centrifuge at 1000 rpm (203 g) for two min and reduce the volume to 200 μl.

Take 50 μl of each drug concentration and make up to 2 ml with distilled water. Dispense 1800 μl of the diluted drug concentration to rows A (Fig. 11.17) on the test plate and place a filter into the well ensuring that the mesh is fully submerged and that there are no air bubbles trapped beneath the mesh.

Mix the larval suspension thoroughly and add the L3 in 200 μl of fluid to each filter by pipetting gently down the inside of the inner collar. NOTE: the suspension must be mixed for every well as L3 settle rapidly in water. Place a cover over the plates and incubate for 2 hours at 37°C in the dark.

Carefully remove the filters and wash any remaining L3 into row B of the cluster plate with distilled water from a water bottle. Add a few drops of helminthological iodine to each well on the culture plate. Using an inverted microscope at ×100 magnification count the number of L3 in each well.

The percentage migration is calculated for each concentration using the formula:

$$\text{Percentage migration} = [(L_m) \div (L_m + L_r)] \times 100$$

where L_m represents number of L3 migrating (row A), L_r the number of L3 remaining on the filter (row B).

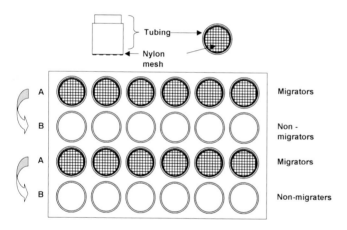

Figure 11.17 Diagrammatic representation of material used in the larval migration inhibition test.

Larval feeding inhibition test

The larval feeding inhibition test allows the examination of feeding behaviour of first stage nematode larvae. If the test substance has been effective at paralysing the pharyngeal musculature, then they are unable to feed and no fluorescence can be seen. If the substance has been ineffective then a clearly defined gut can be seen (Fig. 11.19).

Consumables

Six-well cluster plate, lyophilized *Escherichia coli* (Sigma Chemical Co.), fluorescein isothiocyanate (FITC; Sigma Chemical Co.), 2 ml microcentrifuge tube, bicarbonate buffer (1.5 g/l NaCl, 1.96 g/l Na$_2$CO$_3$, 2.66 g/l NaHCO$_3$ made up in distilled water),

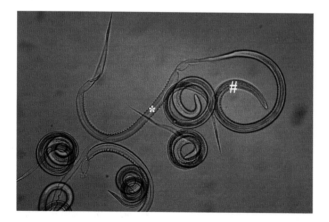

Figure 11.18 Exsheathing *Haemonchus contortus* larvae. Sheath (*), exsheathed larvae (#).

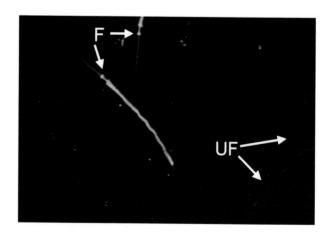

Figure 11.19 Picture of fed (F) and unfed (UF) *Haemonchus contortus* first-stage larvae.

pure anthelmintic powder (macrocyclic lactone or levamisole) is preferable if available although commercially available compounds can be used if necessary, DMSO, PBS (pH 7.2), distilled water, microscope slides.

Equipment
1 μm, 212 μm, 90 μm and 38 μm sieves, mini Baermann apparatus (25 mm mesh), microcentaur, benchtop microfuge, pipettes, inverted fluorescent microscope fitted with UV blue range filter (495 nm).

Protocol
Production of fluorescein isothiocyanate FITC-labelled lyophilized *E. coli* for use in larval feeding inhibition test (LFIT). Incubate 100 μl of concentrated *E. coli* (2250 μg *E. coli*/ml bicarbonate buffer) in 1 ml of bicarbonate buffer containing 1mg of FITC in a 2-ml microcentrifuge tube at 20°C for 2 hours. Centrifuge *E. coli* suspension at 13000 rpm for 2 min. Remove supernatant using a vacuum line. Re-suspend *E. coli* pellet in 1 ml of PBS. Repeat resuspension and centrifugation steps twice. Resuspend *E. coli* in 1 ml of PBS.

Larval feeding inhibition test
Prepare stock drug solutions, suspend in DMSO if using pure compounds (suspend commercial products in distilled water). Extract eggs from test material using differential sieving (1 mm, 212 μm, 90 μm and 38 μm sieves). Incubate eggs at 25°C for 18–24 hours. Following this incubation period, place the embryonated eggs in a mini-Baermann apparatus (mesh aperture 25 μm) and submerged in water in a six-well cluster plate and incubate at 22°C until the eggs hatch and the emerging first-stage larvae (L1) migrate through the mesh. Determine the number of L1 that migrate through the Baermann apparatus. Add 100 L1 in 1498 μl of tap water and 2μl of selected anthelmintic to labelled 2-ml microcentrifuge tubes. For control wells, use 1498 μl distilled water and 2μl DMSO instead of anthelmintic concentration. Run each concentration in duplicate. Incubate tubes horizontally at 22°C for 2 hours. Add 7 μl of FITC-labelled *E. coli* and incubate tubes horizontally for a further 18 hours at 22°C. Following incubation, centrifuge the tubes at 6000 rpm (3000 g) for 20 s and remove 750 μl of the supernatant. Transfer the L1 onto a glass slide for counting and were examined at a magnification of ×100 using an inverted fluorescence microscope fitted with a UV blue range filter (495 nm). Larvae with FITC-labelled *E. coli* visible throughout the gastrointestinal tract are considered to be feeding (Fig. 11.19).

LFI50 or LFI99 estimates, i.e. the concentration of drug at which 50% or 99% of the L1 did not feed, can be determined by performed using a probit model on uncorrected raw data.

The future
Molecular markers for resistance may provide sensitive and relatively rapid ways of screening parasite populations for the presence of resistance genes. In the last 10–15 years much work has been conducted into searching for appropriate markers. Single nucleotide polymorphism markers are well defined for BZ resistance in several species but not for other two broad spectrum anthelmintic drug classes. More research is required into the area before viable diagnostic tests are likely to become both cheap with sufficient specificity to be of use in the field. So in conclusion, the detection and characterization of anthelmintic resistance can be achieved in a number of ways but at present there are no techniques that fulfil all of the criteria that would make them universally applicable such as – cheap to run and set up without the need for expensive equipment, provide reliable, accurate and definitive results, detect resistance even when only present at low levels within a population, provide results in a speedy and expedient manner, be versatile (multiple anthelmintic classes examined), provide added value such as a species profile of the parasites involved or provide objective or non-subjective answers.

Examination of blood and body fluid
Next to faeces, the blood provides the most common medium for recovery of various stages of animal and human parasites. Living protozoa and microfilariae may be seen in fresh blood diluted with saline but their identification requires preparations either as wet films stained with haematoxylin or as dried stained films. From this source a diagnosis is routinely made of malaria, babesiosis, trypanosomiasis, and most types of filariasis.

Protozoa in blood
The standard procedure for diagnosis of protozoa in the circulating blood is to make direct smear preparations. It is important that the slides used for blood films be thoroughly cleaned and grease-free. There are, in general, two types of slide preparations: the thin film and the thick film. The *thin film* ideally is one cell thick, with blood cells lying flat on the glass surface. The haemoglobin as well as other proteins in the blood should be fixed before staining so that after they are stained all elements, including the erythrocytes will remain intact and recognizable. The *thin blood film* is useful for studying details in the blood cells and blood parasites (Fig. 11.20). Its primary disadvantage is that the amount of blood in the sample is small. The *thick film* contains 6–20 times as much blood per unit area as a thin film. It is necessary that the thick film *not* be fixed before staining since the erythrocytes must be de-haemoglobinized during the procedure. The disruption of the erythrocytes and the loss of their haemoglobin from the slide allow the remaining structures, including blood parasites, to be seen microscopically. The thick film is suited for rapid diagnosis of parasitaemia too low to be detected in the thin film.

Microfilariae
Filarial nematodes infect different tissues of the body and produce larvae called microfilaria. Depending on the species, microfilaria may be found in the blood or dermis of the host. Species producing microfilaria that accumulate in the dermis are diagnosed by the skin maceration technique. A biopsy specimen of skin is finely macerated and allowed to soak for at least 6 hours in physiological saline solution at approximately 37°C or about 8–10 hours at room temperature (~21°C). The macerated tissue is strained off,

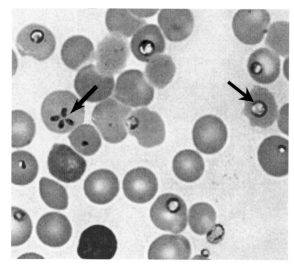

Figure 11.20 Thin blood smear showing developmental stages of *Babesia* sp. (arrows).

the liquid is centrifuged, and the bottom 1 or 2 ml is examined for microfilaria. Histological sectioning of the skin can be used, but is time consuming and less sensitive. For microfilaria of filarial nematodes that occur in the blood, several procedures can be done.

Direct smear
A thin film of blood is smeared on a slide and dried, and the film is stained with Wright's or Giemsa stain (Fig. 11.21). A few drops of freshly drawn blood can also be mixed with physiological saline solution, and the resultant preparation is examined microscopically for motile microfilaria. This technique works only if microfilariae are numerous.

Microhaematocrit technique
The microhaematocrit tube is examined for microfilaria after centrifugation. Microfilaria will be found at the plasma–blood interface (buffy coat).

Membrane filtration technique
This technique is effective in detecting microfilariae when present in small numbers in the blood. It requires 1 ml of blood, which is

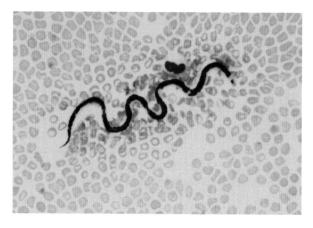

Figure 11.21 *Dipetalonema viteae* microfilaria in a blood smear.

then mixed with the lysing solution (usually 9 ml) to haemolyse the red blood cells. The mixture is then passed through a plastic chamber containing a filter membrane on which the microfilariae are collected. The membrane filter is then removed and placed on a clean microscope slide. A drop of stain is placed on top of the membrane, which is covered with a coverslip for examination under the microscope. Microfilariae collected in this manner may be unsuitable for demonstrating the morphology for species identification.

Knott's concentration technique
One millilitre of blood is added to 9 ml of 2% formalin. The mixture is then shaken until the blood is haemolysed and is centrifuged at 1500 rpm for 5 min, the supernatant fluid decanted, and the sediment examined for microfilariae. These substances may be vitally stained or the film air-dried, fixed, and permanently stained. Measurements are often necessary to distinguish species and must be done to separate *Dirofilaria* spp. and *Dipetalonema* spp.

Urine
Urine sediment is regularly examined for the protozoan *Trichomonas vaginalis* or the eggs of *Schistosoma haematobium*. On rare occasions, *Strongyloides* larvae can be seen in the urine. Also, the swine kidney worm (*Stephanurus dentatus*) lays eggs that pass out in the urine.

Examination of aspirates
Recovery of protozoa or helminths from aspirated materials often constitutes an important diagnostic aid. Duodenal aspiration may be useful in demonstrating infections with *Giardia lamblia*, *Strongyloides stercoralis*, *Fasciolopsis buski* and parasites in the gall bladder or biliary tract. Aspirates from lymph nodes, spleen, liver, bone marrow, and spinal fluid frequently provide diagnostic evidence of African trypanosomiasis, visceral leishmaniasis (kala-azar), Chagas' disease and toxoplasmosis. The aspirated materials can be used as direct unstained preparations to demonstrate motile organisms (trypanosomes), as Giemsa-stained impression smears, and/or for culturing of parasites that may be present.

Skin scrapings for ectoparasites
This procedure is mainly used for detection of ectoparasites, such as mites, louse infestations (Fig. 11.22). Hair may be gently clipped away if the coat is very thick. The scalpel blade is normally held perpendicular to the skin and the scraping should be in the direction of the hair coat. Scrapings should be taken at the periphery of the lesion. Skin scrapes may be taken into either liquid paraffin or 10% potassium hydroxide. When liquid paraffin is used a few drops can be gently added to the sample before a cover slip is added. When potassium hydroxide is used the sample is best left stand for 10–15 min and may be gently warmed before examining as this allows the potassium hydroxide to digest keratin to clear the field. In case of suspected *Demodex*, lesions should be squeezed at the time the skin is scraped to ensure enough sample collections.

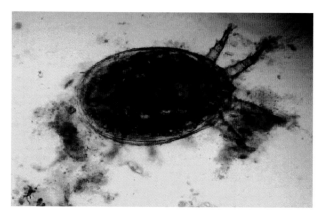

Figure 11.22 Mite isolated from skin lesions of a snake using skin scrapings.

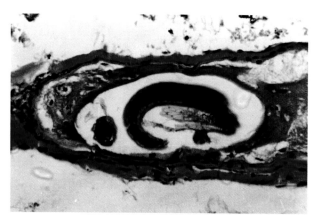

Figure 11.23 Longitudinal section of muscle showing encysted *Trichinella* larva and moderate inflammatory reaction (×400).

Ticks, fleas and lice are all of enough size to see with the naked eye. Sometimes lice are difficult to find; hence a careful examination for nits (louse eggs) attached to the hair may reveal their presence. Dipteran flies are often easily identifiable because they are host and/or site specific (e.g. *Hypoderma* spp., *Gasterophilus* spp., *Oestrus ovis*, and *Cuterebra* spp.). Screw worm larvae can be identified by the presence of two black, pigmented tracheal trunks leading from the spiracle of the body. They can be clearly seen in the living third instar larva with the unaided eye. Other larvae can be identified by the pattern of the spiracle at the caudal extremity of the body. The larval stages of *Wohlfahrtia* spp. can be identified based on the morphological characteristics of the spiracular plates and cephalopharyngeal skeleton of the third instar larva. Accurate identification of ectoparasite requires using taxonomic keys, and best accomplished by a specialist.

Tissue biopsy

Biopsy and histopathology are frequently useful in the diagnosis of parasitic infections, and may be at times the only method of confirming clinical suspicion of an infection (Fig. 11.23). More details are provided in Chapter 12.

Bronchoalveolar lavage

Endoscopy may be used to confirm the presence of upper airway disease and to perform diagnostic tests such as transtracheal aspirate (TTA) or bronchoalveolar lavage (BAL). The latter is a valuable diagnostic tool that becomes more widely used in the diagnosis of veterinary clinical diseases. The test depends on sampling of the cellular and biochemical composition of the lung in a live animal by injecting and retrieving sterile fluids. BAL is done intratracheally by inserting a tube directly into the larynx and bronchi, or transtracheally by inserting a tube via a needle across the skin into the trachea. BAL is used for the diagnosis of lungworm infections.

Immunodiagnosis of parasitic infections

Serological tests have been developed as alternatives to faecal examination, which is labour-intensive and requires a skilled microscopist. Serological tests for the parasites may be divided into two categories; testing for immune response to parasite and

testing for the presence of parasite itself. Tests that look for the presence of immune response to parasite include ELISA, IFA, Western immunoblotting, agglutination testing, and T-cell proliferation assays. It is important to consider what aspect of immune response is being tested. T-cell proliferation assay tests for the presence of cellular immune response, whereas the others test for the presence of humoral immune response. A cellular immune response primarily uses cytotoxic T cells to trigger self-destruction of host cells that are infected with intracellular parasites, e.g. *Toxoplasma gondii*. Cellular and humoral immune response often, but not always are found together. Also an animal may have a cellular immune response without a significant humoral immune response or vice versa. It is also important to consider whether the patient has had time to develop an immune response to a parasite. Monitoring immune response with serological testing could have a considerable impact on the diagnosis and evaluation of therapeutic responses to parasitic infections.

Antigen detection

Antigen detection assays involve the use of parasite-specific antibody to detect or bind to the parasite protein or antigen in the clinical sample (Fig. 11.24).

Antibody detection

Evaluation of the host immunological response involves detection of antibody to a specific pathogen. This provides, at the least, a historical perspective of the parasite to which the animal has been exposed or vaccinated. By doing paired sera testing in the acute and convalescent phases of disease, the infection status can be determined. Serology on herds or flocks can be used to establish the prevalence of the agent in the population. Serological assays may be qualitative or quantitative. The former determines only the presence of antibody, not the level. The assays that are used to detect antibody are similar to ones for antigen detection.

Molecular detection

The assays described above involve detection of whole parasite or its protein components. These microscopic and serological tests are still considered the 'gold standard' for the diagnosis of parasitic diseases. However, if an unequivocal identification of the parasite

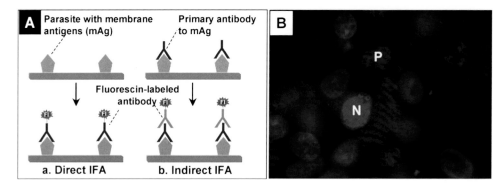

Figure 11.24 (A) Sketch of immunofluorescence assays (a) direct and (b) indirect version of the assay using fluorescein-labelled antibody. (B) Photomicrograph of immunofluorescence assay of parasite-infected cells using fluorescein-labelled antibody. P, parasite; N, host cell nucleus.

can not be made, the specimen should be analysed using molecular techniques. Polymerase chain reaction (PCR), sequencing, recombinant DNA, and hybridization technology are causing a revolution in diagnostic parasitology. They offer rapid, sensitive, and specific diagnostic testing for parasitic diseases. These techniques are designed to identify parasitic infection by detecting specific DNA targets in the parasite genome.

PCR

This technique involves the isolation of nucleic acid from the sample and amplification of a portion of genetic material of the agent of interest. This amplification is accomplished by repeated cycles of DNA synthesis primed by small nucleic acid primers that are designed to target a specific gene from a particular parasite (Fig. 11.25). Amplified DNA fragments are electrophoretically resolved on an agarose gel for analysis of results. PCR amplified fragments can be analysed by using restriction fragment length polymorphisms (RFLP) or DNA sequencing if further species or subspecies characterization is needed. Quality assurance, stringent controls and a high level of expertise are required for accurate results using PCR.

One of the hallmarks of PCR is its superb sensitivity, especially with nested PCR, which can be a double-edged sword. It allows the detection of small amounts of the agent in the sample, which can be advantageous if low amounts are present. But this high sensitivity makes PCR susceptible to false positive results as a result of contamination or carry-over. Real-time or quantitative PCR can provide information on the amount of parasite that is present in the sample. This can assist in distinguishing clinical from subclinical form of infection.

Specificity of PCR also depends upon primer design, but generally, specificity of PCR is high. Depending upon the target, the assay can be family, genus-, species or strain specific. False negative results also can occur and may be due to a variety of reasons. These may include degradation of the sample during transport, presence of PCR inhibitors in the sample that interfere with nucleic acid extraction or amplification, or insufficient genetic homology between the primers that are used and the target DNA. This last reason can be problem with parasites that undergo significant genetic variation. In this case, primers should be designed to target highly conserved regions.

A variety of sample types can be used for PCR; parasites that are shed in faeces can be tested for using faecal material; blood parasites may be tested by using plasma or whole blood; parasites that are shed in urine or sputum may be detected in urine and sputum. Shipment of the sample usually requires refrigeration or freezing to prevent degradation of the genetic material of the parasitic agent.

Culture

Even though culture is the standard for the diagnosis of most infectious diseases, it is not commonly used in the parasitology laboratory settings. Some protozoan parasites, such as *Trichomonas* spp., *Acanthamoeba* spp., *Leishmania* spp., *Toxoplasma gondii*, and other cyst-forming coccidians can be cultured in immortalized cells. However, culture of many other parasites has not been successful due to technical difficulties.

Animal inoculation

Animal inoculation is a sensitive means of detecting infection caused by blood (e.g. Trypanosomes) and tissue parasites (e.g. *Toxoplasma gondii*, *Neospora caninum*, *Besnoitia* spp., *Leishmania* spp.). Although useful, this approach is not practical for most diagnostic laboratories and is largely confined to research settings.

Xenodiagnosis

This technique employs the use of laboratory-based arthropod vectors to detect low levels of parasites in infected hosts. Traditionally, this approach has been used to diagnose Chagas' disease, where an uninfected reduviid bug is allowed to feed on an individual suspected of having the disease. Then, the bug is dissected and examined microscopically for evidence of developmental stages of *Trypannosoma cruzi*.

Perspectives

In this chapter we described numerous laboratory methods for diagnosing parasitic diseases. Some are useful in detecting a wide variety of parasites, and others are particularly useful for only one or a few parasites. The mainstay of diagnostic clinical parasitology is the morphological (usually microscopic) demonstration of parasites in clinical materials. Occasionally, demonstration of a specific antibody response (serodiagnosis) helps in establishing

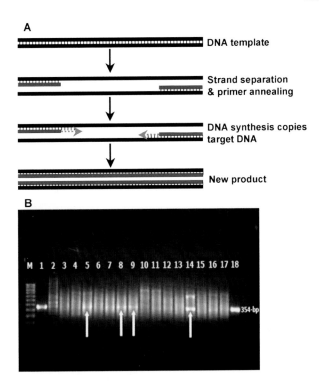

Figure 11.25 (A) Sketch of the main steps of Polymerase Chain Reaction. (B) Agarose gel electrophoresis analysis of DNA products. M; molecular weight markers; lanes 1 and 18 indicate positive controls; lanes 5, 8, 9 weak positive; lane 14 strong positive PCR products. The rest are negative.

the diagnosis, but, proper interpretation of results can be difficult. Molecular methods of detecting and quantifying parasites can be powerful tools to analyse samples for the presence of suspected parasites with far greater certainty than can occur by conventional parasitology methods.

Further reading

Amarante, A.F.T., Pomroy, W.E., Charleston, W.A.G., Leathwick, D.M. and Tornero, M.T.T. (1997). Evaluation of a larval development assay for the detection of anthelmintic resistance in *Ostertagia circumcincta*. Int. J. Parasitol. *27*, 305–311.

Ballweber, L.R. (2006). Diagnostic methods for parasitic infections in livestock. Vet. Clin. North Am. Food Anim. Pract. *22*, 695–705.

Bath, G.F., Malan, F.S. and Van Wyk, J.A. (1996). The FAMACHA© Ovine Anemia Guide to assist with the control of haemonchosis. Proceedings of the 7th Annual Congress of the Livestock Health and Production Group of the South African Veterinary Association, 5.

Besier, R.B. (1998). Field application of the Drenchrite test. In Proceedings of the Australian Sheep Veterinary, Watts, T. ed. (Society AVA Conference, Sydney).

Christie, M. and Jackson, F. (1982). Specific identification of strongyle eggs in small samples of sheep feces, Res. Vet. Sci. *32*, 113–117.

Coles, G.C., Bauer, C., Borgsteede, F.H., Geerts, S., Klei, T.R., Taylor, M.A. and Waller, P.J. (1992). World Association for the Advancement of Veterinary Parasitology (W.A.A.V.P.) methods for the detection of anthelmintic resistance in nematodes of veterinary importance. Vet. Parasitol. *44*, 35–44.

Coles, G.C., Jackson, F., Pomroy, W.E., Prichard, R.K. von Samson-Himmelstjerna, G., Silvestre, A., Taylor, M.A. and Vercruysse, J. (2006). The detection of anthelmintic resistance in nematodes of veterinary importance. Vet. Parasitol. *136*, 167–185.

Duncan, J.L., Abbott, E.M., Arundel, J.H., Eysker, M., Klei, T.R., Krecek, R.C., Lyons, E.T., Reinemeyer, C. and Slocombe, J.O. (2002). World association for the advancement of veterinary parasitology (WAAVP): second edition of guidelines for evaluating the efficacy of equine anthelmintics. Vet. Parasitol. *103*, 1–18.

Eysker, M., Bakker, J., van den Berg, M., van Doorn, D.C. and Ploeger, H.W. (2008). The use of age-clustered pooled fecal samples for monitoring worm control in horses. Vet. Parasitol. *151*, 249–255.

Grimshaw, W.T., Hong, C. and Hunt, K.R. (1996). Potential for misinterpretation of the fecal egg count reduction test for levamisole resistance in gastrointestinal nematodes of sheep. Vet. Parasitol. *62*, 267–273.

Hennessy, D.R., Bauer, C., Boray, J.C., Conder, G.A., Daugschies, A., Johansen, M.V., Maddox-Hyttel, C. and Roepstorff, A. (2006). World association for the advancement of veterinary parasitology (WAAVP): second edition of guidelines for evaluating the efficacy of anthelmintics in swine. Vet Parasitol. *141*, 138–149.

Hubert, J. and Kerboeuf, D. (1992). A microlarval development assay for the detection of anthelmintic resistance in sheep nematodes. Vet. Record *130*, 442–446.

Le Jambre, L.F. and Whitlock, J.H. (1976). Changes in the hatch rate of *Haemonchus contortus* eggs between geographic regions. Parasitology 73, 223–38.

Martin, P.J., Anderson, N. and Jarrett, R.G. (1985). Resistance to benzimidazole anthelmintics in field strains of *Ostertagia* and *Nematodirus* in sheep. Aust. Vet. J. *62*, 38–43.

McKenna, P.B. (2007). How do you mean? The case for composite fecal egg counts in testing for drench resistance. N. Z.Vet. J. *55*, 100–101.

Ministry of Agriculture, Fisheries and Food, (1986). Manual of Veterinary Parasitological Laboratory Techniques. Her Majesty's Stationery Office, London.

Morgan, E.R., Cavill, L., Curry, G.E., Wood, R.M. and Mitchell, E.S.E (2005). Effects of aggregation and sample size on composite fecal egg counts in sheep. Vet. Parasitol. *131*, 79–87.

Sutherland, I. (2003). Fecal mass and parasite strategies. Trends Parasitol. *19*, 68.

Taylor, M.A., Hunt, K.R. and Goodyear, K.L. (2002). Anthelmintic resistance detection methods. Vet. Parasitol. *103*, 183–194.

Van Wyk, J.A., Cabaret, J. and Michael, L.M. (2004). Morphological identification of nematode larvae of small ruminants and cattle simplified. Vet. Parasitol. *119*, 277–306.

Varady, M., Čorba, V.L. and Gabriel, K. (2009). Comparison of two versions of larval development test to detect anthelmintic resistance in *Haemonchus contortus*. Vet. Parasitol. *160*, 267–271.

Vercruysse, J. and Claerebout, E. (2001). Anthelmintic treatment vs. non-treatment in cattle: defining the threshold. Vet. Parasitol. *98*, 195–214.

Von Samson-Himmelstjerna, G. (2006). Molecular diagnosis of anthelmintic resistance. Vet. Parasitol. *136*, 99–107.

Wood, I.B., Amaral, N.K., Bairden, K., Duncan, J.L., Kassai, T., Malone, J.B. Jr., Pankavich, J.A., Reinecke, R.K., Slocombe, O., Taylor, S.M. and Vercruysse, J. (1995). World Association for the Advancement of Veterinary Parasitology (W.A.A.V.P.) second edition of guidelines for evaluating the efficacy of anthelmintics in ruminants (bovine, ovine, caprine). Vet. Parasitol. *58*, 181–213.

Yazwinski, T.A., Chapman, H.D. Davis, R.B., Letonja, T., Pote, L., Maes, L., Vercruysse J. and Jacobs D.E. (2003). World Association for the Advancement of Veterinary Parasitology (WAAVP) guidelines for evaluating the effectiveness of anthelmintics in chickens and turkeys. Vet. Parasitol. *116*, 159–173.

Pathology Associated with Parasitic Infections

Scott D. Fitzgerald

12

Introduction

Parasites may induce a wide variety of pathology in their host tissues. These changes vary from inapparent, to frank necrosis, grossly visible granulomas, and induction of hyperplastic or neoplastic changes in various tissues. The host may exhibit no clinical signs, or develop anaemia, hypoproteinaemia, weight loss, anorexia, even death. A few simple terms need to be defined before we begin our discussion of pathology. *Localized* infection refers to a parasitic infection that is limited to a single host tissue or focal areas of a given organ system. While *generalized parasitic infection* refers to parasites that have widespread migration throughout the host body in many tissues. While we are not going to make the reader a pathology expert, you should understand some basic pathology terms. *Necrosis* refers to destruction of normal tissue cells and organ architecture resulting in accumulations of cellular debris, fibrin, inflammatory cells, and red blood cells. *Granulomatous inflammation* is a chronic form of inflammation which is comprised predominantly of mixed mononuclear leucocytes including macrophages, lymphocytes, plasma cells, and sometimes multi-nucleated giant cells. If a granuloma has central zone of necrosis, this is a *caseogranuloma*. A hyperplastic change involved increased numbers or size of normal tissues, such as thickening of a keratinized layer in the epidermis being known as *hyperkeratosis*. *Neoplastic transformation* means that a true neoplasm consisting of a monomorphic population of cells has developed into a microscopic or grossly visible tumour or mass.

Clinical pathology

Parasitic infections can cause a variety of changes in the leucogram, haemogram, protein levels and urine of affected hosts. While these changes are dependent on level of infection, host immunity, duration of infection, and variation from host to host, they can be useful indicators of parasitic infection. Common changes include eosinophilia or basophilia in the peripheral circulation; anaemia and hypoproteinaemia; and abnormalities in the urine sediment.

Increased eosinophil numbers in the peripheral circulation have been documented in domestic animals including: ectoparasites such as fleas, lice and mange mites; nematodes such as *Aeleurostrongylus*, *Dirofilaria*, *Dipetalonema*, *Habronema*, *Spirocerca*, *Strongyloides*, *Trichuris*, and larval migration of hookworms and roundworms, trematodes such as *Paragonimus*; protozoa such as *Sarcocystis*. Increased eosinophils also accompany hypersensitivity reactions such as in response to flea bite dermatitis. On the other hand, many parasites are generally not associated with increased eosinophils including: blood parasites such as *Haemobartonella*, *Babesia*, *Cytauxzoon* and *Hepatozoon*.

Increased peripheral basophil numbers have been reported in domestic animals for the following parasitic infections: fleas, gastrointestinal nematodes, *Dirofilaria* and *Dipetalonema* within vessels.

Increased mast cell numbers have been found in cases of flea bite hypersensitivity and *Sarcoptes*.

Moving now to the haemogram, blood loss anaemia in domestic animals has been associated with: *Ancylostoma*, *Trichuris*, *Haemonchus*, *Ostertagia*, coccidiosis, ticks, blood-sucking lice and fleas. Hypoproteinaemia, characterized by decreases in both albumin and globulin, frequently accompanies parasitic infections in association with blood loss anaemia. Haemolytic anaemias have been reported associated with the following parasites: *Haemobartonella*, *Eperythrozoon*, *Anaplasma*, *Cytauxzoon*, *Babesia*, *Theileria* and *Trypanosoma*. Obviously, a number of these parasites can be visualized within whole blood smears.

A relatively few parasites can be visualized on examination of urine sediments. This would include nematode ova of *Dioctophyma renale* and *Capillaria plica*, and microfilaria of *Dirofilaria* if haematuria is present.

Post-mortem examination for parasitic conditions

How, then, does one undertake a post-mortem or necropsy examination on an animal suspected of parasitic disease when so many different parasites exist which can lead to subtle or gross pathology in any tissue in an animal's body? Starting with a good history is critical. What clinical signs were noted, such as weight loss, anaemia, dependent oedema, diarrhoea, etc? Were any clinical pathology tests run on the animal while alive? Was there hypoproteinaemia, elevated eosinophils or basophils in the leucogram? Was a faecal exam performed to look for parasite eggs or a faecal smear for *Cryptosporidia*?

Next we approach the animal carcass itself. Needless to say, a live animal for euthanasia or freshly dead carcass will provide far more information to the pathologist than a bloated carcass having undergone severe autolysis. Evaluate the carcass for overall body condition, and hydration states by tenting the skin of the eyelid and checking for whether or not the eyes are sunken in their sockets. Check for dependent oedema grossly, and by slicing open the ventral midline skin of the jaw, brisket and ventral abdomen to check for free subcutaneous fluid. Typically at the start of a post-mortem the animal is positioned in lateral recumbency, and the upper fore and rear legs are disarticulated and removed. Then a ventral midline skin incision is made along the sternum and ventral abdomen, and the hide skinned back up to the dorsal midline along the uppermost side of the carcass. The abdominal cavity is opened carefully without perforating any gastrointestinal viscera and contaminating the carcass with digesta. Shears are used to cut the rib cage near the costochondral junction along the length of the ventral thorax, and near the vertebral bodies along the dorsal thorax, so that one side of the ribcage can be removed intact exposing the thoracic viscera. Careful evaluation of the size, positioning, colour, and consistency of all internal thoracic and abdominal viscera can be done now that the carcass has been opened, but before removing any internal organs.

The ventral intermandibular area is opened, and the tongue removed from between the mandibles while still remaining attached to the trachea and oesophagus. The trachea and oesophagus are freed along the course of the neck and into the thoracic cavity. The attachments around the heart and lungs are dissected free, then the entire tongue, trachea, lungs and heart are removed as one, this is known as removing the pluck. Check the surface of the tongue for the 'whip-stitch' pattern of Gongylonema. Open the entire length of the oesophagus, checking the mucosal surface for evidence of parasites. Now open the entire length of the trachea to the bifurcation of the primary bronchi, again carefully checking the mucosa for attached or encysted parasites. Open all lung lobes be slicing along the major bronchi, this will reveal lungworms much easier than random cross-sections of the lung lobes. The heart should have the pericardial sac removed, and all chambers of the heart opened and examined, following the normal blood flow from right auricle and atrium, through the right ventricle and out the pulmonary artery, then the left atrium and auricle, the left ventricle, and out the aorta. Parasites may be found in the myocardial wall, or free in the various chamber lumens amongst the clotted blood.

Move now into the abdominal viscera. Locate, collect, and open both kidneys, and both adrenals. Follow the descending abdominal aorta and open that with knife or scissors at least to the level of the cranial mesenteric artery, checking for migrating strongyles. Remove the entire gastrointestinal tract intact, by severing the terminal rectum and distal oesophagus, then lay the intestinal tract out on a table or floor in a serpentine manner starting with the stomach(s) and ending with terminal rectum. In this manner, even for a large animal with over 30–40 m of intestines, you can easily survey the entire tract in a thorough and systematic manner in a confined area. By all means, collect a faecal sample from the terminal rectum if a parasitic egg check has not already been done. Now start at the front with the stomach(s) and work your way to back to the rectum, opening all levels of the gastrointestinal tract with a sharp knife or scissors. Don't be afraid to take a close look, many gastrointestinal parasites are quite small. You will need a hose with running water to flush digesta out of the intestinal lumen to properly view the mucosal surface for attached parasites.

Serially section solid organs like the liver, spleen, and kidneys at 1–2 cm intervals to detect encysted parasites. Open luminal organs like the gall bladder, bile duct, and urinary bladder to detect parasites residing there. You need to slice through all major muscle masses of the legs, as well as the tongue and diaphragm if you want to detect encysted parasites there. The skull needs to be carefully opened or at least split in half with hatchet or band-saw if you are to detect meningeal worms, abnormally migrating nematode larvae, or Toxoplasma. Don't forget to remove the spinal cord, no small job but critical if the animal is exhibiting neurological signs and you suspect parasites there. The eyes should also be removed by cutting the extraocular muscles and connective tissue surrounding the eyeball, collected, and fixed in formalin to examine for Toxoplasma and other migrating parasites. And of course, the hide or skin is subject to numerous parasitic infestations, so collect multiple areas of skin especially those that appear thickened, discoloured, ulcerated, alopecic, or otherwise abnormal.

Above all, be thorough and have a written plan of what you want to collect. Many parasitic infections are missed because of a rushed or incomplete necropsy. In fact, most wildlife have multiple parasitic infections, since no one is treating them with anthelminthics, or rotating their pastures to control parasite build-up. If you routinely perform necropsy examinations on wildlife, you are likely to find parasites in close to 100% of the animals you examine. In Michigan where I perform many white-tailed deer necropsies for ongoing surveillance projects, I would estimate 100% of the deer have bots in their retropharyngeal pouches, 40% of the deer have inapparent meningeal worm infections, 90% have inapparent lungworm infections, and 100% have a variety of gastrointestinal parasitism. You need to have multiple containers available filled with 10% neutral-buffered formalin and collect representative samples of most or all tissues. You will not see most protozoal parasites on gross examination, or many migrating larvae, or encysted larval forms of Trichinosis, etc., so it is imperative you take samples for histopathology.

Working with a pathologist

If you are close to a veterinary diagnostic pathology laboratory, it is often optimal to deliver the animal carcass there and have the necropsy performed by a pathologist, and the remains properly disposed in a biologically safe manner. Unfortunately, for reasons of proximity, transportation, cost, or otherwise, many times you may have to perform the necropsy yourself. You may not be a pathologist yourself, or even be able to identify many gross lesions, but taking the proper samples and submitting them to a pathologist is the necessary first step to identifying both pathological changes and the underlying causative parasites. Let your pathologist know what gross lesions you observed, and which parasites you expect may be present. The better information and samples you provide, the better information you will receive back in the histopathology report. Establish a relationship with a specific diagnostic laboratory or with a specific pathologist, so that you can provide optimal specimens and your pathologist can respond to your particular concerns and questions. You will learn what a typically turnaround time for various requests are, and familiarize yourself with the reporting methods.

Beyond standard necropsy examination, and routine haematoxylin and eosin stained histopathology, most pathology services can now provide extensive testing. For parasites, especially protozoa, modern molecular techniques including PCR testing which specifically identify a parasite to genus and even species are now available. *In situ* hybridization or immunohistochemical staining utilizing organism specific antibodies can now be performed on formalin-fixed tissues at many laboratories to again give specific organism identification. Whole parasite worms can be examined and through the use of morphological features and standardized keys, definitive identifications may be reached. Even the routine faecal examination for worms and eggs can be run as a simple qualitative method (eggs are present in low, moderate or high numbers) or a more exacting, time consuming and expensive quantitative counts can also be performed if that information is needed. Of course, parasites are not the only pathogenic organisms that infect animals, and most full service diagnostic laboratories can also provide testing for bacterial, viral, and fungal organisms, as well as nutritional deficiencies, neoplastic conditions, and toxic compounds.

Understanding the pathologist's report

Once you receive your necropsy or histopathology report, be sure you understand and read the entire report. Generally the main body of the report contains a detailed histological description of all abnormalities found in each tissue examined. Next come a series of morphological diagnoses; these start with the tissue (liver, heart, lung, etc.) and are followed by a series of terms which describe the duration of the lesions (acute, subacute, chronic), severity of the lesion (mild, moderate, severe), type of lesion (necrotizing, granulomatous, proliferative), and the histological term for the abnormal tissue (hepatitis, enteritis, pneumonia, etc.). If organisms are found in tissue section, this will usually be noted in the morphological diagnosis as well (bacterial colonies, intranuclear viral inclusions, protozoal cysts, etc.). Next should be a major diagnosis or diagnoses (whole body emaciation; fetal abortion; enteric coccidiosis). The last portion of the histopathology report is generally a summary comments section, in which simple layman's words are used to clarify the principal condition, cause of death, and management recommendations to control further disease in the unit. Not every report from each diagnostic laboratory will be set-up the same way, but these major components should be present if histopathology was requested. If the report is not clear, share the report with your local veterinarian, or call the pathologist responsible for the report and they can explain it further, determine if additional testing or samples are needed, or answer any questions you may have.

Anatomic pathology associated with parasites

Different classes of parasites tend to induce different pathological effects. In general, protists tend to cause cell disruption, necrosis, anaemia, and frequently result in disseminated reactions due to their widespread anatomic distribution in the host and their ability to multiple within host tissues. Helminths, including cestodes, trematodes, nematodes and acanthocephalids, tend to produce localized reactions because of their frequently localized distribution and the fact that many cannot undergo their complete life cycle within a single host. Their pathological effects include tissue necrosis, inflammation, formation of abscesses, formation of granulomas, tissue hyperplasia or metaplasia, and some are associated with neoplastic transformation of host tissues. More specific examples of helminth-induced pathology include obstruction of blood vessels or lymphatic channels; obstruction of bile ducts or the lumens of gastrointestinal, respiratory or urinary tracts; acting as foreign bodies with displacement of normal anatomic structures; invasion and displacement of host cells or tissues resulting in loss of function, tissue necrosis, or hypersensitivity reactions; ingestion of blood leading to anaemia; competing with the host for nutrients leading to weight loss; direct destruction of host tissues by ingestion; serving as a vector of bacterial disease; and secretion of toxic products into host tissues. Arthropods, including mites, fleas, flies, and pentastomes, comprise the final group of parasites. These parasites tend to affect the integumentary tissues, and are classified as infestations rather than infections. While many incite localized reactions of the skin, some invade other tissues and may even result in disseminated reactions.

We will examine a number of specific examples of parasitic conditions in order to illustrate different types of pathological responses in various tissues, and also to see examples of how the host pathological response helps to control the parasitic infection.

Cerebrospinal nematodiasis

A significant number of nematode larval parasites will preferentially or aberrantly migrate through the brain and spinal cord leading to neurological disease in either their primary or aberrant hosts. A partial list includes *Pneumostrongylus* and *Elaphostrongylus* spp. – deer meningeal worms, *Parastrongylus cantonensis* – a rat lungworm, *Setari digitata* – the peritoneal worm of herbivores, *Halicepalobus gingivalis* – a soil saprophyte which aberrantly infects horses, *Toxocara canis* – the dog roundworm which commonly infects the brain of children and occasionally dogs, and *Baylisascaris* spp. – the roundworms of raccoons and skunks respectively which aberrantly affect numerous avian and mammalian hosts including humans. We will examine *Baylisascaris procyonis*, the raccoon roundworm, to illustrate the pathology. Like many roundworms, the adults live in the intestinal lumen of their primary host, rarely producing any detectable effect. *Baylisascaris* sheds enormous numbers of eggs through the faeces and into the environment where they remain infectious for prolonged periods due to their resistance to extremes of temperature and desiccation. As the faeces breakdown, the faeces contaminate the soil, or other substrate which may include bedding, or feed.

Once ingested by a parenthetic host, the eggs release larvae which migrate into virtually any tissue of the body as they search fruitlessly for their normal raccoon intestinal microenvironment. Larvae have been reported in adrenals, spleens, lymph nodes, gonads, etc., all without any apparent detrimental effects. However, if the larvae should migrate to the brain, spinal cord, or eye, then serious neurological disease or blindness may occur. The parasites as they tunnel through the central nervous tissues leave linear tracts of neuropil necrosis or malacia, and attract large foamy macrophages or 'gitter cells' to clean up the cellular and myelin debris, as well as significant numbers of eosinophils (Fig. 12.1). Often on histological section there may appear to be multiple parasite larval cross-sections in a focus, however, in reality there is often only a single parasite, or at least very few, which because of their serpentine coiling appear as multiple individuals (Fig. 12.2). Interestingly, these parasites continue their migratory behaviour even after the host has died or is euthanized. So the parasites may be found within the histological section some

distance away from their path of destruction and inflammation – remember that neither necrosis nor inflammation occur after the host organism is dead. So, with very few migrating larvae about, and not always remaining in place associated with their resulting pathology, it can be extremely difficult to find such larval parasites even with many histological sections.

Another interesting, but markedly different parasitic cause of cerebrospinal disease is *Haliocephalobus gingivalis* (previously *Micronema deletrix*). This filarid nematode normally resides as a non-parasitic soil saprophyte, but for unknown reasons it has been encountered many times in the brains and spinal cords of horses, and less frequently humans. Other tissues sometimes infected include nasal mucosa, oral mucosa, maxillary and mandibular bones, kidney, eye, lung, lymph node, mammary gland, prostate, and adrenal. The small Rhabditiform nematode is distributed in the soil across portions of North and South America, Europe and Asia. An unusual feature of this parasite is that the adult and larval forms are nearly the same size, making separation of the life stages somewhat difficult. It is believed that the parasite larvae are accidentally inhaled or ingested, or even directly inoculated into the skin by contaminated wounds, due to their predominant anatomic locations being located in the horses face and cranium. The parasites incite a markedly granulomatous response, irrespective of anatomical location (Fig. 12.3). Associated with tissue destruction variable numbers of parasite adults (females only), larvae, and eggs, surrounded by macrophages, lymphocytes, plasma cells, eosinophils, and multinucleated giant cells are frequently present. While such granulomatous lesions may be considered incidental in many organs, granulomas of sufficient size and distribution can result in clinical renal disease and more commonly neurological signs when the brain and spinal cord are involved.

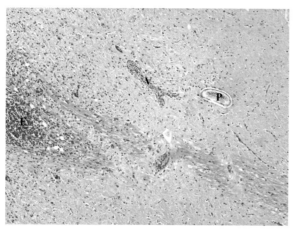

Figure 12.1 Photomicrograph of the brain from a porcupine infected with *Baylisascaris procyonis*. To the left is a massive accumulation of eosinophils (E). The central vessel (V) is cuffed by accumulations of lymphocytes and plasma cells. To the right is a section of the nematode parasite (P) itself. H&E stain (×100).

Echinococcosis

Cestodes are a large group of flattened and segmented worms, which in their adult stages commonly inhabit the gastrointestinal tract, with minor resulting pathology. It is the intermediate

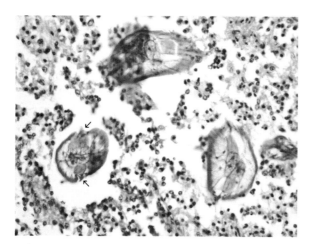

Figure 12.2 Photomicrograph of a different portion of the porcupine brain seen in Fig. 12.1. Here the brain parenchyma is necrotic (malacic), with numerous gitter cells attempting to clean-up the debris, and 3 cross-sections of the same *Baylisascaris* worm displaying their prominent lateral alae (arrows) (×350).

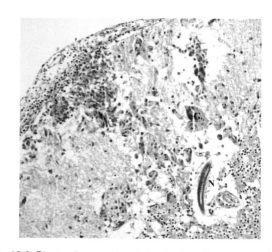

Figure 12.3 Photomicrograph of the brain of a horse infected with *Haliocephalobus*. Note the nematode organism (N), the rarefaction of the neuropile, and the accumulations of lymphocytes, macrophages, and rare multi-nucleated giant cells (G). H&E stain (×175).

forms which tend to cause the greatest harm to their hosts and result in the most interesting pathology. *Taenia* spp. tend to form intermediate cysticerci or bladder worms. While *Echinoccocus* spp. result in larger intermediate form, known as hydatid. Here we will examine the pathology associated with *Echinoccocus granulosus*. The adult cestode is found in various carnivores worldwide, including domestic dogs, dingos, wolves, foxes, and coyotes. The larval stage, known as the unilocular hydatid cyst, which does not have exogenous budding that leads to spread and tissue invasion as occurs with the multilocular hydatid cysts of *E. multilocularis*. Typically the hydatid cysts of *E. granulosus* parasitize the lungs, and occasionally livers, of herbivores including elk, deer, moose, cattle, sheep, kangaroos and rabbits. These larval cysts form a several individual fluid-filled cavities, which compress the surrounding parenchyma, and in severe infections the lungs begin to resemble Swiss cheese due to the numerous cystic spaces (Fig. 12.4). The cyst wall is composed partially of fibrous connective tissue produced by the host, and a multi-laminated parasite-derived membrane which on its innermost surface consists of a germinal membrane from which arise brood capsules. Within the membrane of the brood capsules are numerous protoscoleces and mineralized concretions which form the 'hydatid sand', or white granular material seen when examining the capsules grossly (Fig. 12.5). Surprisingly, other than compression atrophy of the surrounding pulmonary parenchyma, and a mild fibrous connective tissue response, there is very little inflammatory response to the intact hydatid cysts. Over time, as the cysts degenerate and break down, mineralization and granulomatous inflammatory response develops. Tissue responses in the liver are similar to those described in the lung.

Eimeria stiedea

This coccidian parasite of rabbits does not reside in the intestinal tract where most coccidian parasites are found, but instead resides in the bile ducts of the liver. Instead of the typical necrotizing response seen with intestinal coccidiosis, the bile duct epithelium becomes markedly hyperplastic in response to *E. stiedea*. The bile ducts are markedly enlarged, and reduplicated, thus forming

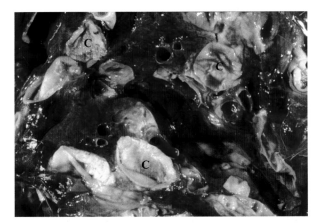

Figure 12.4 Gross photograph of the lung of a white-tailed deer infected with *Echinococcus granulosus*. The large white cysts (C) represent the parasitic capsules and fibrous connective tissue surrounding each unilocular hydatid cyst.

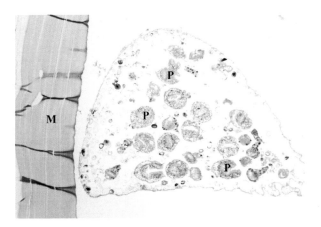

Figure 12.5 Photomicrograph of the lung seen in Fig. 12.4. The multi-laminated parasitic membrane (M) is present on the far left, while the brood capsule to the right contains numerous protoscoleces (P) and smaller basophilic mineralized concretions. H&E stain (×100).

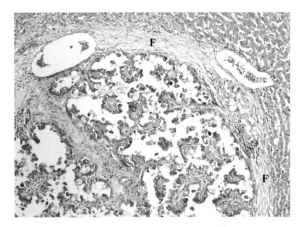

Figure 12.6 Photomicrograph of a liver from a rabbit infected with *Eimeria stiedea*. The normal liver parenchyma is seen to the right and top, while fibrous connective tissue (F) surrounds the markedly hyperplastic bile duct which contains many finger-like projections into its lumen. Numerous oval and brightly eosinophilic oocysts are present in the bile duct epithelium and free in the duct lumen. H&E stain (×40).

grossly visible pale linear lesions in the liver. Histologically, the duct mucosa has increased mitotic activity, may pile up several layers deep instead of the normal single cell thickness, and forms papillary projections into the duct lumen (Fig. 12.6). On close inspection, the bile duct epithelium frequently contains massive numbers of merozoites, macrogametocytes, microgametocytes, and oocysts, which are released into the duct lumen when the host epithelial cell ruptures; travel down the biliary tree, and pass out with the faeces. Other than increased fibrotic tissue surrounding the bile ducts, there may be limited inflammatory response in *E. stiedea* infections.

Equine protozoal myelitis

Equine protozoal myelitis, or EPM, is caused by the apicomplexan protozoa *Sarcocystis neurona*. For many years the definitive host was unknown, but has been shown to reside in Virginia opossums. The adult gastrointestinal parasite appears as typical intestinal coccidian, and produce relatively minor superficial mucosal necrosis. However, when ingested by a horse – an aberrant host – the parasite reaches the brain and spinal cord, resulting in a multifocal, randomly distributed series of non-suppurative and necrotizing lesions. The resulting meningoencephalomyelitis, characterized by lymphocytes and plasma cells cuffing around blood vessels, and widely scattered lesions in the neuropil are necrotic or malacic, with gitter cells, glial cells, and occasional mononuclear leucocytes (Fig. 12.7). Swollen axons, loss of myelin sheaths, haemorrhage, and necrotic neurons are also seen in areas with the inflammatory lesions. Since these lesions are sporadic, it can take many histological sections for the pathologist to identify the lesion, and many more to fortuitously identify the causative protozoa on routine histological section, or with specialized immunohistochemical staining (Fig. 12.8). Because the lesions are so randomly distributed throughout the central nervous system, the clinical syndrome presented by the affected horse can also be markedly variable. Presentation can include lameness, ataxia, paresis, cranial nerve deficits, focal muscle atrophy, to entirely subclinical.

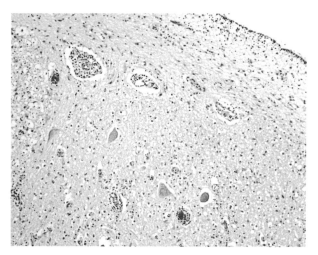

Figure 12.7 Photomicrograph of brain from a horse infected with *Sarcocystis neurona*. There is cuffing around blood vessels by lymphocytes and plasma cells, and generalized gliosis. H&E stain (×40).

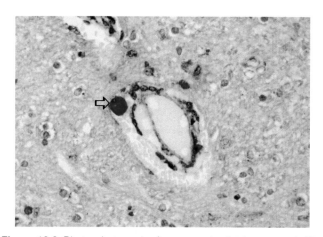

Figure 12.8 Photomicrograph of same equine brain as seen in Fig. 12.7. Note the strong positive immunoreactivity to antibody against *S. neurona* in a tissue cyst (arrow) adjacent to a blood vessel. Immunohistochemical stain (×350).

Equine strongyloidiasis

The strongyles affecting the large intestines of horses include over 50 species, but three large strongyles are particularly problematic: *Strongylus vulgaris*, *S. equinus* and *S. edentatus*. Although all three parasites cause blood loss and protein loss through their blood-sucking behaviour, we will concentrate in this discussion on the larval migration and damage produced by third larval stage of *S. vulgaris*. The adult *S. vulgaris* commonly attaches to the mucosa of the caecum, where it ingests the host's blood. Eggs are released into the lumen, are shed in the faeces, and eventually develop into infectious third-stage larvae. Following ingestion, the larvae penetrate the intestinal mucosa, and after moulting into fourth-stage larvae they enter terminal branches of the intestinal arteries. The wall of the intestine where this larval migration occurs develops multifocal haemorrhage, and small aggregates of neutrophils, eosinophils, and lymphocytes. Larvae continue to migrate along the lumen of the cranial mesenteric arteries and the ileocecal artery within the intima, and eventually reach one of several of the major branches and remain in that location for months. During this stationary period, the larvae cause marked proliferation and hyperplasia of the intima and endothelium, which may be associated with haemorrhage and necrosis. The arterial endothelial lesions initially and most commonly appear as minor tortuous subintimal tracks, caused by fibroelastic thickenings of the vessel lining. These thickened and roughened intimal areas accumulate fibrin and cellular debris, and over long periods fibrous connective tissue forms within both the intimal and adventitial tissues. Inflammatory cells including numerous lymphocytes, macrophages and eosinophils accumulate, as does fibrous connective tissue and smooth muscle cell proliferation from the media of the vessel, resulting eventually in a prominent thickened verminous arteritis lesion (Fig. 12.9). Less commonly, the lesion continues to progress by further thickening and forming a dilated segment, sometimes known as an aneurysmal dilatation, although these

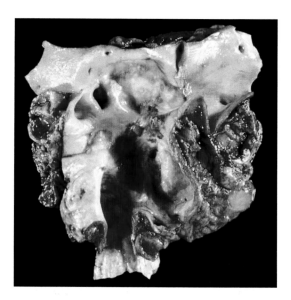

Figure 12.9 Gross photograph of the cranial mesenteric artery from a horse. Notice the roughening of the intimal surface of the opened blood vessel, and the reddened and irregular accumulation of fibrous connective tissue and granulomatous inflammation on the outer adventitial surface of the vessel.

are not generally thin-walled aneurysms but more commonly thick-walled fibrotic and granulomatous arteritis. It is actually relatively uncommon for aneurysms to develop and subsequently rupture, resulting in rapid bleed-out and death. More commonly, the horse exhibits colic due to partial or complete obstruction of arterial blood flow caused by these parasitic lesions, resulting in segmental ischaemia of the bowel. While fourth-stage larvae and young adult worms may remain in these arterial lesions, their chronic time course and the inflammatory reaction resulting in destruction of the worms means that the arterial lesions may or may not contain typical strongyle larvae and adults when examined histologically, or only degenerate parasite remnants (Fig. 12.10).

Larval migration of any of the large strongyles, including *S. edentatus* and *S. equinus* in addition to *S. vulgaris*, are believed to result in the lesion called haemomelasma ilei. This lesion is characterized by large plaques several centimetres wide and sometimes considerably longer on the serosal surface of the small and large intestines, invariably on the antimesenteric aspect of the

gut wall (Fig. 12.11). Lesions vary from bright red to dark brown-black pigmentation. Histologically, these lesions contain oedema, fibrous connective tissue, free red blood cells, macrophages often containing large amounts of haemosiderin and other blood break-down pigments. However, it is rare and requires diligent search to identify any strongyle larvae fragments within these lesions, and so the definitive cause of the lesion remains the subject of debate. In general, hemomelasma ilei is considered an incidental lesion without clinical significance, and rarely if ever is it considered the cause of colic.

Oesophagostomosis

One of the most important gastrointestinal parasites affecting domestic ruminants and swine worldwide are the strongylid parasites of genus *Oesophagastomum*. The ova pass onto the pasture in their host faeces, develop into infective larvae, and are then ingested by another host animal, hence a direct life cycle. Once the larvae penetrate the intestinal mucosa, they become encysted in the submucosa where the predominant pathology is induced. These worms are known as the nodule worms, and in chronic infections result in diarrhoea, anaemia, emaciation, prostration and even death. Grossly, the larvae encyst anywhere between the gastric pylorus and the anus, and encysted larvae moult to the fourth stage and typically return to the intestinal lumen. Sometimes, these fourth-stage larvae invade the intestinal wall a second time, where further development is arrested. As these larval invasions recur over time, a marked tissue reaction develops characterized by a mixed granulomatous response consisting of haemorrhage, lymphocytes, macrophages, multinucleated giant cells and eosinophils (Figs. 12.12 and 12.13). These eosinophilic

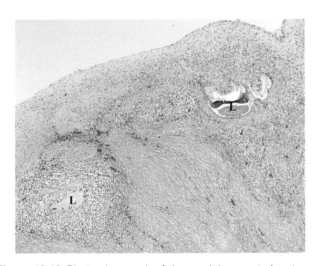

Figure 12.10 Photomicrograph of the cranial mesenteric artery of a horse infected with *Strongylus vulgaris*. The intimal surface (top) is irregular, and massive granulomatous inflammatory reaction extends down from the intima into the vessel wall. The remnants of two degenerate larvae (L) are present in the vessel wall surrounded by inflammatory infiltrates. H&E stain (×40).

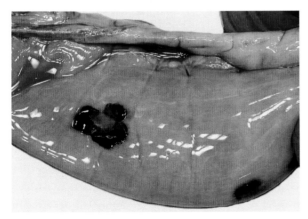

Figure 12.11 Gross photograph of the serosal surface of a loop of equine small intestine. Note the two raised black irregular tracts consistent with haemomelasma ilei.

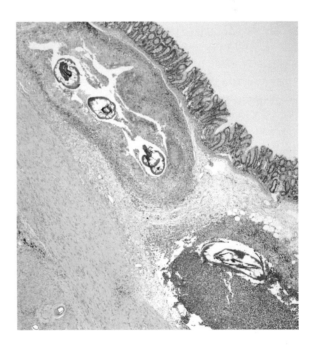

Figure 12.12 Photomicrograph of the colon of a goat. The submucosa tissue is markedly expanded by two granulomas containing cross-sections of *Oesophagostomum* larvae. The left granuloma contains predominantly haemorrhagic contents in addition to the worms. While the right granuloma contains abundant degenerate granulocytes. H&E stain (×40).

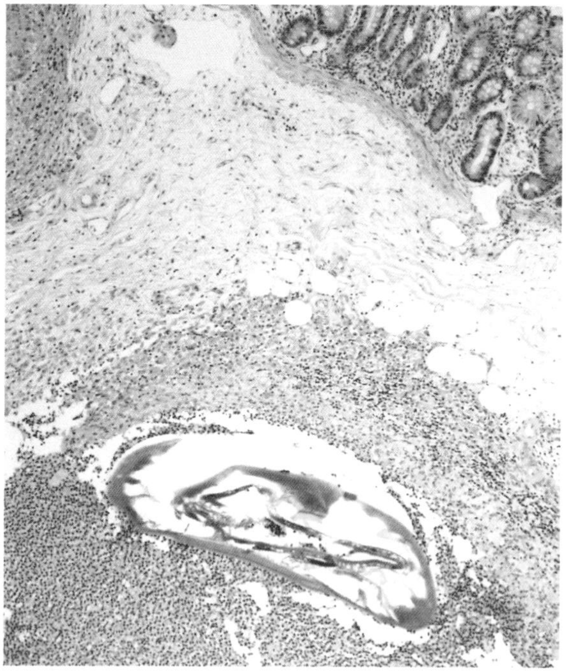

Figure 12.13 Photomicrograph of one granuloma seen in Fig. 12.12. The nematode larva is in the centre of the granuloma associated with numerous degenerate neutrophils and eosinophils. The outer wall of the granuloma is composed of a mixture of lymphocytes, plasma cells and macrophages. H&E stain (×100).

granulomas protrude from the mucosal surface, and may develop caseonecrotic centres. Many of the larvae trapped within this reaction die and degenerate, however, a few live and escape back through the mucosa into the intestinal lumen. Over time, and with continued larval infection, these nodules grow, may become partially calcified, and cause intestinal wall thickening to the point where they become visible as nodules on the serosal surface. These nodules may become infected with bacteria, rupture into the peritoneum, or interfere with intestinal peristalsis and efficient intestinal absorption. The adult *Oesophagostomum* worms induce exudation of mucous and inflammatory cells from the intestinal mucosa on which they feed; and so the adults incite relatively minimal pathology themselves. If not for their larval forms, this particular parasite would not be a significant economic problem.

Paragonimiasis

Trematodes are flatworms that typically have an indirect life cycle, meaning that multiple hosts are required to complete their cycle. Some of the most commonly encountered trematodes are the liver flukes, in which the adult parasites infect the liver and bile ducts of the definitive herbivore host, while the immature forms of the parasite must pass through various invertebrate hosts such as slugs or snails. We will review the pathology associated with *Paragonimus kellicoti*, the lung fluke, which normally parasitizes the lungs of dogs, cats, mink, pigs, and wild carnivores. The intermediate hosts are aquatic snails and freshwater crabs or crayfish. Once the mammalian host ingests the intermediate host, digestion liberates the infectious metacercariae into the host intestine. Eventually the migrating metacercariae reach the pleural cavity, and produces multifocal haemorrhages and fibrinous pleuritis.

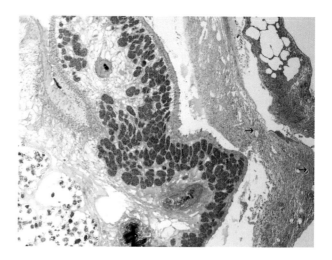

Figure 12.14 Photomicrograph of the lung of a dog with *Paragonimus kellicoti* infection. The compressed lung parenchyma is along the right side, while a portion of the trematode fills the left, with a thin cystic space surrounding the parasite. The cyst wall is composed of mixed granulomatous inflammation with numerous macrophages and eosinophils. Several oval, yellow-shelled fluke ova (arrows) are entrapped within the granulomatous inflammation. H&E stain (×40).

These flukes reach up to 17 mm in length, and form spherical dark red-brown cyst-like cavities in the parenchyma of the lung. The cysts composed of a fibrous connective tissue capsule typically contain two or more adult flukes in order for a patent infection, as well as haemorrhage, haemosiderin-laden macrophages, and numerous eosinophils (Fig. 12.14). In patent infections, numerous 80- to 100-µm-long ova, with yellow shells, opercula at one end, and embryonated larvae are present. In chronic infections, eosinophilic bronchiolitis, granulomatous pleuritis, and hyperplasia of peribronchiolar glands occur in response to degenerate flukes and their eggs. Generally there are no or minimal clinical signs associated with pulmonary infections with these flukes. Occasionally, fluke eggs are found in histological section within the brains of animals with active pulmonary infections; possibly reaching the central nervous system as vascular emboli. Rarely, adult flukes may aberrantly wander into the brain of its host resulting in granulomatous inflammation, neurological signs and even death.

Sarcoptic mange

Sarcoptes scabiei is a ubiquitous mange mite that infests hundreds of mammalian species – including humans, and even reptilian species. The mite produces pathology in three ways: first, by direct damage inflicted by the parasites tunnelling and feeding activity in the stratum corneum; second, by the irritant effects of the parasite secretions and excreta; and, finally, by the host allergic response to components of the mite, or its extracellular products. In normal hosts, the mange mite burrows only as deep as the stratum corneum, unable to penetrate into the deeper living layers of the epidermis. In the stratum corneum the mites result in irritation, itching, a marked hyperplastic response of the epidermis characterized by hyperkeratosis, acanthosis and rete peg formation (Fig. 12.15). The parasite burrows many tunnels

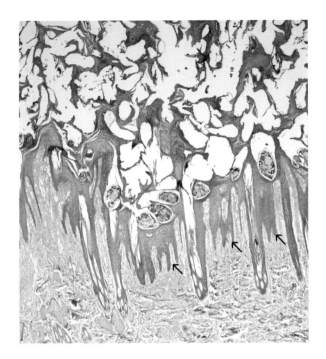

Figure 12.15 Photomicrograph of raccoon skin infested with sarcoptic mange. The upper keratinized layer (stratum corneum) is massively thickened, and contains numerous tunnels containing adults, larvae, nymphs, and eggs of *Sarcoptes scabiei*. The epidermis is hyperplastic forming multiple downward projections into the dermis (rete peg formation) (arrows). The superficial dermis has mild perivascular infiltration by mononuclear leucocytes and occasional eosinophils. H&E stain (×40).

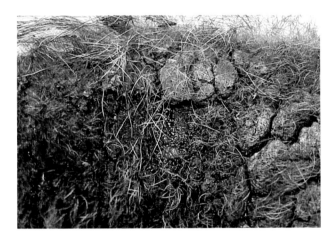

Figure 12.16 Gross photograph of the skin of a raccoon infested with sarcoptic mange. There is severe thickening, crusting, central ulceration, exudation of serum, and marked hair loss, all secondary to pruritus and self-trauma (Image courtesy of the Wildlife Disease Laboratory, Michigan Department of Natural Resources)

within the stratum corneum in which the adults, larvae, nymphs and eggs can be found in histological section. The intense pruritus leads to self-trauma of the host, which subsequently leads to ulcerations, secondary bacterial infections, massive serum exudation and the formation of serocellular crusts (Fig. 12.16). The underlying superficial dermis exhibits congested vessels, and predominantly mononuclear leucocyte perivascular infiltrates. Interestingly, eosinophils may comprise a significant component when immediate or delayed hypersensitivity reactions are present.

Alternatively, eosinophils may be rare to absent in heavy mite infestations which are characterized by a compromised immune system in the host, and are known as crusted scabies in dogs, or Norwegian scabies in humans.

A hyperplastic response of the epidermis to arthropod infestation is a relatively common feature in a variety of mite, lice and flea infestations. Surprisingly, this same hyperplastic epidermal response may be elicited by parasites of a completely different phylum. For example, the nematode free-living parasite *Pelodera strongyloides* produces a nearly identical hyperplastic skin response when it opportunistically invades hair follicles in dogs, cattle, horses or humans. Generally, this skin invasion occurs when the host is laying in damp or filthy bedding, and the skin is moist for prolonged periods of time. Initially a neutrophilic folliculitis develops, but then as the host self-traumatizes its skin, the same proliferative hyperkeratotic lesions as seen in sarcoptic mange. Lesions develop as lichenified skin, with scaling, crusting and alopecia. Recently, we reported a case of dual infection with both *Sarcoptes* and *Pelodera* in a wild black bear, and the overall gross dermal lesions were indistinguishable from *Sarcoptes* alone (Figs. 12.17 and 12.18). The skin appears to have a limited

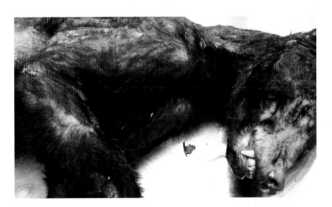

Figure 12.17 Gross photograph of a black bear exhibiting alopecia, thickened crusty and scaling skin over much of its face, legs and body. This animal had infestation by *S. scabiei* and infection with *Pelodera strongyloides*. (Image courtesy of the Wildlife Disease Laboratory, Michigan Department of Natural Resources.)

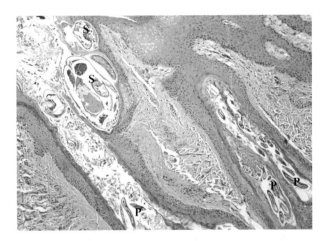

Figure 12.18 Photomicrograph of the skin from the black bear in Fig. 12.17. The opening of the hair follicle contains several sarcoptic mange mites (S), while deeper in the hair follicle lumens are multiple sections of elongated *Pelodera* nematodes (P). H&E stain (×100).

repertoire of patterns of inflammatory response, and self-trauma due to pruritus is a common manifestation of many ectoparasitic conditions.

Spirocercosis

One of the more interesting pathologies associated with parasite infection is the induction of neoplasms. In humans, neoplasms arise in the urinary bladder secondary to *Schistosoma hematobium*; in rats infection with *Cysticercus fasciolaris* is associated with liver neoplasms; and in dogs *Spirocerca lupi* sometimes leads to oesophageal neoplasms. We will examine Spirocercosis more closely to understand the pathogenesis of these lesions. The spirurid nematode *Spirocerca lupi* is found throughout much of the world. The adults live coiled in cystic granulomatous nodules present in the submucosa of the wall of the distal oesophagus and cardia of the stomach of various carnivores including the domestic dog, fox, wolf, and even cats. The complicated life cycle includes dung beetles, and may also include parenthetic hosts (frogs, snakes, lizards, various birds or small mammals). When one of these intermediate hosts is ingested by a definitive canid host, larvae are released and penetrate the stomach wall, then migrate along various arteries through the adventitia or media, until reaching the intrathoracic aorta. After approximately 90 days the larvae then migrate to the adjacent oesophagus, burrow into its submucosa, and form cystic nodules in which they develop into adults. Aortic nodules associated with larvae may become aneurysms which occasionally rupture leading to haemorrhage and death. Oesophageal nodules protrude as plaques into the lumen of the oesophagus. The granulomatous nodules consist of a thick fibrous wall, surrounding a central cavity containing one or more adult worms and inflammatory debris (Fig. 12.19). Many cells types are represented in these oesophageal nodules including red blood cells, neutrophils, lymphocytes, plasma cells, and macrophages, however, eosinophils are generally absent. Highly reactive and pleomorphic fibroblasts with abundant

mitotic figures may develop in the granuloma wall (Fig. 12.20). Occasionally, these fibroblasts undergo malignant transformation into mesenchymal neoplasms including fibrosarcomas or osteosarcomas, which may invade the local tissues and subsequently metastasize to the lungs. The exact carcinogenic substance which initiates tumour development is not known. As these oesophageal sarcomas enlarge, they may incite the paraneoplastic syndrome known as hypertrophic pulmonary osteoarthropathy. In this syndrome, a space-occupying mass in the thorax results in diffuse bony proliferation within the periosteum circumferentially around the diaphyses of bones of the limbs. The exact cause of this new bone formation is obscure, but is associated with increased blood flow to the limbs early in the disease course.

Toxoplasmosis

There are many different protozoal parasites, and many are found in the apicomplexan group, which includes coccidian such as *Eimeria* sp., *Isospora* sp. and *Cryptosporidia* sp., *Besnoitia* sp., *Hammondia* sp., *Sarcocystis* sp., *Neospora caninum*, and *Toxoplasma gondii*. We will select *Toxoplasma gondii* as a representative example for reviewing the pathology produced by an apicomplexan protozoan. Domestic and wild cats are the only definitive host for *T. gondii*, where it undergoes its cycle in the gastrointestinal mucosa releasing oocysts in large numbers into the faeces. Sporulated oocysts may be ingested and cause a variety of pathology in many different intermediate hosts including most mammals and birds. In secondary hosts, *T. gondii* may form slowly dividing bradyzoites, rapidly dividing tachyzoites, or cysts in a variety of tissues. Most infections in secondary hosts are subclinical and never associated with disease; as can be confirmed by serology for toxoplasmosis on human cat owners. However, young or aged animals, and immunocompromised individuals are all more likely to develop acute illness. Typically, infection begins with the ingestion of oocysts excreted in cat faeces, or by the release of bradyzoites from tissue cysts present in infected animals

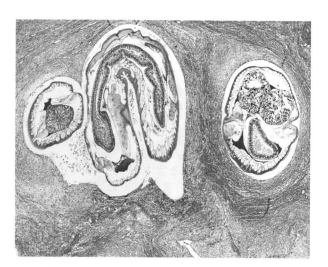

Figure 12.19 Photomicrograph of the oesophagus of a dog with *Spirocerca lupi* infection. This section of the submucosa shows several coiled adults, surrounded by abundant fibrous connective tissue and mixed infiltrates of neutrophils, lymphocytes, plasma cells and macrophages. H&E stain (×40)

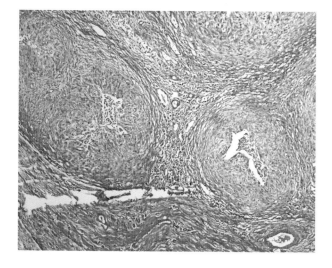

Figure 12.20 Higher magnification of the oesophageal submucosa seen in Fig. 12.19. The fibroblasts form sheets and whorls, and are moderately pleomorphic, suggestive of early neoplastic transformation towards a fibrosarcoma. H&E stain (×100).

which have been consumed by another animal. Once ingested, *Toxoplasma* organisms penetrate the intestinal mucosa, and subsequently become disseminated through blood-borne white cells including lymphocytes, macrophages, granulocytes, and even free in the plasma. Upon reaching tissues the parasite may remain as individual tachyzoites, or become encysted. Tissue cysts remain viable for many months, and relapse or recrudescence can occur following other infectious conditions. For example, dogs suffering from the immunosuppressive effects of canine distemper are at much higher risk for clinical toxoplasmosis then are healthy dogs. If the organisms reach the central nervous system, clinical signs may include incoordination, circling, tremors, seizures and paresis. In the brain and spinal cord the organism results in multifocal necrosis, associated with malacia of the neuropil, recruitment of macrophages, lymphocytes and glial cells resulting in a nonsuppurative meningoencephalitis Vasculitis with lymphocytic and plasmacytic perivascular cuffing is common. Throughout both the white and grey matter of the central nervous system are scattered tachyzoites and cysts which can be found with careful searching of microscopic sections. Many other tissues may also be affected. In the lungs, interstitial pneumonia with thickening of alveolar septae by a predominantly mononuclear infiltrate is common, as is fibrinous and histiocytic alveolitis, and multifocal parenchymal necrosis. In affected livers, randomly scattered foci of coagulative necrosis with minimal inflammatory infiltrates are the most common presentation. In the choroid and retina of the eyeball, *T. gondii* infection results in subacute chorioretinitis, often associated with retinal folding, degeneration and blindness (Figs. 12.21 and 12.22). Immunohistochemical staining can help to locate and positively identify both individual tachyzoites and tissue cysts, since the necrotizing effect of the infection frequently makes microscopic identification of the organisms difficult.

Perspectives

Parasites may produce different forms of pathology in virtually any tissue in the host's body. Certain clinical pathology or histological patterns are fairly typical for certain parasites. In fact, many

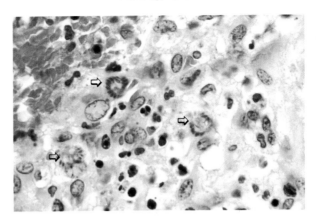

Figure 12.22 Photomicrograph of the same retina seen in Fig. 12.21. Inflammatory neutrophils, macrophages and lymphocytes are present, as well as 3 tissue cysts (arrows) of *T. gondii*. H&E stain (×875).

times a pathologist may suggest a specific parasite may have been responsible for a lesion, even if the parasite itself was not detected in the samples examined. Besides routine gross and histopathology, recently developed techniques including PCR to detect the nucleic acid in protozoa, specific antibodies to some parasites can be detected using ELISA, and immunohistochemical markers can be applied to help confirm a suspected parasite. Identifying the parasite is only the beginning. Since many parasites can be present subclinically, one must determine if they are actually contributing to an animal's illness or death. The degree of pathology produced by a given parasite depends not just on the parasite's deleterious effects on its host, but also on the total parasitic load present, whether the parasitic exposure occurred all at once or by periodic re-exposure, the immune status of the host animal, whether the host was previously exposed to the parasite or this is a naive host, which host tissues are parasitized, and concurrent infection with other diseases or nutritional deficiencies. A thorough understanding of parasite life cycles, hosts, methods of transmission, and control and treatment regimes is also needed to efficiently reduce or eliminate parasitic infections.

Further reading

Bornstein, S., Morner, T. and Samuel, W.M. (2001). *Sarcoptes scabiei* and sarcoptic mange. In Parasitic Diseases of Wild Mammals, 2nd edn, Samuel, W.M., Pybus, M.J., and Kocan, A.A. eds (Iowa State University Press, Ames, Iowa), pp. 107–119.

Dubey, J.P., Odening, K. (2001). Toxoplasmosis and related infections. In: Parasitic Diseases of Wild Mammals, 2nd edn, Samuel, W.M., Pybus, M.J., and Kocan, A.A. eds (Iowa State University Press, Ames, Iowa), pp. 478–519.

Fitzgerald, S.D., Cooley, T.M. and Cosgrove, M.K. (2008). Sarcoptic Mange and *Pelodera* Dermatitis in an American Black Bear (*Ursus americanus*). J. Zoo Wildl. Med. 39, 257–259.

Jones, A. and Pybus, M.J. (2001). Taeniasis and echinococcosis. In Parasitic Diseases of Wild Mammals, 2nd edn, Samuel, W.M., Pybus, M.J., and Kocan, A.A. eds (Iowa State University Press, Ames, Iowa), pp. 150–192.

Jones, T.C., Hunt. R.D. and King N.W., eds (1997). Diseases due to protozoa. In Veterinary Pathology, 6th edn (Williams and Wilkins, Baltimore, Maryland), pp. 549–600.

Jones, T.C., Hunt, R.D. and King, N.W., eds (1997). Diseases caused by parasitic helminthes and arthropods. In Veterinary Pathology, 6th edn (Williams and Wilkins, Baltimore, Maryland), pp. 601–680.

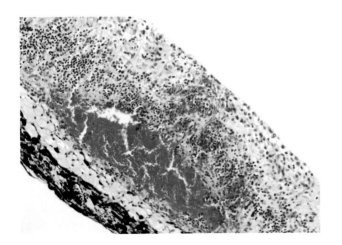

Figure 12.21 Photomicrograph of the retina of the eye of a dog infected with *Toxoplasma gondii*. There is a large focus of intraretinal haemorrhage, as well as degeneration and inflammation of the retina. H&E stain (×175).

Kazacos, K.R. (2001). *Baylisascaris procyonis* and related species. In Parasitic Diseases of Wild Mammals, 2nd edn, Samuel, W.M., Pybus, M.J., and Kocan, A.A. eds (Iowa State University Press, Ames, Iowa), pp. 301–341.

Maxie, M.G. (ed.) (2007). Jubb, Kennedy and Palmer's Pathology of Domestic Animals, 5th edn (Saunders-Elsevier, Edinburgh), vol. 1 pp. 783, vol. 2 pp. 655, vol. 3 pp. 621.

Stockham, S.L. and Scott, M.A. (2002). Fundamentals of Veterinary Clinical Pathology (Blackwell Publishing, Ames Iowa), pp. 610.

Principles of Parasite Control

Controlling Parasites

Hany M. Elsheikha and Gerald C. Coles

13

Introduction

Most animals will carry a few parasites in/on their body and this is normal if kept under control. But, if the infection becomes overwhelming the animal's health will suffer and irreversible damage could result. Indeed, parasite infections continue to be one of the most economically important constraints in raising livestock worldwide, a significant health and welfare issue in companion animals, and an important source of zoonotic infections in humans. Despite tremendous efforts, the number of eradicated parasites is negligible and the perspectives for future eradications would most likely be counteracted by the emergence or re-emergence of other parasite species. Control of parasites can be challenging because parasites can use different immune evasive strategies and/or become resistant to drugs following exposure to the host immune response or to non-judicious use of anti-parasitic therapy, respectively. These challenges necessitate an integrated parasite management approach that encompasses a range of manipulations of the *host* (e.g. increased genetic host resistance through selecting for low faecal worm egg count, improved host resistance through proper nutrition), the *environment* (e.g. pasture management, appropriate husbandry, sound sanitation) and the *parasite* (e.g. sensible use of antiparasitics, maintain susceptible population of parasites, sterile male technologies for insects). This chapter will consider the reasons for parasite control followed by general considerations for parasite control and finally specific considerations for control of endoparasites and ectoparasites in ruminants, horses and companion animals.

Reasons to control parasites

Parasite control is the ability to mange a parasitic infection with the objective to reduce or prevent the spread of a certain parasite. Controlling parasites in the veterinary medicine has been and continues to be a significant goal because of the economic losses and the adverse impact on the animal health and welfare as well as human health.

To reduce economic losses

Efficient parasite control is a key factor in feed efficiency, utilization of available nutrients, immune status, and gut health in all animal species. Economic losses can also be due to abortion caused by *Neospora caninum* in cattle or *Toxoplasma gondii* in sheep. Also, losses can be caused by deaths, failure to gain weight or weight loss, e.g. parasitic gastroenteritis (PGE) in cattle and sheep and coccidiosis in intensively reared poultry. Sometimes the costs are less obvious, e.g. *Anoplocephala perfoliata* is now recognized to cause ileocaecal colic; affected horses may require costly surgical and medical intervention, however this association was inapparent until case control studies demonstrated the association. Sometimes the costs are due to treatment failure due to parasite resistance, which has been seen in every main class of anthelmintic.

To maintain animal health

Effective parasite control is essential for the maintenance of optimal health, performance and productivity in the animals. Animal health can be severely compromised by the presence of parasites and in some cases can lead to death, e.g. high *Toxocara canis* infestation in puppies. Sometimes disease is related to size of parasite burden. In the case of particularly pathogenic parasites the parasitic burden may not be high, but the outcome is severe, e.g. equine protozoal myeloencephalitis in horses.

To maintain animal welfare

Parasitized horses may be thin, hence may be more susceptible to sores from ill-fitting saddles or harnesses. Appetite in PGE is suppressed, hence further exacerbating the impact of infection. Horses with allergy to *Culicoides* rub manes and tail heads and damage themselves (sweet itch). Some ectoparasite infections such as lice or sarcoptic mange may be extremely pruritic so the animal may reduce feeding and concentrate on scratching. Nuisance flies, mosquitoes, and other ectoparasites annoy livestock causing weight loss, reduced milk production and poor reproduction. Besides the nuisance and biting activities of various ectoparasites, there are several species that can transmit diseases to animals. For example, ticks, and the diseases that they transmit, have been a major constraint to the improvement of livestock health and welfare, particularly in the developing countries for the past century.

To minimize parasite zoonoses

Parasite species may jump the species barrier from their natural host to another host species including humans. *Echinococcus multilocularis* infection is transmitted from foxes to humans. *Toxcara canis* infection can cause ocular lesions and visceral migrans in humans. *Toxoplasma gondii* can cause congenital lesions and neurovisual impairments in affected individuals.

General considerations

Failure to control parasite infections in/on animals is due in part to poor understanding of the biology and epidemiology of these organisms. There are some fundamental concepts about parasite biology and pathogenesis that are of critical relevance to parasite control and should be taken into consideration before designing any parasite control programmes.

Knowledge of life cycle

It is important to realize that a basic understanding of parasites and how they replicate and how some produce disease can aid in the management of parasite infections. Knowledge of parasite life cycles can inform pathology, diagnosis, therapeutic 'windows' and provide opportunities to break the life cycle. For example, control of endoparasites in ruminants begins with understanding the life cycle, ecology and epidemiology of problem parasites. Gravid female worms produce eggs that are passed in the animal's faeces. Larvae hatch, and go through several stages of development in the environment before infecting the next host. Continuation of this cycle leads to increasing parasite pasture contamination, which varies according to the location and climate. The success of these parasite stages outside the host depends among other things on the climate. Variable climatic conditions (within and between years), parasite life cycles and survival rates of parasite larval stages outside the host may vary based on geographic localities. Thus, the parasite control programme for helminths needs to be focused on the seasons when infective stages are most available on pasture, usually autumn and spring in all climates, during winter in tropical/subtropical regions and during summer in temperate regions. During the warm, wet months of the year enormous numbers of larvae can build up on pastures in temperate regions, parasite transmission is high, and, susceptible animals are rapidly infected/re-infected with large parasite burdens, particularly in cases of high stocking densities (overgrazing and crowded pens) or low hygiene (faecal contaminated feed bunks and pens). Humidity can promote increased survival of nematode larvae on pasture and promotes increased survival and reproduction of many intermediate hosts such as snails, which are an essential requirement for the ruminant liver fluke (*Fasciola hepatica*). Control programmes need to consider these points and must consider the climatic, topographical, and management conditions of each locality. Limited chemical treatment is indicated when environmental conditions are unfavourable for parasite transmission.

With some exceptions, endoparasites tend to be more problematic in warmer, wetter, temperate areas, while ectoparasites tend to cause the biggest impact in drier warmer areas. However, there is considerable overlap in the geographical incidence of endo and ectoparasites. Endo and ectoparasite infections in combination in/on animal may result in synergistic effects. For example, an animal that is heavily infested with ticks or mites become more severely affected by exposure to nematode parasites than would normally occur if the same animal was free of ectoparasites. It is not uncommon to encounter this combined parasitic exposure in the field. Hence, the use of a broad-spectrum parasiticide (i.e. endectocide) may provide more effective therapy than the use of a product that only treats endo or ectoparasites.

There are two important biological phenomena associated with the nematode parasite's life cycle that we must be aware of (1) hypobiosis and (2) selective pressure/refugia. 'Hypobiosis' is the term used to describe the arrested development of larval stage of nematode parasites in host animals. Many economically important nematode species such as those included in the suborder Strongylida (trichostrongyles and *Dictyocaulus*) undergo hypobiosis. In temperate regions, hypobiosis occurs in late autumn/early winter and is triggered by colder conditions. In tropical/subtropical regions, hypobiosis occurs in late spring/early summer and is triggered by hotter/dryer conditions. However, other factors may be important in triggering hypobiosis such as nematode genetics and host immunity. Hypobiosis of nematode parasites has evolved due to the selective pressures imposed by adverse environmental conditions which would prevent survival of nematode eggs or larvae on pasture. This phenomenon has major epidemiological consequences because arrested larvae are capable of development at a later time stage. In ewes this occurs 1–2 weeks either side of parturition and results in the production of nematode eggs in the ewe faeces at a time when very susceptible hosts (new born lambs) are available to infect. This phenomenon is known as peri-parturient (or spring) rise. This phenomenon also has major clinical consequences because hypobiotic stages besides being difficult to eradicate by therapy they are immature and not detected by faecal egg counts.

While breaking the life cycle using chemotherapy is fundamental to any parasite control programme, this approach implies some risks, most notably, the development of resistance due to the high selective pressure. High treatment frequency has been directly linked to the development of anthelmintic resistance (AR). We should remember that the goal of zero tolerance for parasites is not realistic, environmentally sustainable, or economically justifiable. In fact, accumulating evidence recommends control practices that maintain a proportion of a parasite population in refugia within the animal body. 'Refugia' is a term that describes the proportion of a parasite population that is not exposed to the drug at the time of treatment. For instance, parasitic stages which do not come into contact with the drug, free-living stages on pasture, encysted stages, and parasites in untreated individuals, are all considered to be in refugia. These parasites are not under selection pressure for AR, and, thus, provide a source of susceptible alleles in the population. Leaving of an adequate proportion of the total parasite population in refugia can slow down the development of resistance and has been confirmed by experimental studies with sheep and by computer modelling.

Significance of immunity

Exposure and challenge of animals to parasites is a natural phenomenon in our world. Establishing or maintaining hosts free of nematode infection is not economically feasible or sustainable in livestock production. Preventing livestock from being exposed to parasite via anthelmintic treatment does not allow host immunity to develop. Livestock may develop strong protective immunity to most nematode species following infection. However, in young (susceptible) animals worm burdens may reach clinical levels of significance before immunity develops. It is therefore common practice to manage disease in these animals by the prophylactic use of anthelmintics, for example the administration of anthelmintics prior to turn out and during the first grazing season. Adult animals whose immune systems are compromised by disease, poor nutrition or immune suppression by prolactin (during parturition) are also more susceptible to clinical infections by nematodes.

The immune response to nematodes usually occurs in three distinct phases. The first is suppression of egg laying by female worms before rejection of worms begins. The second occurs when adult nematodes are flushed out of the intestines of their host. This phenomenon is known as 'self-cure' and may be a result of the activation of the innate immune system. The next phase of immunity prevents the host from being infected by newly ingested larvae and may be a result of the activation of the adaptive (acquired) immune response. This latter response prevents subsequent clinical infection but not necessarily some parasite uptake. Immune animals will therefore still shed low numbers of nematode eggs onto pasture. The numbers shed by these immune animals actually serve as a constant source of immune priming, however if young animals or adults that have not previously been exposed to infection are grazed on this pasture they may develop clinical disease. These factors need to be considered during grazing managing and when herds are restocked.

Identifying the host and parasite stage to target for control

Different worm species and life cycle stages affect different age groups of animal. Therefore, it is very important to be aware of the spectrum of parasites expected to be found in a certain host age group. For example, adult horses are commonly affected with small strongyle species, large strongyle species, *Anoplocephala* spp., *Gastrophilus* spp., and pinworm *Oxyuris equi*. Horses under 18 months of age are more likely to be infected by the roundworm, *Parascaris equorum*, but can be infected by other equine parasites too. Horses younger than 6 months of age are more likely to be affected by the threadworm *Strongyloides westeri*. Also, young horses usually show the highest incidence of patent strongyle infections, which is apparently associated with less developed age-dependent immunity. This can lead to an increased infection pressure due to a more heavily contaminated environment of young horses, and result in a higher risk of re-infection and shorter prepatent period.

In sheep, *Nematodirus battus* only affects lambs clinically early in the grazing season (2–3 months after turn out to grass) but as the grazing season progresses other nematode parasites become important. For example, *Teladorsagia* spp. tend to peak in the middle of the grazing season while *Trichostrongylus* spp. tend to peak at the end of the grazing season (late summer/autumn). These 'successions' occur as a result of the different biological and environmental requirements of different nematode species which are ingested and shed at high concentration by hosts at different times of the grazing season.

Because of regional differences in both management practices and climatic conditions, it is unlikely that one rigid regimen will work best for parasite control with anthelmintics. Anthelmintic control of worms on a premise must be based on known faecal egg count reduction test (FECRT) values, stocking density, pasture use, and climatic conditions. Also, it is highly recommended that egg counts be conducted frequently using a sensitive and reliable method to determine parasite status of the animal or the herd before the implementation of any parasite control strategies.

Intervention based on diagnosis or not

Endoparasite infections in dogs and cats caused by helminth parasites present various challenges to small animal practitioners, including parasite identification where there is clinical disease caused by parasitism and defining a rational approach to preventative control. Treatment of pets for parasitic disease is done when animals present with clinical signs of disease, or prophylactically to prevent infection.

In the first situation it is important to reach a specific diagnosis, where diagnosis of parasitic infections relies on a combination of clinical history, physical examinations, laboratory tests, and imaging studies in some cases. For most gastrointestinal infections, in which adult female worms are present, laboratory diagnosis depends on demonstration of eggs or larvae in the faeces using flotation techniques such as the modified McMaster technique or the Baermann technique, respectively. The recently developed FLOTAC technique allows quantification of eggs and/or larvae of nematodes and trematodes as well as cysts and oocysts of intestinal protozoa in up to 1 g of faeces. Also, FLOTAC can be used for fluke eggs with 1 EPG accuracy, and can detect nematode larvae in 15 min. This improved sensitivity along with the wide range of parasites that can be detected makes FLOTAC a very powerful faecal analysis test.

Likelihood of diagnosis of some parasites where daily excretion of eggs or larvae may be intermittent may be increased by sampling over two or three days where necessary. Occasionally where there is a prepatent infection or low-level intermittent shedding, faecal examination may be negative, so a negative result does not necessarily preclude the possibility of a helminth infection. Where 'true' heartworm caused by adult *Dirofilaria immitis* is suspected, which currently in the UK would be associated with a history of travel abroad to warmer countries, then a blood sample for microfilariae, antigen or antibody detection is recommended. Where a specific diagnosis is made then therapy can be initiated. Specific treatments indicated for cats and dogs are shown in the therapy tables within the European Scientific Counsel Companion Animal Parasites (ESCCAP) website (www.esccap.org). Where adult heartworm (*D. immitis*) is diagnosed then current approaches to treatment can be found in the ESCAP vector-borne disease (vbd) guideline and also in the American Heartworm Society website (www.heartwormsociety.org). Where clinical signs are severe then supportive therapy and nursing may also be important.

More commonly the situation is not one of overt clinical signs, rather the presentation is a healthy dog or cat and the question is what is an appropriate management regimen, including treatment, to prevent clinical signs and environmental contamination with eggs or larvae and zoonotic transmission. Here a logical approach is one of risk assessment and then appropriate management of the risk. And the risks are likely to vary from animal to animal with animal-related factors such as the age of the animal, its environment, its nutrition, its geographic location and any previous travel being the important determinants of the likelihood of infection, and indeed what the spectrum of species exposure is likely to have been. Another consideration is the risk of zoonotic infection and its prevention. Thus prevention of worm infections in a puppy living in a household with small children whose personal hygiene may not be well developed may be very critical in prevention of infection by *Toxocara canis*.

Assessment of the risk can be based on faecal examination which will identify patent helminth infections present in sufficient numbers at the time of treatment and/or an assessment of the likelihood of infection based on a knowledge of the animal, the parasites that it is likely to be exposed to and the risk that those parasites pose, either to the animal itself, other animals or humans. Theoretical assessment of the likely exposure is more useful than diagnostics for some parasite species such as cestodes where the current diagnostic methods are very likely to underdiagnose infection, and in situations where prevention of patent infection is highly desirable. Any dogs which feed on sheep carcasses may be infected with *Echinococcus granulosus* (a potentially fatal zoonotic disease). Exposure to carcasses may be the reason why this infection is more prevalent in upland sheep dogs that may scavenge carcasses before a farmer knows that sheep are dead.

Integrated parasite control

For some decades, parasite control in animals has been based on routine use of chemotherapeutic agents, often several times per year. This traditional approach is no longer sustainable; especially with the increasing emerging problem of drug resistance. Thus, it is essential to develop more integrated control strategies. The key to successfully controlling endoparasites in animals and minimizing selecting parasite populations for drug resistance is to rely on different, but complementary approaches, such as targeted drug treatment, proper grazing strategies, use of copper oxide wire particles (COWP), improved nutrition, and environmental management. This integrated parasite control approach must take in account the dynamic interactions between parasite, host, and environment, and must consider interventions that are targeted at these three components. In integrated control it is important to look at each farm individually, use frequent FECR testing to evaluate parasite load status, and plan use of anthelmintic products in consideration of climate and other factors such as grazing schedules.

Monitoring the effectiveness of a control programme

Early detection of resistance is of great importance for parasite control. Evidence indicates that herd testing by faecal sampling at regular intervals is a powerful tool in developing and evaluating a parasite control programme. Indeed, the faecal egg count (FEC) is the only available feasible measure to assess the relative parasite load, to monitor efficiency of the deworming programme, and to make sure that the animal's egg-shedding capacity has not changed. A high FEC means that the pasture will be contaminated with eggs, which subsequently hatch into larvae and infect animals when grazing. Egg count conducted before and after using an anthelmintic will inform end users about the type of anthelmintic to use and the frequency of its usage. Ideally, the FEC should decrease by 90–100% following treatment and if it does not, this may indicate that adult worms are resistant to the anthelmintic.

Egg reappearance period (ERP) is the interval in which faecal egg count returns to 20% of pretreatment values. A shortening of REP of an anthelmintic over time may be an early warning of the development of resistance for the anthelmintic used. Increasing prevalence of AR in ruminant and horse nematodes calls for a regular re-evaluation of the effectiveness of current parasite control programmes to identify factors influencing control efficacy and development of resistance, and any required amendments should be performed whenever possible.

Principles of endoparasite control

Ruminants

Anthelmintics and deworming regimes

Anthelmintics provide an excellent tool for the control of parasitic worms by interrupting the life cycle of the parasite, thus reducing worm burdens and minimizing pasture contamination of infective eggs and larvae. Anthelmintics may eliminate parasites in a variety of ways. For example, by paralysing them and allowing the host to expel them; by halting their ability to metabolize nutrients, thereby killing them; or by limiting their ability to reproduce. Different anthelmintics may act in one or more of these ways (see Chapter 14 for more details).

Deworming is the process of treating animals for endoparasites, such as round worms (nematodes) and tapeworms (cestodes). A proper deworming programme should be carried out in a manner that reduces the number of deworming treatments needed. By reducing the number of treatments, the goal is to reduce the number of worms that are exposed to the drug and reduce the selection for resistance. *Strategic deworming* is used to remove the parasites from their hosts before they enter their reproductive cycle and contaminate the pasture, e.g. early season deworming. *Tactical deworming* means planning the timing when deworming is performed such as when deworming immediately precedes times when worm problems are anticipated. *Selective deworming* means deworming only animals which warrant deworming and only when necessary, e.g. animals with a high number of eggs per gram of faeces. *Opportunistic deworming* occurs during handling other procedures, such as vaccination, castration, or shearing. Although it is convenient it is less effective in the long-term animal health management. *Salvage deworming* is used to save the lives of heavily parasitized animals, e.g. deworming after animals show signs of parasitism. But, by then, the animals have already been weakened. *Suppressive deworming* programme involves the use of anthelmintics at regular intervals, e.g. every 4 weeks. Some of these deworming approaches might appear initially effective, but on the long-term they are labour-intensive, tend to be expensive, fail to identify animals with superior immunity to parasites, and ultimately result in AR. Regardless the pros and cons of each deworming strategy, there is no single deworming programme that suits all animals and all situations. A deworming schedule should be tailored to meet each producer's needs in their respective locations, production strategies and time of year, and must not become a routine.

When to treat?

Although anthelmintics are very powerful tools, there are some measures that need to be considered to maximize their effectiveness and to decrease the rate at which parasites develop resistance.

Proper treatment timing

For worming programmes, timing is key. If you treat too early, targeted worms will be too immature to be affected by the anthelmintic. However, in most cases such as in ruminants several anthelmintics have efficacy against adult and larval stages of parasites. If you treat too late, adult worms will have the opportunity to produce eggs, infecting the animal's environment and raising the animals' risk of exposure. Initial faecal egg counts will determine whether the animal is infected or not, and whether the animal is a high shedder, medium shedder, or low shedder. The range of FEC varies with each animal species and based on the FEC the frequency of treatment can be determined.

Treating animals based on evidence of infection

Parasite infections are over dispersed, the majority of parasites being in the minority of animals due to variation in susceptibility between individuals. Controlling parasites in these animals will have the greatest impact on the risk of infection for the entire herd/flock. In small ruminants, the FAMACHA© system has been used in targeted selective deworming programmes to identify animals who need treatment. This system, pioneered in South Africa by F. Malan and J. van Wyk, uses the colour of the ocular membrane of small ruminants as an indicator of anaemia to identify individuals at risk of haemonchosis.

What to consider when using anthelmintics

Proper dosing

The anthelmintic dosage is based on the animal's body weight, and this needs to be accurately measured because underestimation may result in the administration of insufficient anthelmintic, which may reduce the level of control and increase the risk of developing resistance to the drug. In contrast, applying anthelmintics at high rates prolongs withdrawal times and increases host toxicity. Furthermore, overdosing provides the same level of control as recommended levels, but at a higher cost.

Anthelmintics are not all the same

Just as different antibiotics are active against different bacteria, anthelmintics also have their own spectrum of activity. To control all of the major parasitic species in the animal different anthelmintics must be used. Each type of anthelmintic also has its own recommended dosing interval due to a difference in the period of suppression of the passage of worm eggs.

Be aware of and ready to manage resistance

Anthelmintic resistance should be monitored regularly. Observe and note even the smallest changes in the animal's behaviour, eating habits, dung, coat and general condition. These may be the first clues that there is a parasitic problem. Ensure that the anthelmintics or combination of anthelmintics used on the farm actually works (kills at least 90% of worms). Faecal egg counts before and after deworming using a sensitive technique should be used to check for resistance with current anthelmintics. When a worm becomes resistant to one drug in anthelmintic group (called side resistance) it becomes resistant to all of them. Resistance to most of the currently available anthelmintics has been documented in several animal species and once it occurs reversion to susceptibility will probably not occur. It is a good strategy to identify and select animals naturally resistant to worms. Continuous exposure of a population of worms to the same drug hastens resistance and so rotation of anthelmintic groups is another consideration.

Rotational deworming

The basic concept behind rotational deworming (using a different class of anthelmintic at each deworming, not just switching brand names) is that if worms survive treatment with a particular anthelmintic class, anthelmintics from a different class may control them. However, resistance to two of the three anthelmintic classes, or in some case all three classes, has been documented. These multi-drug resistant strains represent a significant concern and constraint to global livestock farming, and although resistance varies among farms and herds, it's no longer prudent to just assume that simple anthelmintic rotation will kill all worms.

Maintain refugia

An important concept in reducing the current pressure from anthelmintic drugs is to preserve refugia, the proportion of the worm population that are not exposed to the drug when treatment is applied. By maintaining susceptible genes within the population, resistant worms will not have an unfair advantage when they survive anthelmintic therapy. Thus, reducing the amount of used drugs accomplishes two goals: It helps preserve refugia, and it reduces the selection pressure for drug resistance.

Safety to animals and humans

An ideal anthelmintic should exhibit a high level of toxicity to the parasite but not to the host, thus having a wide therapeutic index or margin of safety, be easy to administer to be of practical use, does not leave residual substances in the host that negatively impact humans who consume meat or milk from the treated animal and be cost effective. Virtually all anthelmintics have a meat or milk withdrawal time that must be considered. Drug residues in animal tissues can also potentially compromise trade in food commodities of animal origin. Not all anthelmintics have the same margin of safety. Any anthelmintic used during pregnancy must be safe to the dam and developing foetus.

Pasture and environmental management

Sound pasture management reduces the need for anthelmintics, minimizes re-infection by preventing re-contamination of spring pastures, when over wintered larvae resume their life cycle, and prevents the midsummer build up of infective nematode eggs or larvae on pasture. By predicting the times of the year that large numbers of infective larvae will be on pasture, measures can be taken to reduce the intake of infective larvae.

Safe pasture

'Parasite safe' pastures is a term used to designate pastures with low enough numbers of infective worm eggs or infective larvae to result in a low adult worm load in hosts. Examples of safe pastures would be those permanent pastures not grazed for a long time, pastures used for hay, pastures used for temporary grazing and those protected from the shedding of parasite eggs by properly timed deworming. Pasture that has been renovated or rotated with row crops is considered 'safe'. Pasture grazed by livestock such as horses which do not share parasites with cattle is also considered 'safe'. However, some parasites (e.g. the stomach hairworm, *Trichostrongylus axei*) can infect ruminants and horses grazing on the same pasture.

Safe pastures should be reserved for young animals, when possible, because they are much more susceptible to infection. Severely contaminated pastures can be withheld from grazing for one year, cropped, or tilled and re-seeded. Also, by using controlled grazing methods that allow pastures to rest and soil life to function well, contamination can be reduced. This reduction occurs because soil organisms, such as nematophagous fungi can kill parasite eggs and larvae.

Cull heavy shedders

Eradicate heavily infected animals from the flock/herd to remove the perceived source of infection and control the spread of infections among animals.

Stocking density

The number of animals per acre/hectare should be kept at a level that will prevent overgrazing and reduce pasture contamination with parasite eggs and larvae. Also, avoid overcrowding and any other causes of stress.

Good hygiene and husbandry

Endoparasites are primarily transferred via manure, hence, good management is essential. Pick up and dispose of manure regularly at least weekly from pastures and pens. Avoid spreading uncomposted manure on fields to be grazed by animals; instead, compost it in a pile away from the pasture. Compost manure for at least a year; turn it frequently to produce heat needed to kill the endoparasite eggs and larvae. Use a feeder for hay and grain rather than feeding on the ground.

Copper oxide wire particles (COWP)

These particles can be administered as a gelatin capsule or in a feed supplement. The capsule form is administered into the abomasum of sheep or goats by inserting at the back of the throat using a pill gun. COWP have been shown to reduce the total *H. contortus* counts in young lambs and kids. The antiparasitic properties of COWP might be attributed to the direct effect of copper on worms and/or boosting the animal's immune system. However, the exact mechanism of how COWP control abomasal nematode parasites is not yet fully understood.

In addition to the above approaches, endoparasites control strategies in ruminants should be developed to fit individual production situations and should also take into consideration some important variables (Table 13.1).

Additional resources

Further information on the management and control of parasites in ruminants can be found in published key articles and reviews, and in the two comprehensive technical manuals: SCOPS (Sustainable Control of Parasites in Sheep) and COWS (Control of Worms Sustainably). SCOPS and COWS manuals were devised mainly to ensure more efficient and effective anthelmintic usage by promoting 'best practice' worm control principles for sheep (SCOPS) and cattle (COWS). Both technical guides provide useful recommendations for veterinary surgeons and advisors. Free copies are available in downloadable PDF format from www. nationalsheep.org.uk/images/stories/pdf/scopstechmanthree. pdf (SCOPS) and www.eblex.org.uk/documents/content/ research/cows_manual_2010_plus.pdf (COWS).

Table 13.1 Variables influencing parasite treatment and control programmes

Animal factors, e.g. immune status, physical condition, age, genetic resistance, dose exposure, stress, stocking rate, nutritional factors, and reproductive cycle

Anthelmintics, e.g. efficacy, cost effectiveness, ease of application, and withdrawal time

Weather, e.g. temperature, humidity, oxygen and sunlight

Soil, e.g. nematophagous fungi

Forages, e.g. height, species, and rotation; condensed tannin-rich forages

Husbandry, e.g. regimens of nutrition, sanitation, quarantine, and pasture rotation

Management protocols for the animal species, e.g. herd management, individual management, access to animals, and indoor/outdoor maintenance of animals

Horses

Endoparasites are one of the most common threats to equine health and well-being, especially in young and vulnerable foals and in geriatric horses. Hence, parasite control in equines is essential for the maintenance of optimal health and performance. Worm control in equines has been mainly based on the exclusive and regular use of anthelmintics. However, due to the escalating prevalence of AR this approach is considered unsustainable. Equine ascarids, large strongyles and small strongyles (cyathostomes) have been reported to have developed resistance to at least one class of equine anthelmintics. Key factors contributing to the development of AR in horses are high treatment frequencies, rotation between the same class of anthelmintic, high stocking rates, underdosing and the off-label use of anthelmintics. In some countries, a further problem of equine parasite control is the decreasing involvement of veterinarians in therapy. Instead, worm control is often carried out by horse owners and farm managers. Some European countries (e.g. Denmark) have responded to this problem by making anthelmintic drugs available only by prescription and prohibiting their use for routine, prophylactic treatment.

Current worm control strategies need to take the consequences of spreading AR into account, and should be evaluated for their effects on the development of resistance in addition to the maintenance of horse health. Improved control strategies for equine parasites are needed to ensure a more sustainable use of anthelmintics via implementation of measures that will delay the development of AR in equine nematodes. These measures should include the following.

Avoid underdosing

All of the horse's product dosages are based on animal weight, so animal's weight should be estimated with some accuracy. Relying on visual assessment of horse weight for the calculation of dose is a common mistake, which will often lead to underdosing, which in turn propagates AR. Thus, more precise means of weight assessment like the use of a girth tape should be used where scales are unavailable.

Avoid frequent treatments

Some researchers argue that young horses require more frequent treatments than adult horses. However, such a differentiated management programme for different age groups/the intensive treatment frequency for young horses will probably not be sustainable since a relationship has been demonstrated between the frequency of treatment and the rate of development of AR.

Controlled quarantine treatment

Newly introduced horses should be treated with an effective, ideally larvicidal, anthelmintic drug or a combination of different anthelmintic drugs at arrival since they can introduce AR to a herd. It is also advisable to evaluate the success of any quarantine treatment to avoid introduction of resistant populations.

FEC monitoring

Monitoring of equine ranches and farms for FECR and ERP is essential in determining whether anthelmintic preparations are effectively controlling parasites. FLOTAC is a sensitive technique, which allows both the detection of low levels of resistance and the use of composite samples, reducing the cost of the test for farmers and horse owners. Also, the FECPAK test system can be used on farm by trained owners to monitor faecal egg output from individual animals quickly, cheaply and reliably. This approach will allow treatment of the correct horse at the correct time. Targeted and selective treatment via using anthelmintic only after FECs reach a certain level has been advocated in horse parasite control programmes to decrease the frequencies and amounts of anthelmintics used. Targeted treatment using ivermectin after FEC reached more than 100 EPG and 200 EPG in young horses and in adult horses, respectively, has been shown to be effective in reducing FEC in a population of cyathostomes resistant to fenbendazole and pyrantel salts. However, there is no a consensus among scientists as to what threshold of FEC should be reached before treatment is initiated.

Slow or fast rotational deworming

Conflicting reports exist on which type of anthelmintic rotational regimen should be used to achieve good levels of parasite control simultaneously with the goal of preventing resistance. Many of the recommendations of using fast rotation (i.e. rotation between anthelmintic classes at periods of 3–6 times per year) versus slow rotation (i.e. using a single anthelmintic for a year followed by another class in years 2 and 3) of anthelmintic classes have not been tested clinically or in the field.

Pasture management

Sound management practices, such as pasture rotation, pasture rotation between species of animals, reducing overcrowding, avoiding feeding horses on the ground, composting of manure, and regular removal of faeces – at least once or twice weekly – have been recommended as important additional measures to anthelmintics therapy with the aim of reducing the sole reliance on anthelmintic treatment. Pasture management with responsible use of current anthelmintic regimens (e.g. 4 or less yearly treatments of anthelmintics) has been suggested to be essential to reduce the selection pressure for resistance and to maintain the efficacy of available equine anthelmintics.

Maintain worms in refugia

In horses, refugia is also considered to be of relevance in parasite control programmes via diluting the resistant parasite population, and thus reducing selection for resistance.

Companion animals

Treatment: spectrum and interval

There are a large number of products available to treat worm infections in dogs and cats. Some are endectocides, produced either by having a single active ingredient with a broad spectrum of activity such as selamectin or by combining active ingredients. Such products may be used to control both worms and ectoparasites and the precise spectrum of activity varies according to the active ingredients. Matching the spectrum of activity to the infections present, or the risk for individual animals, is an important part of managing parasite infection. A review of the spectrum of activity of each individual product in the National Office of Animal Health (NOAH) compendium is available under therapies on the ESCCAP website (www.esccap.org). Similarly an assessment must be made of the worms present or likely to be present, hence whether nematocidal treatment or cestocidal treatment or a combination is necessary. Other factors to consider include activity against immature as well as adult stages of parasites and ease of administration.

The appropriate frequency of worming is often debated and is likely to change according to different situations. Where it is critical to minimize risk of patent infection (for example when zoonotic infection control is important), re-treatment at a frequency close to the prepatent period (often monthly for convenience) will help to achieve this, though should not be viewed as a panacea as virtually no treatment can be counted on to have 100% efficacy. In other situations this frequency of treatment would be 'over kill', particularly where other management measures are instigated to reduce the risk of parasite infection. To date there is no hard and fast rule, or much published evidence, of what the frequency of treatment should be in these lower risk situations. Some data has suggested that one or two treatments per year may not have a significant epidemiological impact and generally four treatments per year (or an equivalent number of faecal examinations) are recommended.

What is sought is a balance between minimizing zoonotic and animal health risk whilst managing environmental contamination and minimizing the risk of selection for resistance. Fortunately, AR has been very rarely reported for parasites of pet animals, perhaps because of a decreased intensity of treatment compared with farm animals. However, no sensitive egg counting procedures have been used to look for anthelmintic failures in pets. Nonetheless, the cost of treatment and the potential for resistance selection must be balanced against the health risks to achieve an overall regimen that works for an individual animal or group of animals.

Management and animal factors

Knowledge of the animal and its management can be used to aid the risk assessment of parasitic infection and animal management can also be manipulated to, where possible, diminish the risk of parasitic infections.

Animal factor

The age of the animal, particularly if it is a young puppy or kitten may be significant. *Toxocara* spp. infections are most common in puppies and kittens, and intensity of infection may be highest in these two populations. However, older dogs may repeatedly acquire patent *T. canis* infections throughout their life, usually when they have not been highly exposed as pups. Therefore it is a mistake to believe that *T. canis* is an infection of puppies only, although prevalence in the adult dog population is far lower than in pups at any one time.

Feeding

Good nutrition plays a big part in how well any animal's immune system mounts the proper defences and also in the animal's overall ability to tolerate the presence of some worms. Healthy and well-nourished animals will be best placed to tolerate a parasite burden but access to uncooked meat, offal or prey (by hunting) may increase the risk of parasitic infection. Thus feeding cooked, prepared food will diminish risk of parasitism.

Housing and management including 'poopascooping'

Depending on management, there may be more opportunity for introduction of parasites and accumulation of an environmental burden of immature stages where there are groups of dogs or cats in kennel situations. Worm eggs are not infective to the pet when passed and so if faeces are collected and disposed of appropriately then the risk of infective stages in the environment is reduced. A recent survey including 1023 participants from England, Scotland and Northern Ireland (including cat owners, dog owners, and non-pet owners) revealed that only 41% of respondents were aware that pet faeces could transmit 'worms' to humans, and only a small percentage of those knew the associated symptoms.

Geographical location

Some worms, such as *T. canis* are ubiquitous, whilst the distribution of others is more localized. In the UK, *Echinococcus granulosus* is largely confined to central Wales, the Welsh borders and the Hebrides, which are upland regions in which dogs (particularly sheep dogs) may scavenge sheep carcasses before a farmer realizes that dead sheep are present. Traditionally, *Angiostrongylus vasorum* infection was associated with geographical 'hot spots' in the south-west of the UK and localized regions in the south-east. However, epidemiological evidence is now accumulating which suggests that *A. vasorum* has spread widely from these traditional areas possibly due to the spread of urban foxes. Therefore, it is important to be alert to consistent clinical signs and disease trends, and to consider screening faecal samples for infection.

Travel and risk of introductions

With the recent confirmation that tick and tapeworm treatments are to be continued under the Pet Travel Scheme (PETS) until December 2011, the risk of introducing *Echinococcus multilocularis* infection into the UK is reduced. However this does nothing to protect pets whilst they are staying in the area where infection is endemic in continental Europe. Hence dogs (and cats) that are staying in this area and who have the opportunity to hunt for rodents should be treated at monthly intervals with praziquantel to decrease the risk of them carrying a patent infection. Maps showing the current approximate distribution of this parasite and other species such as *D. immitis* are shown in the ESCCAP worm control guideline.

Putting risk assessment into practice

Scandinavian countries such as Denmark have developed assessment of risk of helminth infection prior to initiating therapy as a formal legislative requirement for small animals as well as farmed species, following concerns about the overuse of antiparasitic drugs, leading to AR. A recent study reported the results of a small survey of practitioners to assess how practitioners approached this in small animals. The main categories where dogs and cats were treated without faecal examination were travelling animals, puppies and kittens and on clinical suspicion. The percentage of practitioners who responded that they treated older dogs and cats without faecal examination was low, thus indicating that most practitioners rationally assess risk before administering anthelmintics.

Additional resources

Further information on the issues raised herein can be found in the worm and vbd guidelines on the ESCCAP website (www.esccap.org). The risk assessment approach is also provided in the British Small Animal Veterinary Association (BSAVA) worm control guidelines available at www.bsava.com. ESCCAP UK has now developed a website specifically for vets and other animal healthcare professionals and this can be found at www.esccapuk.org.uk. There is also a website for pet owners at www.petparasites.co.uk. This provides information and also interactive maps for pet owners planning to travel to continental Europe with their pets.

Principles of ectoparasite control

Livestock and companion animals are exposed to infestations by a wide range of ectoparasites, such as ticks, mites, flies, fleas, or lice. These organisms cause significant economic loss and serious animal health and welfare issues. Ectoparasites exert their deleterious effects by irritating the animal, interfering with growth, and sometimes act as vectors of disease-causing pathogens (see Chapter 10). Some species are associated with myiasis via invasion of the animal's tissue by fly larvae and economic losses at slaughter houses may occur because of skin damage (e.g. hypodermosis).

Control measures of infestation caused by different ectoparasite species are discussed in Chapters 8–10. Further general guidelines which are fundamental to the success of any ectoparasite control programmes are provided (Table 13.2).

Herein, we provide brief outlines for control of major groups of ectoparasites in ruminants, horses and companion animals.

Ruminants

Control of flies and mosquitoes in the recent past has relied heavily on the use of chemicals, such as the arsenicals, chlorinated hydrocarbons, organophosphates, carbamates, formamidines, pyrethroids, macrocyclic lactones, and more recently the insect growth regulators (IGRs). *Control of flies* should be aimed at preventing flies from breeding via regular removal of dung and other breeding habitats, and destroying adult flies within premises using appropriate insecticides and/or traps. The use of fly-traps for the control of sheep blowfly strike caused by *Lucilia sericata* has been considered extensively in the UK. The release of sterile flies into natural populations has been tried with some success in the eradication of the myiasis-causing flies (e.g. screwworm fly), but failed to control hypodermosis in North America due to the lack of feasible techniques for mass production of *Hypoderma* flies for sterilization. *Control of mosquitoes* within the premises is possible by using aerosol spray in the late evening. Chemotherapy

with repellent active ingredients like pyrethroids may considerably reduce the infestation. These products are applied topically as pour-on or spray-on or as ear tags. Also, the breeding ground of the mosquitoes should be identified and eradicated. Aquatic stages (egg, larva, and pupa) can be destroyed by either draining water reservoirs or covering the surface with oil.

Control of warble fly infestation relies on the use of different organophosphorus (OP) insecticide formulations, which, however, have yielded unsatisfactory results in terms of animal and human safety and efficacy. Additionally, the administration of OPs against *Hypoderma* may lead to a massive release of antigens from larvae destroyed by the insecticide, causing occasionally fatal outcomes. Hence, the timing of drug administration against migrating larvae is of paramount importance. In fact, treating animals when larvae are still migrating in the animal could be dangerous when tackling species that migrate in the perirachidian channel (i.e. *H. bovis*) or in the oesophagus (i.e. *H. lineatum*). Medical interference at this time period may cause paresis/paralysis of the hindquarters or oesophagitis and bloating, respectively. Hence, insecticide formulations that have systemic activity should not be applied after the larvae reach these sensitive tissues. OPs have been superseded by macrocyclic lactones, which are formulated as injectables or pour-ons, including ivermectin, eprinomectin, and moxidectin, which have been used successfully for the eradication of warble flies in the United Kingdom, and other European countries.

Control of ticks can be achieved by removing ticks manually if only a few ticks are present and keeping animals away from infested mates/pasture/premises. Tick control can be achieved through the use of acaricides. Many effective medications are available in different formulations. In addition to the use of acaricides, attempts have been made in some countries to achieve a degree of disease control through the use of a vaccine against the *Rhippicephalus microplus* tick, and by farming with cattle breeds that are naturally resistant to tick infestations.

Horses

Several types of biting flies (e.g. stable flies, horse and deer flies, black flies, biting gnats, horn flies), nuisance flies (e.g. house flies, face flies), mosquitoes, lice, and bots can have a tremendous impact on horse health, comfort, and performance. Other arthropods such as mites and ticks can also cause damage and irritation to horses. Management of these bugs through source reduction is impractical because their breeding sites cannot be eliminated or reduced totally. Therefore, control is often focused on a sound farm sanitation programme and treatment of host animal, by ectoparasiticides and/or repellents.

Control of stable flies is directed at larval and adult stages of the fly. Proper sanitation practices around stable and frequent manure management is essential in limiting fly production. When this is not possible, a larvicide insecticide may be applied directly to places where eggs are laid and larvae develop can kill the developing flies. Control of adult flies is achieved by using residual insecticides as surface treatments (provide control for an extended period when sprayed onto sites where the adult flies congregate) and/or knock-down sprays (requires less time

Table 13.2 General recommendations for ectoparasites' control

---

Quarantine measures

Prevent introduction of resistant pests by keeping newly purchased animals in quarantine under supervision and destruction of pests when found

Prevent spread of resistant pests by limiting their multiplication and extension to other districts

Protection of animals from attack of the insects/ticks/mites

Apply double door and wire netting on windows

Do not use instruments or clothing of infested animals

Apply covers when transporting animals

Maintain proper environmental management

Consider using biological controls, e.g. natural predators of ectoparasites

Proper use of pesticides

Monitor and test for resistance on the farm to optimize the timing of pesticide use and to determine the need for additional treatments

Administer the pesticide(s) effectively (i.e. use at the rate recommended and check method of application)

Adopt strategy to preserve susceptible pests on the farm (e.g. ensure that some of the parasite population remains unexposed to drugs 'in refugia')

Improve physical fitness of animals

Maintain good nutrition and exercise

Avoid overcrowding and other stressors

Consider animal environment

Clean and disinfect all infected premises and leave unused for 2 weeks at least

Clean and disinfect all utensils and covers and leave unused for 3–4 weeks until the ectoparasites will have died

Proper husbandry and general sanitation

Reduce dependence on pesticides

---

for application but will only kill flies present at application and thus provides short-term relief) to kill existing adult flies. *Control of horse and deer flies* relies on individual animal treatment using repellents or insecticidal sprays to reduce fly bites. Horse flies and deer flies like sunny areas and usually will not enter barns or deep shade. If animals have access to protection during the day, they can escape the constant attack of these annoying pests. *Black flies* which feed in the ears of horses can be controlled using insecticidal applications or by using petroleum jelly in the interior of the horses' ears. When possible, horses can be stabled during the day and pastured at night because black flies only feed during daylight hours and usually do not enter stable areas. Direct treatment of horses infested with *biting gnats* or *horn flies* using sprays containing insecticides or repellents can provide relief for the horses. *Control of face flies* can be achieved by stabling horses during the daytime when the face fly feeds. In addition, since the face fly feeds predominantly on cattle, pasturing horses separately from cattle will lessen the incidence of these flies on the horses. Topical insecticide applications are usually not effective because face flies spend little time on the horse.

Control of mosquitoes should be directed at both larvae and adult stages. Control of larvae, is the most efficient and effective and should be the backbone of any chemical programme. Mosquitoes' breeding sites (e.g. stagnant shallow, quiet water bodies) must be eliminated or treated. Control of adults, is less efficient and should be used strictly for supplemental or emergency purposes such as in case of active transmission of a mosquito-borne disease. A number of insecticides are registered for mosquito

control. The numbers of mosquitoes on horses can be reduced by treating individual animals using spray insecticides. In stables, sprays, and insecticide impregnated strips can provide useful aids of control.

Controlling the horse sucking and biting lice involves (i) good grooming that provides an opportunity to inspect the horse for lice, (ii) adequate nutrition to maintain the health of the horse, and (iii) insecticidal sprays.

Controlling horse bots should be directed at breaking the fly's life cycle via (i) mechanical removal of eggs via grooming and (ii) chemical control using a variety of preparations to rid horses of bot infestations in the stomach and intestines. Commonly used medications include ivermectin and moxidectin. These medications are available as pastes, gels, pellets, liquids, powders and boluses. Several of these products are effective treatments for other internal parasites as well. Additional measures include using equine insect repellent and fly sheets on the horse during the summer to reduce the level of bot infestation and treatment of egg laying sites with insecticidal washes to reduce the numbers of larvae which can be ingested by the horse.

Mange infestation in horses includes *Sarcoptes scabiei* var. *equi*, *Psoroptes equi*, *Chorioptes equi*, *Demodex*, Trombiculid, and straw itch mite. Old treatment includes organophosphate insecticides or lime-sulfur solution, which has been used by spraying, sponging, or dipping. Treatment should be repeated at 2-week intervals at least 3–4 times. Modern treatment involves the oral administration of ivermectin or moxidectin. Several treatments are required, 2–3 weeks apart. It is important to treat all contact animals.

Amitraz, used in other species to treat demodectic mange, is contraindicated in horses because it can cause severe colic and death. In some species the pruritus can be controlled with glucocorticoids. Repellents may help prevent mite infestation. *Ticks on horses* can be removed by hand, and topical applications of acaricides can be used to prevent infestations.

Companion animals

Management of *ticks, mite and louse infestation* in companion animals is readily achievable because these parasites live on the skin surface. Control involves identification and isolation of the severely affected animals, systemic and regular treatment of all affected animals that carry ticks, mites or lice, protection of the young animals from exposure to older infested ones, treatment of all introduced animals, and segregation of healthy and untreated animals if the entire group is not treated at one time. A variety of compounds have efficacy against ticks. Amitraz, permethrins, fipronil, and selamectin are all used on dogs for tick control. Multiple therapies are effective for mite infestations: ivermectin, milbemycin, selamectin moxidectin, amitraz, and fipronil. Environmental treatment of ticks and mites with pesticides is non-feasible because the off-host stages are usually widely distributed outdoors and in inaccessible locations. Care should be taken to ensure that infestation is not transferred via contaminated brushes or hair combs from one infested animal to other animals in the same or other households. It is worthy mentioning that the introduction of the PETS travel scheme and the growing awareness of endemic and exotic tick-borne diseases have led ticks to become an important target parasite in companion animals.

Control of *flea infestation* has been the primary target for ectoparasite control in dogs and cats because fleas are widespread, cause irritation, blood loss, can provoke allergic dermatitis in affected animals, and act as the intermediate host for the tapeworm *Dipylidium caninum*. Management is based on locating the flea-breeding sites. Treatment involves the use of flea adulticides on the pet as well as control of the immature stages of fleas in the surrounding environment. All pets in the household must be treated. Control of flea eggs, larvae and pupae in the environment is also important in order to minimize the potential level of challenge to animals or humans. Litter, bedding, and dirt should be removed from the premises and burned and the premises thoroughly cleaned. During the past 15 years, topical and oral applications of insecticides such as fipronil, imidacloprid, lufenuron and selamectin have revolutionized flea control in pets. A combination of imidacloprid and moxidectin has been recently developed in a spot-on formulation with the aim of providing a treatment for, and a prophylaxis against ectoparasites and nematodes of dogs.

Perspectives

Parasite control programme should be designed to minimize parasite load in/or animals, prevent contamination of the environment, and to disrupt the parasite's life cycle. Control of parasites primarily rests on the use of chemicals, either applied directly to the animals or to the environment. Problems associated with this are the development of resistance to the chemicals, and issues around the residues in animals and the environment. This means that over reliance on drug therapy needs to be reviewed and monitored more prudently. We need to use antiparasitic drugs more selectively to maintain their efficacy and, better understand at what levels parasites on hosts have productivity, performance and animal welfare implications. While strategic use of antiparasitic drugs or insecticides is a valuable tool in managing the adverse impact of parasitism on animals, grazing management tools, such as provision of clean pastures, alternate grazing by other animal species, alternate grazing by immunologically resistant hosts of the same species, monitoring of parasite transmission, and timing of reproductive events can also influence the effectiveness of drug/insecticide regimes. These interventions must be tailored to control infection/infestation at the animal level (individual and population) and contamination of the environment; a successful outcome depends on the timing and synchronization of these interventions. The effective control of parasites will not only be determined by the effectiveness of a particular method or combination of methods, but also by the sustainability of the control approach. Hence, we must conserve what we have through strategic and focussed treatments of animals, developing viable vaccines against vectors and diseases they transmit, environmental control of parasites breeding sites, proper disease management, and selection of resistant breeds.

Acknowledgements

We would like to thank Dr Anne M. Zajac from The Virginia-Maryland Regional College of Veterinary Medicine, Virginia Polytechnic Institute and State University (Virginia Tech), Blacksburg, Virginia, USA, and Maggie Fisher, the director of Ridgeway Research Ltd and Shernacre Enterprise Ltd, Worcestershire, UK, for their constructive comments and helpful advice on the manuscript.

Further reading

Abott, K.A., Taylor, M. and Stubbings, L.A. (2009). Sustainable worm control strategies for sheep, 3rd edn. Context Publications, UK.

Brady, H.A. and Nichols, W.T. (2009). Drug resistance in equine parasites: an emerging global problem. J. Equine Vet. Sci. 29, 285–295.

Conboy, G. (2009). Cestodes of dogs and cats in North America. Vet. Clin. North. Am. Small Anim. Pract. 39, 1075–1090.

Craig, T.M. (2006). Anthelmintic resistance and alternative control methods. Vet. Clin. North Am. Food Anim. Pract. 22, 567–581.

Cringoli, G., Rinaldi, L., Maurelli, M.P. and Utzinger, J. (2010). FLOTAC: new multivalent techniques for qualitative and quantitative copromicroscopic diagnosis of parasites in animals and humans. Nat. Protoc. 5, 503–515.

Epe, C. (2009). Intestinal nematodes: biology and control. Vet. Clin. North Am. Small Anim. Pract. 39, 1091–107.

ESCCAP (European Scientific Counsel Companion Animal Parasites) (2006). Worm control in dogs and cats. http://www.esccap.org/index. php/fuseaction/ download/lrn_file/001-esccap-guidelines-ukfinal.pdf.

Fisher, M. (2005). Power over parasites. A reference manual for small animal veterinary surgeons. Kingfisher Press, England.

Grant, S. and Olsen, C.W. (1999). Preventing zoonotic diseases in immunocompromised persons: The role of physicians and veterinarians. Emerg. Infect. Dis. 5, 159–163.

Langrová, I., Makovcová, K., Vadlejch, J., Jankovská, I., Petrtýl, M., Fechtner, J., Keil, P., Lytvynets, A. and Borkovcová, M. (2008). Arrested development of sheep strongyles: onset and resumption under field conditions of Central Europe. Parasitol. Res. *103*, 387–392.

Morgan, E.R. and Coles, G.C. (2010). Nematode control practices on sheep farms following an information campaign aiming to delay anthelmintic resistance. Vet. Rec. *166*, 301–303.

Nielsen, M.K., Fritzen, B., Duncan, J.L., Guillot, J., Eysker, M., Dorchies, P., Laugier, C., Beugnet, F., Meana, A., Lussot-Kervern, I. and von Samson-Himmelstjerna, G. (2010). Practical aspects of equine parasite control: a review based upon a workshop discussion consensus. Equine Vet. J. *42*, 460–468.

Presland, S.L., Morgan, E.R. and Coles, G.C. (2005). Counting nematode eggs in equine faecal samples. Vet. Rec. *156*, 208–210.

Pugh, D.G., Mobini, S.M. and Hilton, C.D. (1998). Control programs for gastrointestinal nematodes in sheep and goats. Comp. Contin. Edu. Pract. Vet. *20*, 112–123.

Ramsey, I. (2008). BSAVA small animal formulary. 6th edn. BSAVA, Quedgeley, England.

Ramsey, I. and Tennant, B. (2001). Manual of canine and feline infectious diseases. BSAVA.

Soli, F., Terrill, T.H., Shaik, S.A., Getz, W.R., Miller, J.E., Vanguru, M. and Burke, J.M. (2010). Efficacy of copper oxide wire particles against gastrointestinal nematodes in sheep and goats. Vet. Parasitol. *168*, 93–96.

Stear, M.J., Strain, S. and Bishop, S.C. (1999). How lambs control infection with *Ostertagia circumcincta*. Vet. Immunol. Immunopathol. *72*, 213–218.

Taylor, M.A., Coop, R.L., and Wall, R.L. (2007). Veterinary Parasitology, 3rd edn., Blackwell Pub., Oxford.

Tennant, B. (2005). BSAVA Small Animal Formulary, 5th edn (BSAVA, Quedgeley, England).

Thamsborg, S. (2009). Legal Considerations in creating and applying guidelines: Denmark as an example. (WAAVP conference, Calgary, Canada).

van Wyk, J.A., Hoste, H., Kaplan, R.M. and Besier, R.B. (2006). Targeted selective treatment for worm management—how do we sell rational programs to farmers? Vet. Parasitol. *139*, 336–346.

Vlassoff, A., Leathwick, D.M., and Heath, A.C.G. (2001). The epidemiology of nematode infections of sheep. N. Z. Vet. J. *49*, 213–221.

von Samson-Himmelstjerna, G., Traversa, D., Demeler, J., Rohn, K., Milillo, P., Schurmann, S., Lia, R., Perrucci, S., di Regalbono, A.F., Beraldo, P., Barnes, H., Cobb, R. and Boeckh, A. (2009). Effects of worm control practices examined by a combined faecal egg count and questionnaire survey on horse farms in Germany, Italy and the UK. Parasit. Vectors 2 Suppl 2, S3.

Wells, D.L. (2007). Public understanding of toxocariasis, Public Health. *121*, 187–188.

Windon, R.G. (1996). Genetic control of resistance to helminths in sheep. Vet. Immunol. Immunopathol. *54*, 245–254.

Zajac, A.M. (2006). Gastrointestinal nematodes of small ruminants: life cycle, anthelmintics, and diagnosis. Vet. Clin. North Am. Food Anim. Pract. *22*, 529–541.

Antiparasitic Drugs: Mechanisms of Action and Resistance

14

Hany M. Elsheikha, Steven McOrist and Timothy G. Geary

Background

Parasites such as nematodes and mites can be debilitating and deadly inhabitants of an animal's body. While some parasitic infections can be controlled effectively by preventive biosecurity, vaccines or other non-pharmaceutical intervention measures, for many parasites, these measures are not available, have a limited effect, or cannot be applied in practical settings. Antiparasitic drugs are the commonly-applied pharmaceutical compounds used to reduce, treat or prevent parasitic infections in animals. Starting perhaps with the initial usage of carbon tetrachloride against *Fasciola* in cattle, the strategic use of anthelmintic drugs has drastically reduced gastro-intestinal helminth infections and improved the welfare and productivity of domestic animals. Widespread effective usage of antiparasitics is therefore one of the greatest triumphs of the parasitology discipline, although they are not without problems and shortcomings. One of the most pressing concerns addressed in this chapter is the emergence of strains of parasites that are resistant to the action of an antiparasitic drug.

Selective toxicity principle

Antiparasitic drugs act by interfering with the growth, metabolism, and motor function of helminths, or disrupting the replication and development of protozoa. These compounds except insecticides, act while the parasite is located within the host. Therefore, the drug's effects on the cells and tissues of the host are crucial. The ideal antiparasitic drug kills the parasites without damaging the host; this is the principal of 'selective toxicity'. It may be easier to develop antibiotics that are effective against prokaryotic bacterial cells and that do not affect the eukaryotic cells of the mammalian host, compared with the problem when the pathogen is a eukaryotic organism, such as protozoa, helminths, or arthropods.

> . . . to succeed in identifying the chemoreceptors of parasites that have no analogue in the body.
>
> Paul Ehrlich (1913)

An ideal antiparasitic drug

A successful drug also needs to fulfil one or more of these fundamental requirements, namely (i) effective in removing adult and immature forms of parasites from body, (ii) a wide therapeutic index, (iii) effective after one dose, however, many antiparasitic drugs are given daily or repeatedly, (iv) easy to administer, e.g. in feed, injections, and pour-on, (v) inexpensive or economically justifiable, (vi) no residue problems, especially in food-producing animals, and (vii) 'pharmaceutically optimal' (i.e. provides specific advantages in terms of pharmacokinetics and/or metabolism).

The ideal drug would also have low levels of possible drawbacks, such as selection for the development of resistant strains and adverse health effects.

Common chemotherapeutic targets

The helminth life cycle is often complex, and the adaptation to survival in the mammalian host depends strongly on (1) neuromuscular coordination for feeding, movement, and for maintenance of a favourable location of the parasite within the host; (2) carbohydrate metabolism as the major source of energy, with glucose the primary substrate; and (3) microtubular integrity, because egg laying and hatching, larval development, and glucose transport are impaired when microtubules are modified. Most anthelmintics affect parasites by interacting with their nervous system or by altering their cellular metabolism and structure. Brief examples of the chemotherapeutic strategies that exploit the differences between parasites (helminths, protozoa, arthropods) and their hosts are listed (Table 14.1). These strategies are discussed in more detail as we deal with the major classes of antiparasitics.

Types of antiparasitics

Classification

Antiparasitic drugs are usually classed as endoparasiticides, ectoparasiticides or endectocides. Endoparasiticides (internal antiparasitics) kill parasites living inside the animal, such as gastrointestinal parasites, respiratory parasites and heartworms. Endoparasiticides include anthelmintics (agents lethal to worms) and antiprotozoal (agents lethal or suppressive to protozoa). Ectoparasiticides (external antiparasitics) kill parasites living on the outside of an animal, including fleas, ticks, mites and lice.

Table 14.1 Mechanism of action of some antiparasitics

Paralysis of parasites via mimicking the action of neurotransmitters
Acetylcholine (ACh), gamma-aminobutyric acid (GABA), glutamate (Glu), octopamine (OA), serotonin (5-HT)*

Alteration of metabolic process
Inhibition of microtubule synthesis (disrupt tubulin-microtubule equilibrium) in nematodes
Uncoupling of oxidative phosphorylation in tapeworms
Inhibition of folic acid synthesis or metabolism in protozoa
Alteration of ion gradients/membrane potential in protozoa
Inhibition of thiamine utilization in protozoa
Inhibition of protein synthesis in protozoa
Inhibition of DNA synthesis in protozoa
Simulation of insect juvenile hormones
Inhibition of chitin formation in arthropods

Alteration of parasite reproduction†
Inhibition of egg production in nematodes
Inhibition of multiplication in protozoa

---

*These neurotransmitters (excitatory or inhibitory) can be present in more than one parasite category (i.e. nematodes, cestodes, trematodes, and/or arthropods).

†This is a consequence of an antiparasitic action, not the antiparasitic action.

Endectocides combine the activity against internal and external parasites, offering greater convenience and broader-spectrum metazoan parasite control.

Herein, we will discuss the major classification of antiparasitics, their spectrum of activity, mechanism of action, and adverse effects, if any. For detailed information on dose rates and dosage forms in each animal species, and currently available products by country please consult specialized pharmacology textbooks and drug compendia.

Endoparasiticides

Anthelmintics

The most important nematocidal veterinary drug classes are the benzimidazoles (BZ), imidazothiazoles and tetrahydropyrimidines (LM) and macrocyclic lactones (ML). They are all broad spectrum and highly effective against most parasitic nematode species. Additionally, the MLs have acaricidal and insecticidal activity, while some BZs can be used for treatment of cestode and trematode infections.

Benzimidazoles

BZs are broad-spectrum nematocidal agents with a wide margin of safety and a high degree of efficacy. Several derivatives of the prototypical BZ thiabendazole (mebendazole, fenbendazole, albendazole, and oxibendazole) are available in the USA, while others in this class are available in the EU and elsewhere.

Spectrum of activity

BZs are effective against ascarids, whipworms, and hookworms in most host animals and have some activity against tapeworms and trematodes. In horses, they are effective against large and small strongyles, and pinworms, but migrating larval forms of strongyles are not considered susceptible. Albendazole and fenbendazole

are effective against lungworms in all species. In dogs and cats, fenbendazole is effective against *Taenia* sp., but not the more common tapeworm *Dipylidium caninum*. In ruminants, fenbendazole, albendazole, and oxfendazole are effective against major gastrointestinal worms and lungworms. But, they are ineffective against filariae. Febantel is a pro-benzimidazole metabolized in the liver to the anthelmintically active metabolites fenbendazole and oxfendazole. Febantel is available in combination with other anthelmintics to provide a wide spectrum of activity.

Mechanism of action

These drugs inhibit microtubule synthesis in nematodes. BZs bind to nematode β-tubulin subunit, preventing its dimerization and subsequent polymerization during microtubule assembly. This assembly is essential for cell functions like transport of nutrients, cell structure and cell division. The progressive loss of microtubule function as a result of BZ activity disrupts cell division, depletes energy stores and starves the nematodes, causing death and removal of most parasites within approximately three days of treatment.

Adverse effects

Mebendazole and oxibendazole have been associated with an idiosyncratic hepatotoxic reaction in some dogs. Bone marrow suppression has been reported following treatment of dogs with albendazole. Albendazole is contraindicated in cattle and sheep during early pregnancy because it is teratogenic and embryotoxic. This is a concern for all BZs, which should generally be avoided in pregnant animals unless specifically permitted by the label.

Remarks

Despite the high sequence similarity of nematode and mammalian tubulin genes benzimidazoles show a significantly higher affinity for tubulin of helminths compared with mammalian tubulin, which explain the high safety indices.

Imidazothiazoles

Spectrum of activity
In food animals, levamisole has a broad spectrum of action against adults and many of the larval stages of intestinal (ascarids, hookworms), and extra-intestinal (lungworm) nematodes. It is not effective against whipworms. Levamisole is an immunostimulant and has been advocated as such in a range of host species, unrelated to its antiparasitic activity.

Mechanism of antiparasitic action
The LMs act as agonists at nematode nicotinic acetylcholine receptors, causing worm paralysis. Levamisole is a depolarizing neuromuscular blocker that interferes with neuronal transmission in parasites. Through mimicking acetylcholine action, it changes the permeability of the post-synaptic membranes. This leads to sustained muscle contraction (spastic paralysis) in treated worms and their rapid removal from the host.

Adverse effects
Signs of toxicosis are related to stimulation of mammalian nicotinic (primarily ganglionic) cholinergic receptors. These signs are similar to organophosphate intoxication and include salivation, defecation, respiratory distress, and seizures. Due to its low margin of safety, it is rarely used in horses or small animals. At higher concentrations these drugs also inhibit the function of acetylcholine esterase. These effects are exerted not only at the parasite but also at the host receptors.

Tetrahydropyrimidines

Spectrum of activity
Pyrantel is active against gastrointestinal roundworms in horses and dogs; tapeworms in horses. Morantel is active against gastrointestinal roundworms in ruminants.

Mechanism of action
These drugs interfere with neuromediators in a way that is similar to that of the imidazothiazoles. Pyrantel is a depolarizing neuromuscular blocker that has a cholinergic action on the musculature of the parasite. These drugs are usually formulated as either the tartrate or pamoate salt. Pyrantel tartrate is more water soluble and better absorbed from the gastrointestinal tract. The pamoate salt is less water soluble and more poorly absorbed. This accounts for its increased efficacy against pinworms in the large intestine. And this is the form used in horses, as nicotinic drugs in general are quite toxic in this host and pyrantel pamoate, not being absorbed, maintains an excellent safety profile.

Adverse effects
Pyrantel has a large margin of safety due to its low bioavailability and is considered safe to administer to young, sick, or pregnant animals. Because of its cholinergic/cholinomimetic properties (stimulating cholinergic neurotransmission at the worms' neuromuscular junction), it should not be administered concomitantly with other medications that have a similar mechanism of action such as levamisole or piperazine to avoid host toxicity.

Macrocyclic lactones

Spectrum of activity
MLs are represented by avermectins (such as abamectin, doramectin, eprinomectin, ivermectin, selamectin) and milbemycins (such as moxidectin).

Ivermectin is a semisynthetic derivative of avermectin with broad-spectrum activity against nematodes and arthropods. It has efficacy against all major gastrointestinal and pulmonary nematodes, many ectoparasites, and infective-stage heartworm larvae in dogs and cats. Ivermectin has activity against the adults and many larval stages of nematodes. Doramectin is another avermectin. In cattle, it is effective against nematodes, lungworms, eyeworms, lice, grubs, ticks, mites, and screwworms. Moxidectin is a broad-spectrum antinematodal and anti-arthropod drug marketed for use in dogs, cattle, sheep, and horses. Moxidectin is more lipophilic than other avermectins and tissue concentrations may persist longer than those of other members of this group. Eprinomectin is available in a pour-on formulation for the treatment of endoparasites in cattle. It is specifically useful for dairy cattle because it has a zero-day milk withdrawal. Milbemycin oxime is marketed as a heartworm preventative for dogs. At heartworm preventative doses (0.5 mg/kg), it also controls infection with hookworms, ascarids, and whipworms in dogs. Selamectin is a semisynthetic avermectin compound, derived from doramectin. Selamectin is the first broad-spectrum, single entity endectocide available in a topical formulation for small animals. Selamectin is also 100% effective in preventing the development of heartworm infection in dogs when administered monthly at 6 mg/kg throughout the transmission season. Selamectin can be applied topically, thus avoid the problems associated with oral administration. It is also effective in preventing and controlling some ectoparasite infestations and certain nematode infections.

Mechanism of action
These drugs have a dual mechanism of action. First, they are agonists and potentiate the action of the inhibitory neurotransmitter GABA. This excess binding of GABA to its chloride-channel receptor, results in a rapid influx of Chloride ions, membrane hyperpolarization, and inhibition of neurotransmission in the parasite. Second, they exert an anthelmintic effect by stimulating the permanent opening of ligand-gated chloride channels especially glutamate-gated channels in the membrane of neurones in invertebrates. This leads to the inhibition of nerves responsible for the control of muscles, for example in the pharynx or body muscle. As a result, the worms show flaccid paralysis and can no longer persist in their environment within the host. However, at therapeutic concentrations, the only effect that matters is on glutamate-gated chloride channels. The GABA effects are less significant until higher concentrations are reached, which only happens in the laboratory.

Adverse effects

Mammals have NO glutamate-gated chloride channels; the p-glycoprotein in the blood–brain barrier protects mammalian GABA receptors from ML action. However, the ML affinity is higher for mammalian GABA receptors than for nematode GABA receptors. Ivermectin can irreversibly open GABA chloride channels in mammals, but this is achieved only at high overdose concentrations. Ivermectin (but not milbemycin) has an abnormal safety profile when administered to collie breed dogs for heartworm or other infections. Signs of toxicosis in this breed are mydriasis, depression, ataxia, and coma. In cattle, animals with migrating *Hypoderma* larvae in their spinal cord or oesophagus at the time of ivermectin treatment develop paresis or oedematous oesophagitis.

Other anthelmintics

Piperazine

Spectrum of activity Piperazine is only effective against ascarids and some pinworms. It is only marginally effective against equine strongyles.

Mechanism of action Piperazine is a GABA agonist and stimulates inhibitory GABA transmission at the parasite neuromuscular junction, leading to flaccid paralysis of adult worms and their expulsion. In ascarids, piperazine also inhibits succinic acid production.

Adverse effects Piperazines are considered safe in all species. Occasionally neurological side effects, such as ataxia, tremors, and aberrant behaviour have been reported, most often in cats given an overdosage.

Organophosphates

Spectrum of activity Organophosphates or OPs can be regarded as mid-spectrum drugs. In pigs it is effective against most nematodes including whipworms. In horses, trichlorphon and other OPs have been used primarily for activity against stomach bots.

Mechanism of action OPs inhibit nematode acetylcholinesterase, leading to interference with nematode neuromuscular transmission and paralysis.

Adverse effects They are no longer used in small animals because of their narrow safety margin, but have some application in swine and horses. Signs of OP toxicity are outlined in other sections, where their more common use as insecticidal agents is discussed. OPs should not be used in young, sick, or pregnant animals.

Monepantel

Monepantel is a new molecule that kills sheep nematodes resistant to all other anthelmintic groups. Monepantel paralyses worms by attacking the receptor – Hco-MPTL-1 – present only in nematodes. This is a unique kind of ACh receptor. These drugs are approved for use in NZ, Australia and some European countries, but not in the USA.

Emodepside

Emodepside is a relatively new anthelmintic that belongs to the class of drugs known as the octadepsipeptides. It is effective against a number of gastrointestinal nematodes and is licensed for use as spot-on on all cats, including pregnant and lactating queens.

Emodepside main action is as an opener of a class of potassium channels. Another formulation exists that combines emodepside, effective against ascarids and hookworms, and praziquantel, effective against tapeworms. An oral formulation for dogs has been approved in Europe. The topical formulation for cats works only because licking behaviour results in ingestion.

Antiparasitic drugs for heartworm

Chemotherapeutic management of heartworm infection involve three aspects: (i) removal of adult heartworms using an *adulticide*, (ii) interruption of the full life cycle using a *microfilaricide* to eliminate the source of adult heartworms and (iii) prevention of infection using a *larvicide*.

Adulticides

These preparations eliminate both immature (L3) and adult heartworms. Different treatment protocols are used depending on severity. Care and support should be provided to the animal when treated with an adulticide.

Melarsomine dihydrochloride (MEL)

This is an organoarsenic compound that is used to treat adult heartworms in the USA. It is used solely in dogs. Two intramuscular injections (2.5 mg/kg given 24 hours apart) or three injections (2.5 mg/kg followed 1 month later by two injections 24 hours apart) are the two treatment protocols available for MEL. Melarsomine denatures proteins/enzymes by binding to the sulfhydryl groups of cysteine residues. Overdose may result in distress, restlessness, pawing, salivation, vomiting, tachycardia, tachypnoea, dyspnoea, abdominal pain, hindlimb weakness, and recumbency. Severe overdose cases terminate in circulatory collapse, coma, and death. Compared with the previously prescribed thiacetarsamide, it is more efficacious and less likely to be associated with hepatotoxicity. It is administered by deep i.m. injection in the lumbar epaxial musculature in dogs. It should not be given i.v. or s.c. About one-third of dogs experience muscle pain at the injection sites, which resolves within 1–2 weeks. Rarely, severe myositis has been reported. The drug should not be given to cats. Cage rest and exercise restriction should continue for 1–3 months following adulticidal therapy to decrease the opportunities of thromboembolic events that can be fatal.

Microfilaricides and larvicides

Macrocyclic lactones (macrolides)

Ivermectin preparations are available for larvicidal use because these preparations kill L4 larvae and microfilaria of *Dirofilaria* worms. Ivermectin should not be used in collie breed dogs as a microfilaricide, but milbemycin oxime can be safely used in Collies. Adverse effects include transient weakness, pale membranes, intestinal hyperperistalsis, and tachypnoea may be seen following administration of a microfilaricide, suggesting a mild cardiovascular shock resulting from reactions to dead microfilaria. The higher the microfilaria count, the greater the chances there are of encountering noticeable adverse effects. These adverse effects can be treated or prevented with glucocorticoids. Monthly oral administration throughout the transmission season of ivermectin at 6 mg/kg, milbemycin oxime at 500 µg/kg or moxidectin at 3 µg/kg provides effective protection against heartworm infection in dogs. Selamectin is principally a topical heartworm preventive for use in dogs and cats at a minimum dose of 6 mg/kg monthly throughout the transmission season. Prolonged administration of some of the ML preventatives kills not only young heartworm larvae but also old larvae, immatures, young adults, and old adults. Of the various MLs, ivermectin has the most potent adulticidal activity, milbemycin oxime has the least, and selamectin and moxidectin injectable lie somewhere in between. Milbemycin and sustained-release moxidectin seem to have minimal adulticidal efficacy when administered at the preventive dose. Ivermectin, selamectin and moxidectin at approved doses for heartworm prevention in dogs have also been found to be effective in preventing *Dirofilaria repens* infection.

Anti-cestode drugs

Drugs that kill tapeworms are often called cestocides. The killed worms may then be digested by the host animal, and therefore may not be evident in the faeces. Segments, which are fragile, may not be evident, but eggs can still be shed until gone. Control of intermediate hosts (e.g. fleas for *Dipylidium*, rodents for *Taenia* and *Echinococcus*, and mites for *Anoplocephala* and *Moniezia*) should also be considered.

Praziquantel

Praziquantel is an isoquinolone that is effective against all species of tapeworms and kills both adult and juvenile stages of the worms. However, its activity against hydatid cysts is erratic. It is also available in combination with pyrantel pamoate, ivermectin, and moxidectin to kill nematodes. Praziquantel is approved for dogs, cats, and horses, and has been used in other animals. Praziquantel is administered orally or subcutaneous. Praziquantel is also available as spot-on, different dose rates according to route of administration

Mechanism of action

The primary effects of praziquantel are tetanic contractions of the parasitic musculature and an intense irreversible focal vacuolization and disintegration of the worm's integument. The integumental damage probably results from the interaction of praziquantel with phospholipids and proteins that create an imbalance in the ion transport of cations through the integument membranes. This results in metabolic disorders as well as strong contractions of the tegumental muscles followed by paralysis of the worms. The destabilization of the integument renders the parasites vulnerable to the digestive system and the immune defence of the host.

Adverse effect

Praziquantel has a high margin of safety. It can safely be used in pregnant, breeding, sick, and young animals. Overdose induces anorexia, vomiting, salivation, diarrhoea, and lethargy in less than 5% of animals.

Epsiprantel

Epsiprantel is a praziquantel analogue with activity against intestinal tapeworms, and is approved for use in dogs and cats. Epsiprantel is administered orally. Unlike praziquantel, epsiprantel is absorbed poorly after oral administration and therefore has no activity against extraintestinal cestodes.

Dichlorophene

Dichlorophene is used to treat *Taenia* and *Dipylidium* infestations in dogs and cats. Its efficacy against *Echinococcus* is variable.

Mechanism of action

Dichlorophene causes uncoupling of oxidative phosphorylation to deplete ATP from tapeworms and disrupts the pH difference across the external tegumental membranes

Adverse effects

Vomiting and diarrhoea may be seen after dichlorophene administration.

Benzimidazoles

These can be effective against mature *Taenia* and *Echinococcus* in dogs and cats, and *Moniezia* in ruminants. They may kill intermediate hydatid cysts in infected cattle and sheep. These agents are not effective against *Dipylidium*.

Mechanism of action

The inhibitory effect on microtubule polymerization by benzimidazoles such as mebendazole leads to disintegration of the tegument of cestodes which renders the parasites more susceptible to the immune system of the host.

Pyrantel pamoate

It is effective against the equine tapeworms *Anoplocephala perfoliata* (at 2× doses). It is not as effective as praziquantel as an anticestodal drug.

Anti-trematode drugs

Anti-trematode drugs are often highly lipophilic and most of them are only effective against mature flukes, and not immature flukes.

Clorsulon

Spectrum of activity

Clorsulon is used against *Fasciola hepatica* in beef and dairy cattle. It is considered a very effective drug against *F. hepatica*, killing both mature and immature flukes. However, its activity against *F. magna* is fair to poor; it is not effective against rumen flukes or lung flukes.

Mechanism of action

The mechanism of action is unknown. However, inhibition of 3-phosphoglycerate kinase and phosphoglyceromutase in the glycolytic pathway, depriving the flukes of a metabolic energy source has been suggested.

Adverse effects

When used as directed, adverse effects are rare. Clorsulon is safe in pregnant and breeding animals.

Salicylanilides

Salicylanilides (such as closantel or rafoxanide) are mainly active against mature liver fluke. These drugs collapse proton gradients across mitochondrial membranes as the primary mechanism of action. However, more direct effects, like the rapid spastic paralysis salicylanilides induce in trematodes, may point at a different mode of action, possibly involving calcium ion influxes through pores created by the drug in the integument of the worms.

Albendazole

It is approved for use against mature liver flukes (e.g. *F. hepatica*) in beef and non-lactating cattle. Because albendazole is a teratogen, it cannot be used in pregnant cattle during the first 45 days of gestation or in female dairy cattle of breeding age.

Praziquantel

It is effective against lung flukes in dogs. In trematodes it increases calcium ion flux into the worm and also facilitates phagocytic ingestion of the worm by causing focal vacuolization of the integument.

Triclabendazole

Triclabendazole is active against immature and adult *Fasciola* in horses and ruminants. It is the best flukicide available but is not licensed in the US.

Antiprotozoal drugs

Antiprotozoal drugs are used in treatment of protozoan infections in animals. The strategy for the use of antiprotozoal drugs is quite different from that for the use of anthelmintic ones. Most antiprotozoal drugs are targeted at rapidly proliferating developmental stages of unicellular parasites, whereas with helminths, the targets are generally non-proliferating adult multicellular organisms. Antiprotozoal agents therefore often target nucleic acid synthesis, protein synthesis, or specific metabolic pathways (e.g. folate metabolism) unique to the protozoan parasites. The mode of action of commonly used antiprotozoals is listed in Table 14.2, followed by a description of these processes.

Folic acid antagonists

Dihydropteroate synthetase inhibitors

Although sulfonamides were the first effective anticoccidial agents developed for use, acquired drug resistance, especially in the poultry industry, has limited their use as coccidiostats. They are still effective anticoccidial drugs in small animals and ruminants.

Sulphonamides work by interfering with protozoal folate synthesis. They competitively inhibit the enzyme dihydropteroate synthase, which catalyses the formation of dihydropteroate. Inhibition of folate synthesis results in decreased production of the nucleotides needed by coccidia for DNA synthesis. Mammalian cells usually use preformed folate, thereby conserving selective toxicity.

Dihydrofolate reductase inhibitors

Dihydrofolate reductase inhibitors (trimethoprim, ormetoprim) are almost always combined with sulfonamides to inhibit sequential steps in folate metabolism and increase their antiprotozoal action (this is an example of synergy). These potentiated sulfonamides are effective against *Toxoplasma* and *Neospora* spp. Pyrimethamine is another dihydrofolate reductase inhibitor used in the treatment of toxoplasmosis in small animals and for equine protozoal myelitis. It is often combined with other drugs that share some antiprotozoal action such as clindamycin or sulfonamides. The drug is associated with a higher incidence of gastrointestinal disturbances than trimethoprim particularly in cats. Bone marrow suppression may occur. Concurrent administration of folinic acid prevents the development of mammalian folate deficiency. Very high doses of pyrimethamine are teratogenic in laboratory animals. Pyrimethamine is selective for protozoa, trimethoprim for bacteria.

Ionophores

Ionophore antibiotics are the most widely used anticoccidials. The anticoccidial action of ionophores is related to their ability to form lipophilic complexes with cations and to facilitate their transport across biological membranes. The intracellular accumulation of these ions interferes with parasite metabolism. These drugs include monensin, lasalocid and salinomycin. Ionophores, particularly monensin, can be toxic to muscle tissues in mammals and birds. Ingestion of monensin causes fatal cardiotoxicity in horses. Monensin is used in prophylaxis of coccidiosis in poultry and as a dietary additive to improve feed conversion efficiency, growth rate, and reproductive performance in cattle. Monensin has also been used to reduce the incidence of frothy bloat in cattle grazing wheat pasture or alfalfa successfully.

Thiamine antagonists

Amprolium is an analogue of vitamin B_1, thiamine. It acts on the first-generation coccidial schizonts to prevent development to the merozoite stage. It prevents coccidia from utilizing thiamine, a co-factor for a number of essential enzymes. It has some activity against the sexual stages and the sporulating oocysts of coccidia. Prolonged use can lead to the development of thiamine deficiency and the development of CNS dysfunction.

Other anticoccidials

Diclazuril

Diclazuril is a benzeneacetonitrile, a class with potent anticoccidial activity. It is effective against various stages of the life cycle by inhibiting nuclear division. It is used for the treatment and

Table 14.2 Mechanisms of action and indications for the major antiprotozoal agents

Drug class	Mechanism of action	Parasite
Folic acid antagonists (sulphonamides, pyrimethamine, trimethoprim)	Inhibit dihydropteroate synthetase and dihydrofolate reductase (parasites unable to use exogenous folate)	*Toxoplasma*, *Cyclospora*
Ionophores (lasalocid, monensin)	Act at ion transport across mitochondrial membrane	*Eimeria*
Nitroimidazoles (metronidazole)	Disrupts DNA synthesis	*Giardia*, *Trichomonas*
Macrolide (azithromycin)	Block peptide synthesis at level of ribosome	*Cryptosporidium*, *Pneumocystis*, *Toxoplasma*
DNA synthesis inhibitors (allopurinol)	Inhibit enzymes in purine salvage pathway	*Leishmania*
Aromatic diamidines (imidocarb, pentamidine)	Inhibition of topoisomerase II	*Trypanosoma*, *Leishmania*

prevention of coccidial infections in lambs caused in particular, by the more pathogenic *Eimeria* spp. *E. crandallis* and *E. ovinoidalis*. Also, it is used to aid in the control of coccidiosis in calves caused by *Eimeria* bovis and *E. zuernii*.

Toltrazuril

Toltrazuril is triazinetrione derivative that has activity against all intracellular coccidian stages. The mode of action is unknown, but could be similar to diclazuril. It is used for the treatment of coccidiosis in broilers and broiler breeders. It is also widely used for the effective prevention and control of neonatal isosporosis in piglets.

Quinolones

Decoquinate, buquinolate, and nequinate are coccidiostats. These agents permit the coccidial sporozoites to enter the host, but interfere with further development. They work by inhibiting coccidial respiration by interfering with electron transport system within the coccidial mitochondria. Also, it may block DNA synthesis by inhibiting DNA gyrase. Primaquine is an 8-aminoquinolone used to treat hepatozoonosis.

Nitroimidazoles

Metronidazole is one of the most widely used antiprotozoal drugs. It is probably unique in having activity not only against parasitic protozoa but also against anaerobic bacteria. Metronidazole is effective against *Giardia* sp. Metronidazole is well absorbed from the gastrointestinal tract and reaches high tissue concentrations, making it effective against tissue and gastrointestinal protozoa. Once metronidazole enters the protozoan, its nitro group is reduced which results in the generation of toxic intermediates that disrupt the parasites' DNA synthesis (among many other actions). Metronidazole is generally well tolerated, but may cause gastrointestinal upset, and at high doses, neurotoxicity manifested by ataxia, tremors, and weakness may become apparent. There is concern about possible mutagenicity.

Macrolides

The macrolide antibiotic azithromycin is used to treat infections with *Toxoplasma*, *Cryptosporidium* and *Pneumocystis* in dogs and cats.

DNA synthesis inhibitors

Allopurinol is usually administered in combination with meglumine antimonite for the first month of treatment of leishmaniosis and thereafter alone as maintenance for the dogs' life. The mechanism of action of allo-purinol against leishmaniasis is thought to be due to its incorporation into the parasite purine salvage pathway. This leads to the formation of a toxic analogue of adenosine triphosphate which is incorporated into ribonucleic acid. Adverse affects may include erythema, hypersensitivity and predisposition to xanthine calculi.

Aromatic diamidines

Imidocarb dipropinate has activity against *Babesia*, *Hepatozoon*, *Cytauxzoon*, and *Ehrlichia*. The drug interferes with DNA formation and parasite proliferation. Imidocarb has a low therapeutic index. Parenteral administration consistently causes vomiting. Other side effects are pain on injection and signs of cholinergic stimulation (hypersalivation, tachycardia, vomiting, restlessness, and diarrhoea). These latter signs may be due to inherent anticholinesterase activity and can be controlled with atropine. Imidocarb should not be used concurrently with other cholinesterase inhibitors. Imidocarb is also associated with dose-dependent increases in liver enzyme activity and hepatic damage.

Diminazene diaceturate is available for parenteral administration for treatment of trypanosomiasis, babesiosis, and cytauxzoonosis. The drug undergoes hepatic metabolism and gradual urinary excretion over several weeks. Side effects include CNS signs, acute haemorrhages, diarrhoea, and cardiomyopathy.

Pentamidine is an aromatic diamidine derivative that has been used against some species of *Leishmania*. It can be extremely hepatotoxic and nephrotoxic. It acts by interfering with DNA and folate transformation and by inhibiting RNA and protein synthesis.

Antimonials

Sodium stibogluconate and meglumine antimonate are used in the treatment of leishmaniosis. Their exact mechanism of action is unknown. They are seldom effective in curing the disease. Side effects include gastrointestinal disturbances, nephrotoxicity, and cardiac arrhythmias.

Buparvoquone

Buparvoquone and parvaquone are hydroxynapthoquinones. Both act by inhibiting mitochondrial respiration and used in Africa for theileriosis.

Furazolidone

Furazolidone is a nitrofuran derivative that interferes with parasitic enzyme systems, although its exact mechanism of action is unknown. It is effective against *Giardia* sp., coccidia, *Trichomonas*, and some enteric bacteria. It is available as a liquid suspension, which facilitates administration to puppies and kittens. Side effects include anorexia and vomiting. The nitrofurans are suspected mutagens and carcinogens and their use in food animals is prohibited.

Paromomycin

Paromomycin is an aminoglycoside antibiotic used in the treatment of cryptosporidiosis. It is poorly absorbed orally. However, nephrotoxicity has been described in cats. Hence, it should not be used in patients with renal disease.

Nitazoxanide

Nitazoxanide is a synthetic nitrothiazolyl-salicylamide derivative. It has been shown to be very effective against cryptosporidiosis and giardiasis. Nitazoxanide acts by interfering with the pyruvate–ferredoxin oxidoreductase (PFOR) enzyme dependent electron transfer reaction which is essential to anaerobic energy metabolism. Side effects are mostly gastrointestinal.

Benzimidazoles

The anthelmintics, fenbendazole and albendazole, have some activity against *Giardia* sp in dogs and cats. Fenbendazole is not appreciably absorbed from the gastrointestinal tract and is not associated with toxicity. Albendazole may be toxic to liver and bone marrow and is a teratogen.

Ectoparasiticides

Ectoparasites of veterinary importance include insects (fleas, lice, flies) and acarines (mites and ticks). Ectoparasiticides are clinically used (i) on animals to control mites, ticks, lice, fleas, and flies, (ii) on the premise to control flies and other insects, and (iii) on feedstuffs to inhibit developmental stages of flies.

Ectoparasiticides can be classified according to their chemical constituent or their mode of action. Based on chemical structures they include botanical compounds, synthetic pyrethroids, chlorinated hydrocarbons, organophosphates, carbamates, formamidines, macrocyclic lactone endectocides, fipronil, imidacloprid, insect growth regulators and development inhibitors, and spinosad.

Ectoparasiticides are presented here based on their mode of action. To understand ectoparasiticides' mechanisms of action, it is necessary to understand how the ectoparasite body systems normally function. Ectoparasiticides generally target the nervous system, energy production, or growth and development of the parasite. Table 14.3 is a summary of the mode of action of the commonly used ectoparasiticides.

Interference with the parasite nervous system

Macrocyclic lactones

The avermectins and milbemycins are very potent against a broad range of economically important endoparasites and ectoparasites; hence the name endectocides can be used for these drugs. The target parasites include nematodes in the heart, lung and intestinal tract; arthropods; mange mites, grubs, biting and sucking lice, fleas and ticks.

Mode of action

Avermectins bind to and activate glutamate-gated chloride channels, causing an inhibitory effect, which, when excessive, results in preventing muscles from contracting or neurons from firing by lowering the ion gradient across the muscle or neuronal membrane; it is a strong inhibitory effect.

Adverse effects

They are approved for use in food animals, but require long withdrawal times. Selamectin is safe to use in avermectin-sensitive breeds of dogs.

Phenylpyrazoles

Fipronil is a broad-spectrum phenylpyrazole insecticide/acaricide that is active against fleas and ticks in dogs and cats.

Mode of action

Fipronil blocks the passage of chloride ions through the GABA receptor and glutamate-gated chloride channels (GluCl), components of the central nervous system. This causes inhibition of contaminated insects' nerves and muscles. Insect specificity of fipronil may come from a better efficacy on GABA receptor but also on the fact that GluCls do not exist in mammals.

Adverse effects

No toxicity has been reported with the drug. Fipronil should not be used in pregnant, sick, or debilitated animals or in dogs or cats < 10 or 12 weeks old, respectively. Although fipronil is effective against mite infestation in rabbits, it should be used with extra care in rabbits due to the high incidence of toxicity in this host.

Chlorinated hydrocarbons

The chlorinated hydrocarbons in use today are lindane and methoxychlor. These agents lack the environmental persistence that was characteristic of earlier chlorinated hydrocarbons (e.g. DDT). Lindane is used in tick sprays for horses and methoxychlor is a common ingredient in products to treat fleas, ticks, and lice.

Mode of action

Although the exact mode of action is unknown, these drugs may target the nervous system by affecting sodium channels or potentiate GABAergic neurotransmission, which paralyse the insects.

Adverse effects

Clinical signs of toxicosis may be immediate or, since the drugs are stored in body fat, they may be delayed for days. These signs

Table 14.3 Summary of mode of action of common ectoparasiticides*

Class of pesticide	Mode of action	Examples
Target the parasite nervous system (neurotoxic)		
Macrocyclic lactones	Chloride channel activator	Selamectin
Phenylpyrazoles	Chloride channel modulator	Fipronil
Chlorinated hydrocarbons	GABA-gated chloride channel antagonist	Endosulfan, lindane, methoxychlor
Botanical compounds (pyrethroid and pyrethrins)	Sodium channel modulator	Deltamethrin, Cypermethrin
Organophosphates	Acetylcholinesterase (AChE) inhibitor	Dimpylate
Carbamates	Acetylcholinesterase (AChE) inhibitor	Carbaril, propoxur
Neonicotinoids	Nicotinic acetylcholine receptor (nAChR) agonists	Imidacloprid
Formamidines	Monoamine oxidase inhibitor	Amitraz
Macrolides	Nicotinic acetylcholine receptor (nAChR) agonists	Spinosad
Interference with parasite energy production		
Botanical insecticides	Electron transport inhibitor – site I	Rotenone
Interference with parasite growth and development		
Insect growth regulators (IGR)	Juvenile hormone mimics/analogues	Methoprene
Insect growth inhibitors (IGI)	Inhibitors of chitin biosynthesis	Lufenuron

*Traditional ectoparasiticide agents such as organophosphates, carbamates, pyrethroid and pyrethrins and others have largely been replaced by newer drugs that are discussed in the following section. They are no longer used for ectoparasite control with the frequency they once were. However, they still remain as active ingredients in some ethical and over-the-counter animal products and in many environmental products.

include apprehension, exaggerated response to stimuli, vomiting, muscle twitching, tremors, and seizures.

Botanical compounds

Pyrethrins are naturally occurring compounds derived from members of the chrysanthemum flower family. While they have a quick knock-down effect against insects, they are unstable in the environment, so may not last long enough to kill the insects. *Pyrethroids* are synthetic analogues of pyrethrins, designed to be more stable in the environment, thus provide longer-lasting control. The pyrethrins and pyrethroids have efficacy against flies, fleas, lice, and ticks. Pyrethroids have repellent activity. Dog preparations should not be used in cats because cats are unable to metabolize permethrin in the same way as dogs. Hence, they cannot tolerate the high permethrin concentrations used on dogs and if a cat accidentally ingests such a product then potentially toxic levels may result.

Mode of action

These compounds act on voltage-sensitive ion channels through which sodium is pumped to cause excitation of neurons. They prevent the sodium channels from closing, resulting in continual nerve impulse transmission, tremors, and eventually, death.

Adverse effects

These compounds are relatively safe insecticides. Adverse reactions, which are rare, include depression, hypersalivation, muscle tremors, vomiting, ataxia, dyspnoea, and anorexia. They are commonly used in combination with synergists to increase their potency. These synergists inhibit the enzymes responsible for

degradation of the pyrethrins or pyrethroids. However, products containing synergists should be used with caution in cats because they increase the likelihood of a toxic reaction. Permethrins have a high incidence of toxic reactions in cats and should not be used in this species.

Organophosphates

Organophosphates are a large group of drugs with insecticidal, acaricidal, and helminthicidal properties. Commonly used organophosphates include chlorpyrifos, coumafos, cythioate, fenthrothion, dimpylate (diazinon), dichlorvos, fenthion, malathion, phosmet, tetrachlorvinphos, and trichlorfon. These products are effective on flies, fleas, ticks, mites, and lice.

Mode of action

These drugs work by binding to and inhibiting the enzyme acetylcholinesterase (AChE), which degrades acetylcholine (ACh). ACh thus accumulates at the neural synapse, resulting in continuous neuronal stimulation and paralysis of the parasite. The binding of AChE by an OP results in phosphorylation and inhibition of the enzyme. The phosphorylated enzyme is capable of reactivation, but this reaction proceeds so slowly that the OPs are considered irreversible AChE inhibitors.

Adverse effects

The OPs have a low margin of safety. They should not be used with other agents that inhibit AChE or block neuromuscular transmission, and care should be taken when used in combination with CNS depressants. OPs should not be used in young, sick, or pregnant animals or in greyhounds, whippets, Persian cats, and certain breeds of cattle (Chianina, Charolais, Simmental, Brahman) due to high sensitivity.

Clinical signs of OP toxicosis are due to interference with muscarinic or nicotinic neurotransmission. Muscarinic side effects include miosis, lacrimation, salivation, diarrhoea, frequent urination, bradycardia, and hypotension. Nicotinic effects are manifested as muscle twitching and fasciculations followed by severe weakness and paralysis. CNS signs such as depression and seizures may also be noted. Toxicosis is treated with anticholinergics (atropine) and antihistamines. Pralidoxime chloride (2-PAM) can be given in an effort to promote the reactivation of AChE.

Like insects, humans also use ACh as a neurotransmitter and AChE to break it down, and cholinesterase poisoning in humans can be very severe. Upon each exposure to an OP or carbamate insecticide, more AChE becomes bound and is unavailable to function. Cholinesterase inhibition due to OP poisoning is not reversible. This means the insecticide is not released from the bound cholinesterase. Fortunately, the body continually produces AChE, although it may take several weeks to again reach the desirable circulating level. Ops have adverse impact on humans of long-term exposure to sheep dips.

Carbamates

The most commonly used carbamates are bendiocarb, carbaril and propoxur.

Mode of action

Carbamate insecticides inhibit ACh breakdown by inhibiting AChE via carbamylation. They bind to the enzyme that is normally responsible for inactivating ACh in the synapse. When an insect has been poisoned by a cholinesterase inhibitor, the cholinesterase is not available to help break down the ACh, and the neurotransmitter continues to cause the neuron to 'fire,' or send its electrical charge. This causes overstimulation of the nervous system, and the insect dies. The effects of carbamates are more spontaneously reversible than those of OPs, since the binding between carbamate and AChE is non-covalent.

Adverse effects

The clinical signs of toxicosis are similar to those seen with organophosphates.

Neonicotinoids

Neonicotinoids are a class of neuroactive insecticides modelled after nicotine. The commonly used neonicotinoids are Imidacloprid and nitenpyram. Imidacloprid kills fleas, but not ticks. Imidacloprid is topical and exerts its action primarily topically not systemically. Nitenpyram kills fleas on dogs and cats.

Mode of action

Neonicotinoids act specifically on the insect nicotinic ACh receptors, leading to rapid inhibition of insect nervous system function. These drugs are not degraded by AChE.

Adverse effects

Neonicotinoids can be used safely in animals because of unique and structural differences between vertebrate and insect Ach receptors. Transient pruritus and salivation may be observed if the animal licks the application site immediately after treatment. Imidacloprid should not be used in animals < 16 weeks old and its use in pregnant and sick animals is not recommended.

Formamidines

Formamidines are a group of acaricides-insecticides that have a direct effect on the parasite's CNS. The formamidine amitraz is used to treat local and generalized demodectic mange and sarcoptic mange in dogs. It is also marketed for use in cattle and swine to control ticks, mange mites, and lice.

Mode of action

Although their exact mechanism of action is unknown, they may inhibit the monoamine oxidase activity, which is responsible for metabolism of neurotransmitter amines, and/or activate the inhibitory neurotransmitter octopamine.

Adverse effects

Signs of toxicosis include sedation, bradycardia, CNS depression, hypotension, mydriasis, and vomiting and diarrhoea. Amitraz should not be used in horses or cats.

Spinosad

Spinosad is a fermentation-derived macrolide insecticide produced by the soil bacterium *Saccharopolyspora spinosa*. Spinosad is indicated for the prevention and treatment of flea infestations. It is for dogs 14 weeks of age or older. Also, it is used to control chewing and sucking lice on cattle in the USA.

Mode of action

Spinosad works by activating nicotinic ACh receptors in the flea nervous system, causing an overload of the flea nervous system, leading to involuntary muscle contractions, prostration with tremors, and finally paralysis and death of the fleas. Spinosad also has effects on GABA receptor function that may contribute further to its insecticidal activity.

Adverse effects

Spinosad is relatively low in toxicity to mammals and birds, and, although moderately toxic to fish, this toxicity represents a reduced risk to fish when compared with many available insecticides. Side effects are rare but may include vomiting, decreased appetite, lethargy, diarrhoea, cough, excessive thirst, redness of skin, hyperactivity or drooling.

Interference with parasite energy production

Botanical insecticides

Rotenone is a botanical insecticide, an alkaloid derived from the root of the derris plant.

Mode of action

Rotenone inhibits the respiratory system of the parasite by blocking NADH oxidation and subsequent ATP generation. As a result, oxidation of lactate, glutamate, and other substances is reduced and nerve conduction is inhibited.

Adverse effects

Although it is more toxic than the pyrethroids or pyrethrins, it is still used in dogs and cats. Signs of toxicosis include gastrointestinal upset, respiratory stimulation, seizures, coma, and death. Do not use in reptiles.

Interference with parasite growth and development

Insect growth regulators (IGRs)

Insect growth regulators are used in dogs and cats to control fleas and to control flies in cattle. These drugs include methoprene, fenoxycarb, and cyromazine. These preparations maintain persistently the larvae in an immature stage and interfere with reproductive organ differentiation. They are used to control faecal maggot in poultry and for flea control.

Mode of action

IGRs are analogues and mimic the effects of an endogenous insect growth hormone, juvenile hormone. Juvenile hormone maintains the larval stage of the insect and inhibits maturation to the pupal and adult stages. In a normal insect, juvenile hormone is circulated throughout the insect's body and 'tells' the insect to stay in its current stage. After a certain amount of time, the insect stops producing juvenile hormone, and the insect mature into its next life stage. When an insect is exposed to an IGR that mimics juvenile hormone, the insect does not receive the signal to develop because, even though the insect may have stopped producing juvenile hormone, the IGR is still circulating throughout its body and sending the signal to stay in the current stage. Hence, insects poisoned with IGRs cannot moult or reproduce, and eventually die. Another hormone important in metamorphosis is ecdysone. The insecticide tebufenozide interferes with the production of ecdysone, causing the insect to be unable to moult.

Adverse effects

IGRs have very low toxicity for mammals when used as directed because they do not make or use the hormones insects use in moulting.

Insect growth inhibitors (IGIs)

Insect development inhibitors include diflubenzuron and lufenuron. Lufenuron is marketed as an oral and parenteral flea-control product for dogs and cats. Lufenuron, a very lipophilic compound, accumulates in adipose tissue and is subsequently released slowly into the bloodstream. Adult fleas ingest lufenuron when they feed on the host and the drug is passed transovarially to the flea egg. Most flea eggs exposed to lufenuron fail to hatch and the ones that do die during the first moult.

Mode of action

Chitin is an important constituent of exoskeleton and egg shell. Lufenuron interferes with the development of the insect's exoskeleton by inhibiting chitin synthesis or deposition in larvae and eggs. They have no effects on adult insects.

Adverse effects

The drug is very safe and can be used in nursing, breeding and pregnant animals and can be given to animals as young as 6 weeks.

Resistance to antiparasitic drugs

Potential reasons for lack of antiparasitic efficacy

Users often point to resistance, early in the course of an apparent case of a failure of efficacy of antiparasitic usage. However, therapeutic failure can be due to several common and non-resistance-related reasons: (i) interaction with another drug or health condition in the patient that diminishes the drug efficacy, (ii) the failure to diagnose and treat the presence of mixed infections of parasites or of other infectious agents, (iii) patient immunodeficiency, (iv) quick re-infection/infestation due to contaminated environment, (v) failure to deliver or receive the correct dosage or form of product, such as compliance failures, usage of out of date products etc. However, this chapter will assume that these confounder issues have been ruled out from the situation and instead considers the biology of resistance to antiparasitic drugs.

Anthelmintic drug resistance

Anthelmintics will continue to play a key role in the control of gastrointestinal helminths in domestic animals in the foreseeable future. However, increasing problems with parasite populations that have developed resistance against anthelmintics threaten to limit the continued reliance on this drug tool. Parasitic nematodes have now evolved the ability to survive the waves of anthelmintic drugs developed during the last five decades.

Anthelmintic resistance arises when a greater frequency of individuals in a parasite population no longer responds to the normal clinical dose of treatment. This impacts agricultural incomes and poses a clear threat to animal health and welfare. A critical aspect of resistance is that it is a heritable trait. It is genetic in essence.

The extent of the resistance problem

In small ruminants, anthelmintic-resistant nematodes represent a serious problem. Resistance has developed to all of the major families of broad-spectrum anthelmintics, the BZs, LMs, and the MLs. In cattle, the situation is less severe, but there are cattle nematodes resistant to multiple anthelmintic classes in New Zealand and the Americas. In horses, BZs resistance is widespread among the cyathostomes; MLs are still effective for cyathostomes. This could change as their usage increases and selection pressure increases.

The lack of effective alternatives of worm control indicates that we should understand how resistance develops and thus predict effective methods for limiting the development of resistance as much as possible. Unfortunately, current evidence clearly shows our incomplete understanding of the mechanisms of resistance. Therefore, it is imperative that research initiatives studying mechanisms of resistance are maintained, and that all those involved in the control of helminths remain abreast of the latest developments.

Development of anthelmintic resistance

Nematodes have a range of different strategies to achieve a state of reduced susceptibility towards a given anthelmintic drug. These include:

- modification of drug target (e.g. binding site), so that the drug is no longer recognized by the target and is thus ineffective;
- increasing target site numbers (e.g. neuronal receptors) or amplification of target genes to overcome the drug action;
- increasing drug efflux (e.g. through transmembrane pumps), for instance, up-regulation of P-glycoprotein exporter in the helminth;
- a change in the distribution of the drug in the target parasite that prevents the drug from getting to its site of action (e.g. increased sequestration of the drug).

For each anthelmintic, resistance to one member usually confers resistance to others of the same chemical class. It is possible to have multiple simultaneous resistances in which parasites sequentially develop resistance to several anthelmintic classes.

Detection of resistance

This usually involves the treatment of infected hosts with a recommended dose of drug followed by a *faecal egg count reduction test* that compares pre-treatment egg counts with those of untreated controls. Reductions of less than 90–95% (based on group arithmetic means) score as clinical resistance. Please refer to Chapter 12 for more details on methods of detection of anthelmintic resistance.

Management of anthelmintic resistance

Proper understanding of the modes of action of the antiparasitics is fundamental to prevent development of resistance in the target pest(s). Using antiparasitics with the same modes of action contributes to this problem by killing the susceptible parasites and leaving only those with resistance to the entire class of antiparasitics that work through similar mechanisms. Development of resistant parasite can be avoided or delayed by rotating pest control chemicals that work through different modes of action. However, this regimen is not thought to be in the patients' interest. Better results are obtained if two drugs with different mechanisms are combined. Because resistance to insecticides is often due to metabolic inactivation, the situation for ectoparasites is more complex. Some factors affect the development of resistance and, thus, should also be considered. These factors include:

- use of other control methods to complement anthelmintics, or use alternative anthelmintics with a different mechanism of action;
- avoid under-dosing and insure that treatments are fully efficacious;
- treatment planning, through timing and management, to reduce the survival of free-living resistant stages in the environment. Where possible, the access of free-living resistant stages to the next host should be reduced by measures such as regular removal of faeces and alternative grazing of different hosts;
- some anthelmintics allowing resistance to emerge faster than others (e.g. fenbendazole is likely to be faster than ivermectin due to its ability to select for resistance);
- parasites that have a short generation time and high fecundity increase the speed of resistance development. Production of many individuals of several generations in a short time increases the spread of resistance alleles through the population;
- parasite populations that are mobile, especially if the hosts are moved, increase the spread of resistance;
- use of drugs in a manner that maintains 'refugia' to reduce resistance (see Chapters 14 and 15 for more details).

Antiprotozoal drug resistance

Drug resistant protozoa have been documented and, there is sound evidence that resistance does occur in protozoal species such as *Plasmodium* spp. (the agent of malaria) and *Eimeria* spp. (the agent of coccidiosis). The appearance of drug resistant strains is a potential health risk and the identification and spread of these strains need to be monitored. Several techniques for strain identification are now available and include DNA fingerprinting, electrophoretic karyotyping and isoenzyme typing. The use of these techniques will allow the differentiation of truly drug resistant strains from those which are derived from cases where treatment failures have occurred for other reasons. Future epidemiological studies should be designed to identify and assess the spread of drug resistant protozoa and to ensure that drug resistant strain does not become a major health issue.

Resistance to ectoparasiticides

Some ectoparasites can develop resistance to the lethal effects of ectoparasiticides following continuous exposure to them. Ectoparasiticides may lose their efficacy due to (i) diminished penetration into target organism, (ii) increased detoxication (metabolism) of ectoparasiticides, or (iii) decreased sensitivity of the target site (i.e. receptor). Some of the factors that affect the rate at which ectoparasite populations become resistant include lack of refugia for maintaining of susceptible genes, and the persistence of residues (the more persistent the residues, the sooner resistance develops).

Management of resistance to ectoparasiticides

The following factors should be considered when designing a treatment strategy using ectoparasiticides, where resistance is to be prevented, as far as possible.

Reduction in the number of treatments

Resistance to pesticides is still relatively uncommon in the UK and other countries; use pesticides only when necessary. This is best achieved by an integrated approach to parasite management in which chemicals are combined with other means of controlling parasites.

Limited exposures with pesticides

Increased frequency of interactions of target ectoparasites with pesticides may accelerate the development of resistance. It is prudent to consider reducing dependence on pesticides (long-term goal) and to integrate procedures for managing animal ectoparasites to avoid promoting resistance against currently effective agents.

Resistance monitoring

It can be useful in determining continuing efficacy of agents or the effectiveness of resistance management programme. Continuous monitoring to optimize the timing of pesticide use and to determine the need for additional treatments.

Appropriate selection of ectoparasiticides

Use narrow-spectrum pesticides where possible.

Other management issues

Be aware that adult arthropods may be killed by a single treatment, but eggs and larvae may persist in the environment, necessitating additional treatments. Administer the pesticides effectively (use at the rate recommended, do not mix, check method of application). Avoid introducing resistant arthropods – use quarantine treatments. Adopt strategy to maintain refugia (i.e. susceptible individuals), which by mating with resistant individuals, reduce the resistance level of the population.

What do you need to know before using antiparasitic drugs?

Proper use of antiparasitic drugs is critical to the success of the treatment and prevention programmes. Therefore, to ensure a better outcome of the chemotherapeutic intervention the following points should be taken into account before embarking on the use of antiparasitic drugs.

Know the mechanism of action of the drug that you are using

Compounds belonging to one class generally act by the same mode of action, so that, for example, MLs can be considered to be neuronal toxins, whereas BZs are metabolic toxins.

Is it toxic to the host?

The overdose level varies with species and within species in different breeds.

Are there special concerns?

Collies are sensitive to ivermectin due to a mutation in the multidrug resistance gene (MDR1). This gene encodes a P-glycoprotein that is responsible for pumping many drugs and other toxins out of the brain. About 25% of collies have the mutant gene and, thus, cannot pump some drugs out of the brain as a normal dog would, which may result in abnormal neurological signs that require an extended hospital stay or can be fatal. So, collies do not have a proper transport system and become intoxicated and may die when exposed to ivermectin at high doses.

Teratogenicity

Some drugs, such as albendazole, have been shown to be teratogenic and should never be given to pregnant animals.

Age-related toxicity

Organophosphates are not given to very young animals because of the narrow margin of safety.

Dosage

This information is always available on the package insert and so there is no excuse to make a mistake. Always be sure that you are using the correct dosage for the species. Make sure scales are accurate and that weights are obtained and recorded properly.

How is the therapeutic dosage related to the therapeutic index?

You cannot tell from the label. It could be different for different species and related to mechanism of action and bioavailability of the drug.

What does extra-label usage imply?

Use at a different dosage or use in a different species than covered by the approved label. Extra-label usage in feeds is prohibited in food animals and horses. In the UK, 'Cascade' is a route through choices of drugs not licensed for a species.

What are refugia?

They are subpopulation of parasites that are not exposed to drug treatment. Refugia are parasite stage in the environment such as larvae on pasture or inhibited larvae that are not susceptible to the effects of drugs. They are important because the higher the proportion of the population in refugia, the slower the selection for resistance.

Formulation or route of delivery of anthelmintic

Anthelmintics may be administered by various routes or in various formulations. While this may have some effect on efficacy by altering bioavailability or drug concentration, there is no difference in the spectrum of activity per se.

Kinetics in the host

Are there residues in the host? What is the withdrawal time?

Resistance

Are any resistance issues known in the literature?

Scope of the drug activity

Effective parasite control depends on the correct use of the most appropriate anti-parasitic for any given infection. Therefore, understanding the spectrum of activity of anti-parasitic families used to control those parasites is a key aspect of successful control. The spectrum of activity varies considerably across parasite species, stage of the life cycle and site of infection. Hence, it is critical to understand the specifics of each infection and consider these variations when recommending antiparasitic treatments to clients as inappropriate use will not only be ineffective, but may also encourage the development of resistance. In general, anthelmintics can be classified into two classes based on their activities:

- *Class 1* includes drugs that their activities are limited to the gastrointestinal tract, such as piperazine, pyrantel pamoate.
- *Class 2* includes drugs for which activity extends to tissues (can kill migrating larvae), such as fenbendazole, oxfendazole, ivermectin.

Products available

Several products are available to treat worm infections. Some are endectocides, produced either by having a single active ingredient with a broad spectrum of activity or by combining active ingredients. Such products may be used to control both worms and ectoparasites: the precise spectrum of activity varies according to the active ingredients. Matching the spectrum of activity to the infections present or the risk for individual animals is an important part of parasite control. A review of the spectrum of activity of each individual antiparasitic product is available in the NOAH compendium and under therapies on the ESCCAP website (www.esccap.org) for companion animals.

Know the target species

There is little variability in the range of target species for anthelmintics in either sheep or cattle, although the relative importance of particular species may vary with factors such as climate.

Combination therapy

The use of two or more antiparasitic drugs with different mechanisms of action may increase the spectrum of activity by including more target species. Also, it often leads to more effective killing of the parasite, hence circumventing the appearance of parasites resistant to one compound or the other (i.e. helps combating the resistance problem). However, combination therapy does not always clear an infection, such as in case of a combined drug-resistant strain.

Perspectives

Despite more than 50 years of research, our arsenal of antiparasitic drugs remains modest. There are many reasons for this, but a key reason is that antiparasitic drugs must be safe. This may be difficult to attain due to the close similarities between parasites and their mammalian hosts as they are both eukaryotic organisms; consequently, compounds interfering with parasite survival often have adverse effects on the host. For this reason, developing safe and effective anti-parasitic drugs based on differences between the parasite and host has been challenging. Differential toxicity is commonly achieved by preferential uptake or differences in the susceptibility of functionally equivalent sites in the parasite and host. Additionally, treating parasitic diseases is difficult, mainly because of the chronic and prolonged course of infection and the complex life cycles and multiple developmental stages of many parasites.

In recent years, our level of knowledge about the mechanism of action of antiparasitics has significantly and steadily increased. The continuation of this process will be a prerequisite to maintain the successful and sustainable use of chemical compounds as key instruments in the control of parasitic infections in animals and humans. Unfortunately, the problem of anthelmintic resistance has reached an emergency level. Dealing with this crisis will require both intensified educational campaigns to promote the wise use of existing anthelmintics and extra-efforts towards the development of new ones. Antiparasitic drugs are not the only means to prevent parasitic infections. Effective public health measures in the veterinary context, proper nutrition, and proper management and husbandry remain fundamental contributors to the prevention of parasitic infections.

Further reading

Alvarez-Pellitero, P., Sitja-Bobadilla, A., Bermudez, R. and Quiroga, M.I. (2006). Levamisole activates several innate immune factors in *Scophthalmus maximus* (L.) Teleostei. Int. J. Immunopathol. Pharmacol. 19, 727–738.

Bishop, J. (2005). The Veterinary Formulary, 6th edn (BVA/Pharmaceutical Press, Cambridge), pp. 171–179; 181–220.

Durden, D.A. and Wotske, J. (2009). Quantitation and validation of macrolide endectocides in raw milk by negative ion electrospray MS/MS. J. AOAC Int. 92, 580–596.

ESCCAP (European Scientific Counsel Companion Animal Parasites) (2006). Worm control in dogs and cats. http://www.esccap.org/index.php/fuseaction/download/lrn_file/001-esccap-guidelines-ukfinal.pdf.

Harder, A., Holden-Dye, L., Walker, R. and Wunderlich, F. (2005). Mechanisms of action of emodepside. Parasitol. Res. 97, S1–10.

McCall, J.W. (2005). The safety-net story about macrocyclic lactone heartworm preventives: a review, an update, and recommendations. Vet. Parasitol. 133, 197–206.

Sajid, M.S., Iqbal, Z., Muhammad, G. and Iqbal, M.U. (2006). Immunomodulatory effect of various anti-parasitics: a review. Parasitology 132, 301–313.

Wolstenholme, A.J. and Rogers, A.T. (2005). Glutamate-gated chloride channels and the mode of action of the avermectin/milbemycin anthelmintics. Parasitology 131, S85–95.

Biology and Management of Anthelmintic Resistance

15

Ray M. Kaplan

Introduction

Anthelmintic resistance is defined as a heritable genetic change in a population of worms that produces an alteration in the chemical sensitivity of that population. This change enables some individual worms in that population to survive drug treatments that are generally effective against the same species and stage of infection at the same dose rate. In practical terms anthelmintic resistance is present in a population of parasites when the efficacy of the drug falls below that which is historically expected, when other causes of reduced efficacy have been ruled out. These types of genetic changes occur slowly, usually over many years, and are the direct result of natural selection on parasite populations in response to drug treatments. Precise molecular mechanisms have not been clearly elucidated for any of the anthelmintics, but some important mutations have been identified that are involved in resistance to benzimidazole drugs.

Many parasitic nematodes have biological and genetic features that favour the development of anthelmintic resistance. Short life cycles, high reproductive rates, rapid rates of nucleotide sequence evolution, and extremely large effective population sizes combine to give many parasitic worms an exceptionally high level of genetic diversity. In addition, most nematode species demonstrate a population structure consistent with high levels of gene flow, suggesting that host movement is an important determinant of nematode population genetic structure. Thus, it seems that many parasitic nematodes, including most of the species important in livestock, possess both the genetic capacity to respond successfully to chemical attack, and the means to assure dissemination of their resistance alleles via host movement.

Anthelmintic resistance first arises in individual worms as a set of alleles of particular genes that render the parasite less sensitive to a specific anthelmintic drug. Before a drug is ever used, rare resistance alleles exist within the midst of a genetically diverse population, which may number in the hundreds of millions or billions. Included within this population are all the various parasitic stages living within hosts, but the greatest proportion consists of preparasitic stages – eggs and larvae in the environment. When resistant individuals reproduce, they confer unique biochemical traits to their offspring via various genetic mechanisms. However, resistant individuals and their offspring will remain rare within a worm population unless they gain a survival advantage over their parasitic competitors as a result of anthelmintic treatment.

Parasiticidal treatment per se does nothing positive for resistant individuals, but by killing the sensitive worms, which comprise the majority of a parasite population, resistant individuals are able to reproduce for a given interval in the relative absence of competition. As a result, the genotypic frequency of resistant worms increases incrementally within the population as a whole. Amplification of resistance alleles within a worm population is a slow and gradual process, requiring numerous generations under drug selection (usually taking many years) before gene frequencies for resistance reach levels that can be detected by diagnostic assays. Even further amplification is then necessary before resistance becomes clinically apparent in the form of therapeutic or prophylactic failures. Thus from a practical perspective, the genetic phase of resistance develops slowly over time during which it is impossible to detect, but then increases very rapidly in its later phase, where it is then perceived as a clinical event. This has great clinical relevance because resistance can transition from undetectable, to clinically important levels over a very short period of time. Consequently, unless a surveillance programme is in place that closely monitors the effectiveness of drug treatments over time, resistance will not be noticed clinically until levels of resistance are extremely high. This is a major problem because once resistance reaches phenotypically detectable levels, irreversible changes in the genetic structure of the worm population have already occurred, ensuring that 'resistance' alleles are fixed in that population forever. Thus, once resistance is diagnosed as a clinical problem 'reversion' to susceptibility likely will never occur. In theory, reversion to susceptibility might occur if use of a drug is discontinued and worms resistant to that drug suffer from a decrease in fitness. However, there is scant evidence that resistant worms have any measurable decrease in fitness or that true reversion occurs in the field. In a few instances where reversion to greater susceptibility has been demonstrated, it has proven to be short lived once the drug is reintroduced.

History of anthelmintic resistance and potential for new drugs

The problems posed by anthelmintic resistance in helminth parasites of veterinary importance are not new. In fact resistance to thiabendazole (considered the first modern anthelmintic) was first reported in 1964 in the sheep nematode *Haemonchus contortus*, just a few years following this drugs' introduction. Shortly thereafter, thiabendazole resistance was reported in equine cyathostomin (small strongyle) nematodes, and then in the other major gastrointestinal trichostrongylid nematodes of sheep; *Teladorsagia* (*Ostertagia*) *circumcincta* (brown stomach worm), and *Trichostrongylus colubriformis* (black scour worm). By the mid-1970s multiple-species resistance to benzimidazole anthelmintics was common and widespread in nematode parasites of both sheep and horses throughout the world. This same pattern repeated itself in the 1970s and 1980s following the introduction of the newer imidazothiazole–tetrahydropyrimidine and avermectin–milbemycin (macrocyclic lactone) classes of anthelmintics. By the early 1980s, reports of multiple-drug-resistant (MDR) worms appeared for the first time, and presently, a high prevalence of MDR (to all three major anthelmintic classes) *H. contortus*, *T. circumcincta*, and *T. colubriformis* are documented throughout the world.

Similar problems exist in parasites of horses. In 2001–2002, a large multi-state study was performed to determine the prevalence of anthelmintic resistance on 44 horse farms in the southern United States. In this study the percentages of farms found to harbour resistant cyathostomins were: 97.7% for fenbendazole, 53.5% for oxibendazole, 40.5% for pyrantel pamoate and 0% for ivermectin. In terms of actual faecal egg count reductions (FECR), the mean per cent reductions for all farms were 24.8% for fenbendazole, 73.8% for oxibendazole, 78.6% for pyrantel pamoate and 99.9% for ivermectin. With the exception of ivermectin, these values are far below the levels achieved when the products were first licensed, and are far below what is needed for effective treatment (i.e. > 90%). Surveys for drug resistance performed in Italy, Germany, Sweden, Australia, and a recent study performed in Italy, Germany and the United Kingdom, confirmed high levels of benzimidazole resistance (38–85%), and low to moderate levels of pyrantel resistance (0–30%), but no compelling evidence of ivermectin resistance. It is interesting to note that the high prevalence of resistance to pyrantel pamoate found in the US study has not been detected in studies performed outside the United States. Many parasitologists have suspected that low-dose daily feeding of pyrantel tartrate may lead to resistance. Because the United States and Canada are the only countries in which daily feeding of low-dose pyrantel tartrate is practiced, one must wonder whether this regimen of administration is having a major impact on the selection for resistance to other pyrantel compounds.

Furthermore, numerous reports strongly suggest that avermectin/milbemycin resistance is fairly common in *Parascaris equorum* of horses. This demonstrates that avermectin/milbemycin resistance is already becoming a significant concern in an important nematode parasite of horses. Altogether, there is no biological rationale to believe that cyathostomins will not develop avermectin/milbemycin resistance. This has most recently been underlined by several reports of greatly shortened egg reappearance periods (ERP) of cyathostomins after treatment with ivermectin. It is suggested that shortened ERP represents the first sign of developing anthelmintic resistance. This recently was

confirmed in a study demonstrating that the reduced ERP for ivermectin was due to a lack of efficacy against L4 larval stages within the intestinal lumen. Thus, cyathostomin resistance to avermectin/milbemycin drugs is certainly developing and could reach levels producing therapeutic failures at any time. Given the published evidence that avermectin/milbemycin resistance in *P. equorum* is already an important problem, that resistance to benzimidazoles and pyrantel in cyathostomins is quite common, and that resistance to avermectin/milbemycin drugs in cyathostomins is emerging, it is clear that no single drug class can be regarded as a safe choice for controlling equine nematode infections any longer. Horses are always co-infected with several nematode species at a time, thus faecal egg count surveillance and testing for drug resistance should be a routine component of equine health programmes.

Few studies have been performed to establish the prevalence of resistance in parasites of cattle so it is impossible to know how severe and widespread the problem is. However, available evidence suggests that avermectin/milbemycin resistance in *Cooperia* spp. is relatively common and widespread in the major cattle producing regions of the world. Recently published data indicates that resistance is becoming a very serious problem in New Zealand and in South America; a study in New Zealand reported that ivermectin resistance was evident on 92% of farms and resistance to both ivermectin and albendazole was evident on 74% of farms. However, *Cooperia* spp. generally are not viewed as serious pathogens, and currently it is not known to what extent resistance in *Cooperia* impacts animal health and productivity. Nonetheless, there is clear evidence that uncontrolled *Cooperia* infections can have a significant negative effect on growing cattle. Other parasite species, particularly *Ostertagia* are considered to be much more important, and there is still no evidence suggesting that resistance in *Ostertagia* is a problem anywhere in the world. Should avermectin/milbemycin resistance emerge in *Ostertagia*, the problem of resistance in cattle parasites will reach a new level of importance and concern.

The problem of anthelmintic resistance could theoretically be mitigated by the introduction of new classes of anthelmintic drugs with novel modes of action. However, in the past several decades, there has been limited investment in antiparasitic discovery by pharmaceutical companies, and the current trend is towards declining investment in research and development. The great cost associated with the development of new drugs and the modest size of the anthelmintic market, have created an environment in which few animal health companies are heavily committed to the discovery of new antiparasitic drugs. This is important because virtually all new drug classes are developed first for humans where the market potential is extremely large, and then only later are used in animals when the cost is less. In contrast, anthelmintics are developed first for the veterinary market and then later are used in humans, because the human anthelmintic market is small. New anthelmintic classes represented by emodepside (2005), monepantel (2009), and derquantel (2010) are being developed and marketed, but these drugs are quite expensive and so far have very limited label claims for efficacy. For instance, emodepside is labelled only for treatment of intestinal worms in cats, and monepantel and derquantel (in combination with abamectin) are labelled only for use in sheep. Though it is likely that some of these drugs will be labelled for use in more species in the future, the cost of these drugs will be much higher than products of the older drug classes. Thus, it seems most probable that the development of resistance will continue to outpace the introduction of new anthelmintic drugs, and any new drugs will be much more expensive. As a result, the management and prevention of resistance will become increasingly more important.

Factors affecting the rate of development of anthelmintic resistance

It is easy to understand how resistance may evolve when anthelmintics treatments are administered frequently. But what factors regulate the rate with which resistance develops? Why does resistance develop so much quicker in some parasites and in some hosts than in others? We don't fully know all the answers to these questions but there is much we do know. It is generally recognized by parasitologists that the most important factor affecting the rate of development of anthelmintic resistance is the proportion of the worm population under drug selection. 'Refugia' is a term used to describe the portion of a parasite population which is not exposed to an anthelmintic during a treatment event. Because such nematode stages thereby escape selection pressure, the population in refugia constitutes a reservoir of susceptible genes. Examples of refugia include eggs, infective third-stage larvae (L3) and pre-infective larvae (L1, L2) in the environment; these stages often comprise > 99% of the total parasitic nematode population on a farm. Other examples of refugia include parasitic stages in those individual hosts that are not dewormed whenever other herd members are treated. A final example are parasitic stages within the host at the time of a deworming treatment that are not affected by the anthelmintic (do not come into contact with therapeutic levels of the drug). To illustrate this point, consider the case of horses where cyathostomin larvae are encysted within fibrous capsules in the caecal and colonic mucosa. Only moxidectin and a 5-day regimen of fenbendazole have demonstrable efficacy against such encysted larvae, so these stages can be considered to be in refugia whenever the selected anthelmintic is ivermectin, a member of the pyrimidine class (i.e. pyrantel), or a single-dose benzimidazole. Similarly, pyrimidine anthelmintics are poorly absorbed from the gut, and only minimal quantities are distributed systemically. Thus, migrating stages (e.g. large strongyles, ascarids) which are not present in the alimentary system at the time of a pyrimidine treatment could be considered in refugia as well. It is important to note that refugia are composed of both susceptible and resistant worms; whatever the base population of nematodes is on that property will make up the refugia. But by maintaining adequate refugia, the susceptible worms will continue to remain in the majority.

The bottom line is that maintaining refugia on a farm preserves genetic diversity within the worm population. Thus, susceptible worms and alleles are preserved, which will help to reduce the frequency of resistant worm mating events, as well as dilute the frequency of resistant alleles in the overall population. This should significantly slow the evolution of resistance on the farm.

It is a logical conclusion that the most effective way to maximize refugia and thus prevent the development of anthelmintic resistance is simply never to deworm. However, the primary goal of a parasite control programme is not to prevent the development of resistance, but rather it is to maintain the health of the herd. Thus a reasonable compromise must be sought in the form of an effective and sustainable control programme that takes into account the need for maintaining refugia, so that the few remaining effective drugs will stay that way.

Why resistance develops more slowly in some hosts and parasites than others is a complex question, which is dependent on many factors. These factors relate to the parasite biology and epidemiology, the dynamics of the host–parasite relationship, and the pharmacokinetics of the drugs. Some factors relating directly to the parasite biology include: life history (generation time, direct or indirect life cycle), fecundity of female worms, lifespan of mature worms, survival of free-living stages in the environment, level of genetic diversity, manner of inheritance of resistance traits, number of genes involved, frequency of the 'resistance' alleles in the population prior to the first use of the drug, actual dose level required to kill susceptible worms of a particular species as compared with label dose level, and worm pathogenicity (and therefore need for treatment). Host factors include: levels of innate and acquired immunity, behavioural differences effecting exposure rates, and differences in anthelmintic pharmacokinetics between host species. In livestock species, anthelmintic drugs generally demonstrate highest bioavailability in cattle, and lowest bioavailability in goats. It is frequently suggested that the extremely high prevalence of anthelmintic resistance in nematodes of goats is associated with this unique pharmacokinetic profile. All of these factors combined with treatment frequency, means of drug delivery (affecting pharmacodynamics and kinetics), dose rate, drug persistence, quality of drug used (e.g. expired drug) and levels of refugia at time of treatment interact to effect the rate of resistance development. It is difficult to know with precision or certainty how large a role each of these different factors play in the development of resistance, and most likely they change with each host/parasite relationship. However, the fact that the important nematodes of cattle and sheep/goats are extremely closely related, (both phylogenetically and biologically) but resistance is much slower to evolve in nematodes of cattle, gives strong evidence that many factors other than the genetics of the worms are involved in the dynamic process of resistance selection.

Practices that promote the development of resistance

A number of common and widely used practices can be regarded as risk factors for accelerating the development of anthelmintic resistance. Some of the most important are briefly mentioned here.

Frequent treatment

Frequent anthelmintic treatments are perhaps the single greatest risk factor for anthelmintic resistance, as this will greatly diminish refugia and cause parasite populations to be under continuous selection pressure for resistance.

Treating all animals at the same time

Parasite populations are never evenly distributed in a group of animals. Rather, parasites are greatly overdispersed, and, as a rule of thumb, 20–30% of the animals harbour approximately 80% of the parasite population at any given time. Thus a majority of animals tend to harbour low parasite burdens, while a minority will harbour relatively higher burdens. Animals with low parasite burdens will gain minimal benefit from anthelmintic treatment; however, the small number of eggs they produce will serve as an important source of refugia. If all animals are treated, this source of refugia is eliminated. Thus, the only infective stages shed into the environment for a prolonged period following treatment (until a new cycle of infection and patency occurs) will be from those worms that survived treatment. Furthermore, until reinfection occurs, resistant individuals are able to breed and reproduce in the absence of competition from susceptible worms. These factors cause whole-herd treatments to greatly increase the selection pressure for resistance as compared with targeted selective treatments, where only animals with clinically significant worm burdens are treated.

Treating when there are low levels of refugia on pasture

The size of parasite refugia is greatly influenced by climatic conditions. During times of the year that are too cold, too hot, or too dry for development and survival of eggs and larvae, there will be few free-living parasitic stages on pasture. Anthelmintic treatment during these times will greatly increase the selective pressures for resistance because the majority of the parasite population is concentrated in the animals. Thus a much larger proportion of the total parasite population is placed under selection pressure. Furthermore, eggs shed onto pasture by survivors of treatment will not be diluted by other worms. As a result, anthelmintic resistance will evolve much more rapidly than when treatments are given when pastures contain significant levels of refugia.

Frequent use of larvicidal drugs

This is most relevant in horses, since most important worm species infecting ruminants do not have encysted or migrating stages that are refractory to single dose anthelmintic treatments. In adult horses, the majority of the total cyathostomin burden is in the encysted stages which are not affected by most anthelmintic treatments. These encysted stages thus serve as an important source of refugia. Treatments targeting these stages using moxidectin (single dose) or fenbendazole (5-day regimen) will therefore place selection pressure on a much larger proportion of the total worm population, thus promoting the development of resistance. Similarly, only the avermectin/milbemycin drugs ivermectin and moxidectin kill tissue migrating stages of *P. equorum*. Thus, when using these drugs all parasites in the animal are under drug selection for resistance. This is likely an important factor in the frequent diagnosis of resistance to ivermectin and moxidectin in populations of *P. equorum*. As a consequence, larvicidal

treatments should be used prudently and in a targeted selective manner.

Underdosing

Administering anthelmintics at dosages which are substantially less than label recommendations may contribute to selection for resistance. Underdosing can be intentional, as an ill-advised cost-cutting measure, but most instances are inadvertent, and result from under-estimation of a patient's body weight or spillage during dosing. The genetic mechanisms which determine the magnitude of resistance are highly complex and appear to involve multiple genes. Accordingly, if an individual worm has some genetic changes that make it less susceptible to a drug (e.g. a subset of alleles necessary for resistance or is heterozygous for resistance at a particular loci), but does not have the complete complement of alleles required for full resistance, then it may survive a treatment if it is administered at a reduce dosage. Allowing these 'partially' resistant worms to survive will increase their mating probabilities, with the outcome being more worms with a larger subset of resistance alleles and/or homozygote resistant worms.

Treat-and-move strategies

The very first strategic parasite control strategy developed, and one which has been advocated in ruminants for several decades is termed 'treat-and-move'. In this management scheme, parasitized animals are treated with an effective dewormer and then moved promptly to a new pasture, which has few infective stages and thus provides a minimal risk of reinfection. Since the only parasites moving to the new pasture are those that survived the treatment, and there are few parasites in refugia on the new pasture, treat-and-move strategies can lead to the rapid development of a resistant population. Rather, many parasitologists are recommending a move-then-treat strategy. By moving the animals a few days before treating them, the pasture will be contaminated with a limited number of infective stages that will serve as an important source of refugia. Alternatively, if utilizing a treat-and-move strategy, then a portion of the animals should be left untreated.

Purchasing resistant worms

Anthelmintic-resistant worms come from only two sources: either they are produced on the farm or they are purchased. Unfortunately, resistant worms commonly infect new additions to the herd; this is a very common means of spreading the resistance problem. It is therefore important for veterinarians to recommend quarantine of all new additions to the herd or flock, with aggressive treatment upon arrival. This is especially important for sheep and goats, but is a good practice for all livestock species, perhaps with the exception of horses. Upon arrival, all new additions should be placed in a dry lot (without any grass) or on concrete, held without feed for 24 hours, and then dewormed sequentially on the same day with drugs of each of the main three anthelmintic classes. In the United States it is recommended to use moxidectin, levamisole, and albendazole, however the choice of drugs will differ depending on the country. A FEC should be performed at the time of treatment and again after 14 days together with a centrifugal faecal floatation, and the animal should be allowed to enter the herd only if the faecal is negative. If a 14-day quarantine is not possible, animals should be confined to pens for a minimum of 48 hours following treatment before being moved to pasture. However, this is a risky approach. After the animal is released from quarantine, it should be placed on the most contaminated pasture available (large refugia) and should never be placed on a clean pasture.

Diagnosis of resistance

From a clinical standpoint it is important to appreciate that the prevalence of resistance only tells you what you can expect across many farms; it tells you nothing about which drug(s) are effective on any particular farm. Therefore, it is not possible to make medically sound recommendations regarding drug choice for an individual farm without first doing a test to determine whether resistant worms are present there, and if present, to which drugs and at what levels. Given this reality, resistance testing should be performed on every farm as a standard component of herd health management every 2–3 years. This can be done in one of two ways: (1) by performing a faecal egg count reduction test (FECRT); or (2) by performing an *in vitro* bioassay such as the larval development assay (LDA). The FECRT presently is considered the most definitive means of determining whether resistance is present on a particular property, and is the only test available for horses and cattle. *In vitro* bioassays have been evaluated for parasites of cattle and horses; however, currently there are no properly validated and standardized assays available. A good alternative to the FECRT in sheep and goats is the LDA, which is available as a commercial product (DrenchRite®). However, this and other *in vitro* bioassays are not suited for in-clinic use and can only realistically be performed in a parasitology diagnostic lab. The great advantage of the LDA is that it can detect and measure resistance to benzimidazole drugs, levamisole, ivermectin and moxidectin, all from a single pooled faecal sample in a single assay. In addition, because efficacy is measured at multiple drug concentrations, and the data is analysed such that the relative drug susceptibility of the population is quantified with an LC50 value, the development of resistance can be monitored over time. In contrast, the FECRT is typically performed at a single dosage, so the results can only indicate whether or not full-fledged resistance is present. However, the LDA is only useful where *H. contortus* and *Trichostrongylus* spp. predominate, because avermectin/milbemycin resistance cannot be accurately measured in *T. circumcincta* with the LDA.

Faecal egg count reduction test (FECRT)

Sheep and goats

Guidelines for FECRT in sheep are published by the World Association for the Advancement of Veterinary Parasitology (WAAVP) and it is recommended that these be followed in principle. Briefly, animals that have not been treated with anthelmintic within the past 8 weeks are divided into groups of 10–15 and treated with anthelmintic or left untreated to serve as controls. If enough animals are present on the farm, multiple drugs can be tested simultaneously, but a control group of equal size must always be included. Fewer than 10 animals per group can be tested, but because of the wide variation in faecal egg count (FEC) between animals, results will be less accurate and there is a greater chance for an erroneous result. Consequently, if fewer than 10 animals are included per group it is necessary to balanced the groups on the basis of FEC. This can be done one of two ways. Pre-treatment FEC can be performed, or if *Haemonchus* is the primary parasite, animals can be assigned to treatment based on FAMACHA© score. Using pre-treatment FEC has the disadvantage of requiring a considerable amount of extra labour and expense; since the animals need to be worked an additional time and an additional set of FEC must be performed. In contrast, when using FAMACHA©, allocation to treatment is made on the spot at the time of treatment so that faecals only need to be collected and analysed one time. If using pre-treatment FEC for allocation, animals are ranked from highest to lowest eggs per gram (EPG) of faeces and then blocked into groups of 2, 3, 4 or 5 depending on how many drugs are being tested. Then within each block, animals are randomly assigned to treatment or control groups. If using FAMACHA©, the same approach is used but animals are blocked by their FAMACHA© eye score. For example, if 4 drugs are being tested, of the first 5 animals to come through the chute with the same FAMACHA© score, each of the 5 will be assigned randomly to one of the 5 treatment/control groups. Therefore for each FAMACHA© score, a group of 5 animals will each be assigned to a different treatment group, and then the process repeats itself for the next 5 with the same eye score. If > 10 animals are included in each group, it is likely that random allocation will produce groups that are sufficiently balanced to obtain useful data, but assigning treatment based on FAMACHA© score will increase this likelihood and is recommended as a routine practice no matter how many animals are tested (but only when *H. contortus* is the primary parasite of concern).

Faecal egg counts need to be performed only one time 10–14 days after treatment using the McMaster method, and calculations for faecal egg count reduction (FECR) are made using the following formula:

$$FECR\% = 100\left[1 - (X_t/X_c)\right]$$

where X_t and X_c are the arithmetic mean eggs per gram (EPG) in the treated (t) and non-treated control (c) groups, respectively.

Free software (RESO FECR4) is available that performs all calculations and provides accurate data interpretation according to WAAVP standards.[1] If the RESO calculator is used, the assignment of resistance status is based both on per cent reduction and the 95% confidence intervals. If the RESO calculator is not used, the following guidelines can be applied: reductions of greater than 95% indicate sensitivity, reductions of 90–95% indicate low or suspected resistance, and reductions of < 90% indicate

[1]Cameron, A. RESO faecal egg count reduction analysis spreadsheet. AusVet Animal Health Services, University of Sydney, Sydney, Australia 2000 (Based on calculations developed by Martin, P.J., Wursthorn, L., 1991. RESO faecal egg count reduction test calculator, CSIRO, Animal Health, Melbourne, Australia).

resistance. Control group mean FEC should be at least 150 EPG for the FECRT to yield reliable results. This is rarely an issue with animals infected with *H. contortus*, but group mean FEC of less than 150 EPG is common in adult ewes infected primarily with *T. colubriformis* or *T. circumcincta*. Therefore when FECRT is performed on a sheep farm it is preferable to use weaned lambs if available. Low FEC are less common in goats, but the same issues should be considered before performing a FECRT. Lastly, because animals are almost always infected with multiple species of nematodes, it is extremely important to perform pre- and post-treatment coprocultures to identify the relative abundance of the different species. Because resistance to a drug is species specific, failing to determine which species survived treatment may lead to an incorrect interpretation of the data. This is also important for cattle, but much less so for horses because cyathostomins almost always account for virtually 100% of the eggs shed post-treatment.

Cattle

Standardized methods for FECRT in cattle have not yet been developed. Although the methods recommended for sheep can be used, it is important to appreciate that those methods have not undergone any scientific validation in cattle. Until there are published guidelines for FECRT in cattle, individual investigators or veterinarians can choose among several different methods. However, there are a few specific procedural details that should be adhered to when planning a FECRT in cattle. These include:

1 Use a more sensitive method for FEC than McMaster; the modified Wisconsin centrifugal floatation method with a detection sensitivity of 5 EPG or less is usually recommend.

2 Use an injectable product; with pour-ons there is great variation in drug levels between animals, due both to differences in absorption and the fact that a substantial amount of the dose is ingested as a consequence of licking. If a pour-on product is used, the treated animals must be kept in a separate pen/paddock from the rest of the cattle.

3 Cattle selected should be uniform in age, breed, grazing history and anthelmintic exposure.

4 Weaned animals < 16 months of age are preferable, as older animals tend to have very low FEC.

5 It is suggested to use 20 cattle per treatment group. If 15 or more animals are tested then the mean FEC of treated and control groups can be used to calculate the per cent reduction (using the formula provided for sheep above). If 10 or fewer are tested then FEC should be performed both at the time of treatment and again 14–21 day post treatment on the same animals and FECR should be calculated for each animal separately using the formula:

$$FECR\% = 100[1 - (post\text{-}Tx/pre\text{-}Tx)]$$

where post-Tx and pre-Tx are the eggs per gram (EPG) in the post-treatment and pre-treatment FEC, respectively.

The mean FECR of the group should then be calculated. If mean FEC reduction is < 90% then there is evidence for resistance.

Horses

As with cattle, there are currently no established guidelines for conducting or for interpreting results of the FECRT in horses. However, many of the same general recommendations for cattle apply to horses. One major difference with horses compared with ruminants is that most commonly, there are only small numbers of horses available to test on a farm. In addition, many adult horses will have very low EPG. Therefore, it is always recommended that each horse serve as its own control, and a method for FEC be used that has a detection sensitivity of 5 EPG or less. FEC should be performed both at the time of treatment and again approximately 14 days post-treatment, and FECR should be calculated for each animal separately using the formula:

$$FECR\% = 100[1 - (post\text{-}Tx/pre\text{-}Tx)]$$

where post-Tx and pre-Tx are the eggs per gram (EPG) in the post-treatment and pre-treatment FEC, respectively.

The mean FECR of the group should then be calculated. Because of variability in the measurement of FEC, when the true FECR falls below 95% it is common to see a wide range of FECR for different horses. The smaller the number of horses that are tested, the more impact this variability will have on the calculated FECR. Thus when testing small groups of horses (< 10), care must be used when interpreting the results of the FECRT. Also complicating interpretation of FECRT in horses is the fact that the different drugs have different expected efficacies. Thus, the FECR cut-offs used for declaring resistance to the different drugs should be different. These issues and more are currently being investigated for the purpose of establishing proper guidelines for FECRT in horses. Thus it is recommended that the current literature be examined for the most up to date recommendations before conducting a FECRT in horses.

Strategies for when there is resistance to most or all available drugs

In the past few years it has become increasingly common to find sheep and goat farms that have resistance to all three classes of anthelmintics plus moxidectin. So what can be done to deal with this situation? First, since resistance exists in gradations, it is important to know what the actual level of resistance is. Some drugs that are declared resistant may still be achieving 90–95% reductions in FEC. If this is the situation, then using a two-drug combination with the two most effective drugs would be a rational choice. However, if the situation has deteriorated even further, a triple combination with 3 different drug classes may be needed. In either case, it is critically important to absolutely minimize the frequency of treatment. Unless selective therapy and other strategies to maintain significant refugia are instituted, the worms will fairly rapidly develop higher-level resistance, rendering these combinations ineffective. In addition to using drug-combinations, it is critical that the overall management of the farm be evaluated. Reduced stocking rates and improved level of nutrition will be critical to helping to reduce the need for treatment. Furthermore, novel non-chemical worm control strategies should be implemented wherever practical. Without making the necessary management changes and adjustments to worm control strategy, it is not realistic to expect that the use of drug-combinations will be anything more than a quick and temporary fix.

In horses and cattle the resistance situation is not as dire, but the situation seems to worsening. It is not uncommon on many horse farms in the United States and elsewhere to have resistance in the cyathostomins to two of the three major drug classes. On most farms ivermectin and moxidectin remain effective against cyathostomins. However, there are recent reports of resistance and greatly shortened egg reappearance periods, so resistance to these drugs may finally be emerging in the cyathostomins. In contrast, ivermectin and moxidectin are often the least effective drugs against *P. equorum*. Thus, when treating foals where both parasites are of concern, using combinations may be necessary to restore the broad spectrum effect of the treatment. In cattle most reports of resistance are in *Cooperia* spp., and with this parasite it appears that the avermectin/milbemycin drugs are often the least effective. However, *Cooperia* generally is not considered a very important pathogen. Thus, many parasitologists are recommending that in cattle, a combination of an avermectin/milbemycin drug with either a benzimidazole drug or levamisole be used to provide optimal broad-spectrum activity.

Perspectives

Development of anthelmintic resistance is a logical and inevitable consequence of anthelmintic treatment. However, how the drugs are used has a large bearing on the rate with which resistance will develop. Over the past few decades, there has been a great deal of over and irrational use of anthelmintics. There are several reasons for this. First, and most importantly, these drugs can provide an important benefit to the health and productivity of animals. Due to the relatively low cost compared with the potential benefit, and the quest for maximizing productivity (ruminants) and health (horses), frequent and consistent use of anthelmintics became the norm. However, we now have learned the consequences of these behaviours. Given that development of anthelmintic resistance will almost certainly outpace the introduction of new novel drug classes, now and in the future, parasite control programmes must be designed to be more sustainable and much less intensive. Only by taking a rational evidence-based approach to parasite control with sustainability as a goal can the livestock industry ensure that the few anthelmintic drugs we have available will remain efficacious into the future.

Further reading

Blouin, M.S., Yowell, C.A., Courtney, C.H., and Dame, J.B. (1995). Host movement and the genetic structure of populations of parasitic nematodes. Genetics *141*, 1007–1014.

Geary, T.G., Conder, G.A. and Bishop, B. (2004). The changing landscape of antiparasitic drug discovery for veterinary medicine. Trends Parasitol. *20*, 449–455.

Jackson, F. and Coop, R. (2000). The development of anthelmintic resistance in sheep nematodes. Parasitology *120*, S95–107.

Kaplan, R.M. (2004). Drug resistance in nematodes of veterinary importance: a status report. Trends Parasitol. *20*, 477–481.

Kaplan, R.M., Klei, T.R., Lyons, E.T., Lester, G.D., French, D.D., Tolliver, S.C., Courtney, C.H., Vidyanshankar, A.N., and Zhao, Y. (2004). Prevalence of anthelmintic resistant cyathostomes on horse farms. J. Am. Vet. Med. Assoc. *225*, 903–910.

Lyons, E., Tolliver, S. and Collins, S. (2009). Probable reason why small strongyle EPG counts are returning 'early' after ivermectin treatment of horses on a farm in Central Kentucky. Parasitol. Res. *104*, 569–574.

Roos, M.H., Kwa, M.S.G. and Grant, W.N. (1995). New genetic and practical implications of selection for anthelmintic resistance in parasitic nematodes. Parasitol. Today *11*, 148–150.

Sangster, N.C. (1999). Pharmacology of anthelmintic resistance in cyathostomes: will it occur with the avermectin/milbemycins? Vet. Parasitol. *85*, 189–204.

Van Wyk, J.A. (2001). Refugia – overlooked as perhaps the most potent factor concerning the development of anthelmintic resistance. Onderstepoort J. Vet. Res. *68*, 55–67.

Waghorn, T.S., Leathwick, D.M., Rhodes, A.P., Jackson, R., Pomroy, W.E, West, D.M., and Moffat, J.R. (2006). Prevalence of anthelmintic resistance on 62 beef cattle farms in the North Island of New Zealand. N. Z. Vet. J. *54*, 278–282.

Abomasum: The fourth and final compartment of the ruminant's stomach.

Acanthella: Acanthocephalan larva following the acanthor and prior to the cystacanth.

Acanthor: Acanthocephalan larva with bladelike hooks and develops inside the egg capsules.

Acetabulum: Ventral muscular sucker or holdfast of digenetic trematodes; a sucker on a tapeworm scolex.

Acoelomate: A condition in which a body cavity is lacking, as in the members of the phylum Platyhelminthes, where the organs lie embedded in parenchyma.

Ala (-ae): Wing-like projection such as the cuticular expansions in certain nematodes.

Alveolus (-i): The air sac in the lung where gaseous exchange occurs.

Ametabolous: A type of metamorphosis in insects in which there is no external change as they proceed through a series of molts to the adult; *ametabola* refers to the taxonomic group.

Amphid: Anterior sensory structures of nematodes.

Anaphylaxis: A strong hypersensitivity reaction in which the individual may collapse, stop breathing, and die.

Anapolysis: The process in which terminal, gravid proglottids are not shed in certain tapeworms.

Anisogamete: Morphologically different male and female gametes.

Anterior station: Protozoan development in the anterior part of an insect vector, for example, Salivaria of the genus *Trypanosoma*; transmission takes place by biting.

Anthroponoses: Human diseases that are transmissible to animals.

Antibody: Serum protein (immunoglobulin) synthesized by lymphoid cells in response to an antigenic stimulus.

Antigen: Any substance that can stimulate an immune response.

Antigenic mimicry: Acquisition of or production of host antigens by a parasite so that it is not recognized as non-self, as in *Schistosoma*.

Apical complex: Organelles characteristic of members of the phylum Apicomplexa. It encompasses polar rings, subpellicular microtubules, conoid, rhoptries, and micronemes.

Apolysis: The process in which terminal, gravid proglottids are detached and shed by certain tapeworms.

Autoinfection: A process in which the progeny of a parasite reinfect the host without passing out of it, for example, *Taenia solium*.

Axostyle: A longitudinal rod-like or tube-like structure in members of the protozoan order Trichomonadida; probably serves as a cytoskeleton.

Biramous: Divided into two branches; typical of the terminal segments of the legs of Crustacea.

Bladder worm: Infective stage of *Taenia* tapeworm (Cysticercus). The name refers to the fluid filled bladder which surrounds the larval scolex (*Taenia*) or scolices (*Coenurus*). Bladder worm is also a common name of *Capillaria plica*, found in the dog urinary bladder.

Bothrium (-ia): Shallow, sucking groove on the scolex of tapeworms of the order Psuedophyllidea.

Bots: Larvae of several fly species, particularly *Gastrophilus* (horse bot), *Oestrus* (sheep bot), and *Dermatobia* and *Hypoderma* (affect cattle and other species).

Bottle jaw: Fluid accumulation under the lower jaw (submandibular oedema).

Bradyzoite: Slow-growing zoite or meront of the pseudocyst of *Toxoplasma* and related cyst-forming coccidian protozoa.

Buccal capsule: Mouth cavity of a nematode.

Bursa (copulatory bursa): A cuticular copulatory structure at the posterior end of males of the order Strongylida. It is useful in nematode taxonomy and species identification.

Capitulum: Pseudo-head of a tick; bears the mouthparts and the probing and sensory structures. Its shape is characteristic of the tick species.

Cellular immunity: A specific response to an antigen in which lymphoid cells are the primary effectors.

Cercaria (-iae): A free–living larval trematode which develops from a sporocyst or redia in snail intermediate hosts.

Cercomer: Tail-like appendage, which often retains the hooks of the hexacanth embryo, on procercoid and cysticercoid larvae of certain tapeworms.

Chemokines: Small proteins that attract and stimulate cells of the immune defense; produced by many cells in response to infection. Also called chemotactic cytokines.

Chemotherapy: Use of a chemical that has a specific action in removing or killing a microbial agent.

Coenurus: Fluid-filled metacestode of some tapeworms of the family Taeniidae. It has a non-laminated wall that produces protoscolices, but without brood capsules.

Conjugation: A temporary union of two ciliated protozoans for the exchange of nuclear material.

Conoid: Spirally coiled filaments in the anterior tip of the zoite of certain apicomplexan protozoa.

Control: General term comprising therapy and prevention. *See* prophylaxis.

Coprophagous: Feeding on manure.

Coracidium (-ia): Free-swimming, ciliated embryophore of tapeworms of the order Pseudophyllidea.

Costa: A striated, rod-like structure that lies just under the recurrent flagellum of certain protozoa of the order Trichomonadida; composed of carbohydrate and protein.

Cuticle: A secreted surface covering that is generally considered to be non-living.

Cyst: A general term used when an organism has a membrane surrounding it, whether the covering is of its making or of host origin. Cystic stage is a common resistant stage in protozoa.

Cystacanth: A juvenile acanthocephalan that is surrounded by a capsule of host origin.

Cysticercoid: A tapeworm larva which develops in an invertebrate intermediate host; characteristic of many cyclophyllidean families such as Hymenolepididae, Dilepididae, or Anoplocephalidae.

Cysticercus: A tapeworm larva in which the scolex develops in an inverted form and which has a fluid-filled bladder surrounding it. It is characteristic of the cyclophyllidean family Taeniidae. *See* Bladder worm.

Cytokines: Soluble proteins produced by cells in response to various stimuli, including parasitic infection; they affect the behavior of other cells both locally and at a distance, by binding to specific cytokine receptors. *See* Chemokines.

Didelphic: Having two ovaries and hence a uterus with two horns; usually applied to nematodes.

Dioecious: Separate sexes.

Disease: Abnormal performance of physiological functions as a result of injury to cells performing those functions.

Ectoparasite: A parasite that lives on the external surface or in the integument of a host.

Egg: The germ cell of a female, an ovum.

Emerging parasite: A parasite population responsible for a marked increase in disease incidence, usually as result of changed societal, environmental, or population factors.

Endemic: A disease or disease agent that present continually in a region or among a certain human population.

Endodyogeny: A special form of merogony in which two daughter cells are formed, each with its own pellicle, while still in the mother cell; occurs in certain members of the phylum Apicomplexa such as *Toxoplasma*.

Engorgement: Distension of a feeding female tick with blood; cannot occur in male hard ticks, because their back is covered completely by a hard scutum.

Enzootic: A disease or disease agent that occurs in an animal population at all times. *See* Endemic.

Epidemic: A disease or disease agent that spreads rapidly through a human population.

Epidemiology: The study of the causes of disease; the complex of factors that lead to disease outbreaks. It is usually used for diseases in humans; epizootiology is used for diseases in animals.

Epizootic: A disease or disease agent that spreads rapidly through an animal population. *See* Epidemic.

Euryxenous: Having a broad host range.

Exflagellation: Process of formation of microgametes in certain apicomplexan protozoans such as *Plasmodium*.

Feral: Wild; a feral cycle of a parasitic agent is one that takes place in the wild as opposed to an urban site.

Festoon: Rectangular raised areas separated by grooves; occurs on the posterior edge of hard ticks of certain species.

Fomites: Inanimate objects that may be contaminated with microorganisms and become vehicles for the transmission of infectious agents.

Gamogony (= gametogony): Formation of gametes.

Granuloma: A swelling composed of leukocytes, fluid, and connective tissue; often a foreign-body reaction.

Gubernaculum: A sclerotized plate located on the dorsal surface of the cloaca of certain male nematodes; serves as a guide when the copulatory spicules are protruded.

Gynecophoral canal: The longitudinal groove on the ventral surface of male schistosomes in which the female worm lies.

Haematophagous: Bloodsucking; usually refers to the feeding habits of various insects and acarines such as mosquitoes and ticks.

Haematuria: Blood in the urine; a condition seen in some individuals infected with blood parasites e.g. *Plasmodium falciparum.*

Hemimetabolous: A type of development in insects in which there is a gradual change in the external structure as development proceeds to the adult stage; *hemimetabola* is the name of the taxonomic group. *See* Ametabolous.

Hermaphroditism: The presence of both male and female reproductive organs in the same organism that is capable of reproducing on its own.

Hexacanth: The motile, six-hooked, first-stage larva of certain tapeworms; stage which hatches from the cestode egg and infects the intermediate host.

Haemorrhage: Escape of blood from vessels.

Heterogenic: Reproduction in which sexual and asexual generations alternate, as in the nematode *Strongyloides.*

Heteroxenous: Having more than one host required to complete a life cycle, such as in the digenetic trematodes.

Holometabolous: A type of development in insects in which there is a distinct change in the morphology of the stages; the cycle usually includes several larval stages, a pupa, and the adult; *holometabola* is the name of the taxonomic group. *See* Ametabolous.

Homoxenous: An adjective referring to a parasite that has a direct life cycle or one in which only a single host is required for its completion.

Horizontal transmission: Transmission of a parasitic agent among members of a group.

Host range: The number of species of hosts which can be infected by a parasitic agent.

Humoral immunity: A specific response to an antigen in which the principal effectors are antibodies that circulate in the blood.

Hyperemia: An abnormally large amount of blood in a tissue.

Hyperplasia: An abnormally high number of cells in a tissue.

Hypersensitivity (= allergy): A condition in which a mammal is sensitized to a particular substance and has an abnormally strong reaction when the substance is encountered again.

Hypertrophy: An abnormal increase in the size of a tissue or an organ.

Imago: The adult stage of an insect.

Immune memory: A property provided by specialized B and T lymphocytes (memory B and T cells) that respond rapidly on reexposure to the parasitic infection that originally induced them.

Immunopathology: Pathological changes partly or completely caused by the immune response.

Incidence (of infection): The proportion of a defined population infected or developing the disease during a specific time-period.

Inflammation: A general term for the complex response by a vertebrate to physical, chemical, or biological insult that gives rise to local accumulation of white blood cells and fluid; characterized by pain, reddening, increased temperature, and swelling at the site.

Innate response: The first line of defense; able to function continually in the host without prior exposure to the invading parasite. This complex system comprises, in part, cytokines, sentinel cells, complement, and natural killer cells.

Instar: A developmental stage in the life cycle of an insect, such as a larval or nymphal instar.

Integrated control: The use of several measures to control different parasites or parasite stages present on the animal and stages present in the environment.

Juvenile: An organism similar to the adult of the species but is sexually immature.

Killed vaccine: A vaccine made by taking an authentic disease-causing parasite and treating it with chemicals to reduce infectivity to non-detectable level.

Kinetoplast: An organelle characteristic of protozoa of the order Kinetoplastida.

Koch's postulates: Criteria developed by the German physician Robert Koch in the late 1800s to determine if a given agent is the cause of a specific disease.

Larva: An embryo that becomes self-sustaining and independent before it has developed the characteristic features of the adult form.

Lemniscus (-i): One of a pair of lateral, fluid-filled sacs at the base of the proboscis in members of the phylum Acanthocephala.

Live, attenuated vaccine: A vaccine made from parasitic mutants that have reduced virulence and lacks the capacity to cause a disease.

Lumen (-ina): The central cavity of an organ such as the lumen of the intestine.

Mammillated: Having many small nipple-like protrusions.

Memory cells: A subset of B and T lymphocytes maintained after each encounter with a foreign antigen; they survive for years and are ready to respond and proliferate upon subsequent encounter with the same antigen. *See* Immune memory.

Merogony: A type of asexual reproduction in which there is nuclear replication without plasmotomy and then two to many merozoites or daughter cells are produced simultaneously; a type of schizogony in which merozoites are formed; examples are found in many members of the Apicomplexa such as *Eimeria* and *Plasmodium*.

Merozoite: Product of merogony; usually an elongate organism that infects another host cell to undergo either merogony again or gamogony.

Metacercaria (-iae): The infective stage of a fluke enclosed in a protective cyst that resists adverse environmental conditions. This stage develops from the cercaria and is infective for the definitive host.

Metacestode: Immature tapeworm which develops from the hexacanth embryo (oncosphere) and grows in the intermediate host (mammal).

Microfilaria: Stage of filarial worm transmitted to the biting insect from the definitive host.

Microneme: Slender, chord-like bodies in the anterior of zoites of certain members of the phylum Apicomplexa.

Miracidium: The first developmental stage larva of a fluke which hatches from the egg and penetrates the snail intermediate host.

Monoclonal antibody: An antibody of a single specificity made by a clone of antibody-producing cells.

Moulting (= ecdysis): Shedding of an external covering such as integument or exoskeleton; in arthropods and nematodes, shedding the external covering allows the parasite to expand in its new skin.

Monoecious: Both male and female sex organs in one individual; hermaphroditic.

Monoxenous: Having a single host in the life cycle.

Monozoic: Refers to a condition in members of the tapeworm subclass Cestodaria in which there is only a single set of reproductive organs.

Mucous membrane: Any of several moist surfaces in the body of vertebrates in which there are mucus-secreting or goblet cells; examples are the orbit of the eye, nasal passages, inside the mouth.

Mucosal immunity: Immune responses expressed at mucosal surfaces. These include BALT (bronchial associated lymphoid tissues e.g. Retropharyngeal lymph nodes, harderian gland) and GALT (gut associated lymphoid tissues e.g. Lymph nodes draining the gut, Peyer's patches, lymphoglandular complexes).

Myiasis: Invasion of healthy body tissues by parasitic larvae of Diptera (two winged) fly.

Natural killer cells: An abundant lymphocyte population that comprises large, granular lymphocytes; distinguished from others by the absence of B and T cell antigen receptors; these cells are part of the innate defense system. *Also* called NK cells.

Nymph: The preadult stage of an insect, which has hemimetabolic development in a terrestrial environment.

Occult infection: Hidden infection; one in which no eggs or larvae are produced. For example, infections can be occult when only worms of one sex are present of a species that requires mating to produce eggs or larvae.

Oedema: Abnormal accumulation of fluid in cells, tissues, or tissue spaces resulting in swelling. *See* Bottle jaw.

Oncomiracidium: A free-swimming, ciliated larva of members of the class Monogenea.

Oncosphere: The six-hooked embryo that is contained in the egg membranes of members of the Cestoda. *See* Hexacanth embryo.

Oncotic pressure: The force exerted by proteins to draw tissue fluids into the blood.

Oocyst: A stage in the life cycle of certain members of the phylum Apicomplexa in which the zygote secretes a wall around itself; often highly resistant to environmental conditions.

Ookinete: The term most often refers to the motile zygote stage of *Plasmodium* which is seen in the midgut of the mosquito shortly after syngamy.

Operculum: Lid or cap-like structure at one or both ends of certain worm eggs, i.e., *Trichuris* and fluke; the larval parasite emerges from the egg at the operculum.

Opisthaptor: The highly specialized, posterior hold-fast of members of the class Monogenea.

Ornate: Colored; patterned. (Ant. inornate tick)

Ovum (-a): The female germ cell. *See* Egg.

Papilla (-ae): A nipple-like structure.

Parabasal body: An organelle that is part of the mastigont apparatus of certain members of the protozoan order Trichomonadida.

Parameter: A quantity whose value varies with the circumstances in which it is applied.

Parasite evolution: The constant change of a parasite population in the face of selection pressure.

Parasitophorous vacuole: A clear space between an intracellular parasite and the host cell cytoplasm.

Parenchyma: A reticulum of cells between the organs of an animal; also, the cells that perform the main functions of an organ.

Parthenogenesis: The laying of fertile eggs by a female without the need for fertilization by a male. It is common in some nematodes such as *Strongyloides*.

Passive immunization: Direct administration of the products of the immune response (e.g., antibodies or stimulated immune cells) obtained from an appropriate donor(s) to a patient.

Pathogen: A disease-causing parasite or other microorganisms.

Pellicle: A double external membrane.

Persistent infection: An infection that is not cleared by the combined actions of the innate and acquired immune response.

Petechia (-iae): Pinpoint haemorrhage in a tissue or organ.

Phasmid: Sensory pit located on the posterior part of nematodes of the class Secernentea.

Plasma: The fluid portion of the blood.

Plasmotomy: Fission of a multinucleated protist into two or more multinucleated daughter cells without direct relationship to nuclear division.

Plerocercoid: A larva or metacestode developing from a procercoid in the life cycle of tapeworms of the orders Proteocephala and Pseudophyllidea; this type of tapeworm larva is solid and has a rudimentary holdfast at the anterior end.

Polar filament: A coiled filament or tubule in the spore of the phyla Myxozoa and Microspora; the filament is extruded when the spore is ingested by a host and serves to inject the sporoplasm into the tissue of the host.

Premunition: A type of immunity in which the continued presence of the parasite in the body of the host is necessary for the maintenance of effective immunity.

Prevalence: The proportion of a defined population affected by a disease at a particular point in time.

Prevention: Measures taken prior to any infection/infestation of the animal with parasites, to prevent the establishment of an infection/infestation.

Primary antibody response: The initial response of B cells when first exposed to an infection.

Procercoid: A larva or metacestode that does not have a scolex similar to that of the adult; commonly found in members of the tapeworm orders Proteocephala and Pseudophyllidea.

Proglottid: A body segment of a tapeworm containing a complete set of reproductive organs.

Prohaptor: The anterior holdfast of members of the class Monogenea.

Professional antigen-presentig cells: Dendritic cells, macrophages, and B cells; defined by their ability to take up antigens and present them to T lymphocytes in the groove of a major histocompatibility complex class II molecule.

Proinflammatory cytokines: Cytokines produced predominantly by activated immune cells; responsible for amplification of inflammatory reactions.

Prophylaxis: Prevention; measures that are carried out to prevent the transmission of the parasitic agent or the occurrence of disease.

Protoscolex (protoscolices): A holdfast of tapeworms of the order Cyclophyllidea which forms from a germinal epithelium in a coenurus, hydatid, or alveolar cyst.

Pseudocoelom: A body cavity of a metazoan that is not completely lined with mesoderm.

Pyriform apparatus: The inner membrane of the eggs of certain tapeworms (e.g. *Monezia*), which often is pear-shaped and bears hooks.

Quarantine: Restriction in the freedom of movement of humans or animals in order to contain the spread of a parasitic disease; the length of time is slightly longer than the longest known incubation period of the disease in question.

Rays: Finger–like hypodermic structures which support the copulatory bursa.

Redia: Trematode stage in the snail intermediate host which develops from the sporocyst, and which becomes the cercaria.

Recrudescence: The recurrence of signs or symptoms of a disease after an abatement of days or weeks.

Relapse: The recurrence of signs or symptoms of a disease after an abatement of weeks or months.

Repellent: Compound, which makes a host unattractive to a parasite and thus can prevent attack or establishment.

Reportable disease: A disease that, by law, must be reported to a health authority In general, such diseases are of special concern to the health of the human or animal population; examples are malaria, foot and mouth disease, and tuberculosis.

Rhoptry (-ies): Sac-like, electron-dense structure in the anterior portion of a zoite of a member of the phylum Apicomplexa; involved in the penetration of host cells.

Rostellum: A prominence on the anterior end of the scolex of certain tapeworms of the order Cyclophyllidea. It is usually fitted with rows of hooks.

Schizogony: A type of asexual reproduction in which there are multiple nuclear divisions and then plasmotomy takes place, giving rise to a large number of daughter cells; occurs often in members of the phylum Apicomplexa; merogony, sporogony, and micro-gametogony are types of schizogony.

Scolex (scolices): The holdfast or organ by which a tapeworm attaches to the intestine of its host.

Scutum: A hard plate or shield on the dorsum behind the capitulum of hard ticks. The scutum is much more extensive in male than in female ticks.

Secondary antibody response: The antibody response produced after a subsequent infection of challenge with the same antigen or parasite.

Sequela (-ae): A diseased condition resulting from a previous disease.

Serum: The fluid part of vertebrate blood after the fibrin has been removed.

Sign: Any objective evidence of disease e.g. fever, diarrhea, or skin rash.

Sparganum (-a): A plerocercoid or larval tapeworm usually of the order Pseudophyllidea.

Spicule (= copulatory spicule): An elongate, sclerotized structure of male nematodes used in holding open the vulva of the female during copulation and transfer of sperm.

Spore: A resistant stage that is formed internally by the mother cell.

Sporogony: A type of schizogony in which the product is the sporozoite.

Sporozoite: The infective stage in some members of the phylum Apicomplexa.

Spring rise: The increase in egg production from worms in the spring months; leads to increased numbers of infective larvae on the pastures.

Strobila: A chain of tapeworm proglottids or segments.

Swimmer's itch (= cercarial dermatitis): A skin hypersensitivity reaction to the penetration of cercariae of certain members of the non-human schistosomes.

Sylvatic: Refers to forest or a wooded area; used as an adjective to describe the location of a disease cycle in the wild. *See* Feral.

Systemic infection: An infection that results in spread to many organs of the body.

Tachyzoite: Rapidly growing meront or zoites characteristic of the early stage of infection with *Toxoplasma* and related organisms of the phylum Apicomplexa.

Therapeutic index: margin of safety of a drug; the difference between the dose that kills parasites and the dose that harms the host.

Therapy: any medical intervention to cure a disease; this includes the use of veterinary medicinal products, to eliminate an existing parasite infection/infestation.

Treatment: application of medicinal products (medication) as deemed necessary based on any given diagnosis.

Trophozoite: The growing, feeding stage of a protozoan. It is also called the vegetative stage.

Vaccination: inoculation of healthy individuals with attenuated or related microorganisms, or their antigenic products, to elicit an immune response that will protect against later infection by the corresponding pathogen.

Vertical transmission: transmission of a parasite from one generation to the next through the egg or in utero. *See* Horizontal transmission.

Virulence: The relative capacity of a parasite to produce pathogenic effects or to invade.

Warbles: Swellings under the skin produced by larvae of *Dermatobia* and *Hypoderma* flies.

Zoonosis (-es): Diseases that are transmitted from animals to humans.

Zoonotic agent: An organism that causes a zoonosis.

Index

Current Books of Interest